Praise for *Emergency Nursing*

"This book will entice future emergency nurses to love emergency nursing. Jeff Solheim's passion as a nurse, instructor, and leader in emergency nursing will engage and carry you through this everlasting specialty nursing career to better take care of yourself, your patients, and their families."

–Matthew F. Powers, MS, BSN, RN, MICP, CEN
2015 President
Emergency Nurses Association

"Jeff Solheim and his team of talented contributing authors have brilliantly captured the past, present, and future of emergency nursing. It is exciting and reassuring to know the essence of our profession will be preserved in published print. The book portrays the richness, breadth, and diversity of emergency nursing practice. Reading it is like having a chance to sit down and soak up the institutional knowledge of some of the most experienced nurses in our profession."

–Mary Jagim, MS, RN, CEN, FAEN
Chief Nursing Officer and Director of Clinical Services
Infinite Leap, LLC

"This book is an eloquent and honest account of the profession of emergency nursing, guiding readers throughout the independent and collaborative nature of this specialized practice into their own journeys to emergency nursing."

–Sherri-Lynne Almeida, DrPH, MSN, MEd, RN, CEN, FAEN
Senior Consulting Manager, Philips Healthcare
Past President, Emergency Nurses Association (2002)

"Filled with concrete information, skill enhancing tips, professional leadership advancement practice, and overall career opportunities, this book will answer all your questions and concerns about a future in emergency nursing. A must-read for students of all levels!"

–Cammy House Fancher, ACNP
University of Florida, Division of Cardiothoracic Surgery
CEO, Critical Care Advanced Medical Institute

"Jeff Solheim has written a useful guide to students contemplating emergency department nursing as a career. Emergency Nursing explores additional fields available to ED professionals—including global health nursing services in underdeveloped countries along with preparation for the emotional and physical challenges of working abroad. Solheim's discussion about legacy explores what nurses hope to achieve and how those achievements contribute to their profession."

–Judith Harris, DNP, FNP-BC, RN
Assistant Professor
University of New Mexico College of Nursing
Albuquerque, New Mexico

"The perfect emergency nursing guidebook, both pertinent and practical. Definitely the #1 book addressing the past, present, and future issues related to emergency nursing."

–Gwyn Parris-Atwell, MSN, RN, FNP-BC, CEN, FAEN
New Jersey Emergency Nurses Association Past-President

EMERGENCY NURSING

THE PROFESSION · THE PATHWAY · THE PRACTICE

Jeff Solheim, MSN, RN-BC, CEN, CFRN, FAEN

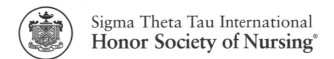

Sigma Theta Tau International
Honor Society of Nursing®

The Honor Society of Nursing, Sigma Theta Tau International (STTI) is a nonprofit organization founded in 1922 whose mission is advancing world health and celebrating nursing excellence in scholarship, leadership, and service. Members include practicing nurses, instructors, researchers, policymakers, entrepreneurs, and others. STTI's roughly 500 chapters are located at approximately 700 institutions of higher education throughout Armenia, Australia, Botswana, Brazil, Canada, Colombia, England, Ghana, Hong Kong, Japan, Kenya, Lebanon, Malawi, Mexico, the Netherlands, Pakistan, Portugal, Singapore, South Africa, South Korea, Swaziland, Sweden, Taiwan, Tanzania, Thailand, the United Kingdom, and the United States. More information about STTI can be found online at http://www.nursingsociety.org.

Sigma Theta Tau International
550 West North Street
Indianapolis, IN, USA 46202

To order additional books, buy in bulk, or order for corporate use, contact Nursing Knowledge International at 888. NKI.4YOU (888.654.4968/U.S. and Canada) or +1.317.634.8171 (outside U.S. and Canada).

To request a review copy for course adoption, email solutions@nursingknowledge.org or call 888.NKI.4YOU (888.654.4968/U.S. and Canada) or +1.317.634.8171 (outside U.S. and Canada).

To request author information, or for speaker or other media requests, contact Marketing, Honor Society of Nursing, Sigma Theta Tau International at 888.634.7575 (U.S. and Canada) or +1.317.634.8171 (outside U.S. and Canada).

ISBN: 9781940446462
EPUB ISBN: 9781940446479
PDF ISBN: 9781940446486
MOBI ISBN: 9781940446493

Library of Congress Cataloging-in-Publication data

Names: Solheim, Jeff, 1967- , editor. | Sigma Theta Tau International, issuing body.
Title: Emergency nursing : the profession, the pathway, the practice / [edited by] Jeff Solheim.
Other titles: Emergency nursing (Solheim)
Description: Indianapolis, IN, USA : Sigma Theta Tau International, [2016] | Includes bibliographical references.
Identifiers: LCCN 2015042809| ISBN 9781940446462 (alk. paper) | ISBN 9781940446479 (epub) | ISBN 9781940446486 (pdf) | ISBN 9781940446493 (Mobi)
Subjects: | MESH: Emergency Nursing. | Emergencies--nursing. | Emergency Service, Hospital.
Classification: LCC RC86.7 | NLM WY 154.2 | DDC 616.02/5--dc23 LC record available at http://lccn.loc.gov/2015042809

First Printing, 2016

Publisher: *Dustin Sullivan*
Acquisitions Editor: *Emily Hatch*
Editorial Coordinator: *Paula Jeffers*
Cover Designer: *Rebecca Batchelor*
Interior Design/Page Layout: *Rebecca Batchelor*

Principal Book Editor: *Carla Hall*
Development and Project Editor: *Rebecca Senninger*
Copy Editor: *Erin Geile*
Proofreader: *Todd Lothery*
Indexer: *Joy Dean Lee*

Dedication

I want to dedicate this book to my incredible family, who has been so supportive of me and my career over the years. With each new venture I have taken on, my time has become more precious. Sadly, that has often meant less time with those I love the most. This written work is but one testament of the appreciation I have for my entire family and for the support they have shown me.

To my parents, Dr. Allen Solheim and Dorthy Solheim, thank you for setting the example of professionalism and hard work that has guided my life and career. You have set the example that I have followed. It is unlikely I could accomplish everything I currently do without your support, and you hold a special place in my heart.

To my son, Brandon, I know that my busy life has often meant we are apart more than I would have liked. But I have watched you grow up with the greatest of pride and admiration and can't wait to see where life takes you next. Thanks for being willing to share me with so many others. I hope the example I have set will be a guiding light for you in life.

To Sue, you were so supportive of me early in my career as I entered into emergency nursing. I have never forgotten the sacrifices we made as a young family so I could do what I loved.

Aside from my family, there are many other incredible individuals who have shaped my emergency nursing career. Sandy Broderick, who was a patient and supportive preceptor when I first entered into the emergency nursing field, thank you for your patience and guidance. And to Jean Belbeck—my first charge nurse who provided a lifeline when I was the victim of terrible lateral violence in my first emergency department job. I doubt I would have survived those horrible months if not for your moral support.

It's important for me to recognize the incredible staff who allow me to pursue all of my passions in emergency nursing, working behind the scenes to make me look good and allow me to balance all the facets of my professional and personal life. Special recognition goes to my personal assistants over the years: Shaun Willis, Doug Peterson, and Thom Larkin. It's no small task to keep tabs on my incredibly busy life and to put up with all the demands that come your way, but you have done so with professionalism and unparalleled patience. And to Ken Weaver, the amazing director of operations at Project Helping Hands who has selflessly taken the reigns of my organization and grown it over the years, thank you for not only allowing Project Helping Hands to flourish but for freeing up time for me to pursue the multitude of projects that comprise my life.

And last, but not least, I would be remiss if I did not dedicate this book to the very individuals for which it is written, my colleagues in the emergency nursing field. You have dedicated your life to the selfless care of others. You spend countless holidays away from your own family. You work hours that few others would work to ensure that patients receive care around the clock. You put yourself in harm's way every time to report to work. May this book serve as inspiration and guidance in recognition of the career path you have chosen.

Acknowledgments

I want to thank all the authors who have been integral in putting this book together. We all live busy lives these days, and taking time out of a busy schedule to author a chapter constitutes great sacrifice. Thank you for agreeing to take time away from your personal life for this project, for meeting tight deadlines, and for putting up with all my queries and edits.

Thank you to Emily Hatch at Sigma Theta Tau International for inviting me to take on this project and for patiently working with my busy schedule to initiate the project. Thank you to the entire production team (including but not limited to Carla Hall, Dustin Sullivan, Paula Jeffers, Rebecca Batchelor, Rebecca Senninger, and Erin Geile) at Sigma Theta Tau International for taking this idea and developing it into a reality.

About the Author

Jeff Solheim, MSN, RN-BC, CEN, CFRN, FAEN, is founder and executive director of Project Helping Hands and president of Solheim Enterprises. Solheim is well known in the emergency nursing field. He has been a nurse since 1989 and an emergency nurse since 1993. He has worked in nearly every facet of emergency nursing including staff nurse, charge nurse, manager, director, trauma coordinator, flight nurse, educator, state surveyor, and pre-hospital nurse. Since 2004, Solheim has been traveling around the world speaking on a variety of clinical and motivational topics. He has also authored more than 20 books and written several chapters for other books as well as being published in numerous journals and magazines. Aside from Solheim's work in the emergency nursing field, he is founder and executive director of Project Helping Hands, a Third World humanitarian medical organization that places short-term medical teams in countries around the world. He has personally led more than 50 different medical teams to countries in all but one continent.

Contributing Authors

Pamela D. Bartley, BSN, RN, CEN, CPEN, CCRN, is president of PDB Nurse Education LLC and has more than 30 years' experience as an emergency nurse and educator, teaching courses as diverse as Basic Life Support, Advanced Cardiac Life Support, Pediatric Advanced Life Support, Trauma Nursing Core Curriculum, and the Emergency Nurse Pediatric Course, as well as preparation courses for the Certified Emergency Nurse and Certified Pediatric Emergency Nurse exams. Bartley has served on the South Carolina LLR Nursing Advisory Board and as an NCLEX item reviewer. She was selected for the AACN Wyeth Nurse Fellow Award in May 2002 and published "The Evolution of ACLS" in the *American Journal of Nursing*. She was elected as the South Carolina Emergency Nurses Association's president in 2001 and in 2013. In 2014, Bartley was honored as the South Carolina Area Health Education Center Educator of the Year and was selected for the 2014 ENA Board Mentoring Program and the Academy of Emergency Nursing's EMINENCE Mentoring Program. She currently serves on the ENA State Achievement Award Committee.

Patricia L. Clutter, MEd, RN, CEN, FAEN, is an ED staff nurse, an independent educator, a journalist, and a ship nurse. She has spent 41 years of her 43-year career in emergency nursing. Clutter has lectured nationwide on a variety of topics, including the Certified Emergency Nurse review course, cultural aspects of care, and triage, and has presented internationally. She has written numerous articles, chapters, and books related to patient care and serves as co-section editor for international nursing in the *Journal of Emergency Nursing*. Clutter was director of education for more than 10 years for a Third World humanitarian medical mission group, Project Helping Hands, and is presently regional education director for South America with this organization. She also has been a team member on multiple medical mission trips to Bolivia. Clutter continues to work part time as a cruise ship nurse, which has afforded her many unique patient care situations. She is also active in the Emergency Nurses Association at the local, state, and national level and was inducted into the Academy of Emergency Nursing in 2005.

Debra Delaney, MS, RN, CEN, is owner and proprietor of Delaney Healthcare Consultants. She has more than 20 years of experience as an emergency nurse and nursing leader. Her roles in the ED have ranged from transporter to director. Delaney's experience also includes more than 8 years as a consultant, traveling across the United States to help emergency departments with redesign and process-improvement opportunities. Her expertise in improving throughput and hospital crowding has gained her national recognition, and she is a sought-after speaker on the topic. She has published several articles and lectures on strategies to improve emergency care, best practices, and current trends in nursing. Delaney is a certified emergency nurse and an active member of the Emergency Nurses Association. She has represented nurses in Massachusetts as a delegate at the ENA General Assembly annual nursing conference. Her nursing honors include Sigma Theta Tau International and Alpha Sigma Lambda. She is also a member of the American College of Healthcare Executives and the American Organization of Nurse Executives.

Darin L. Durham, BSN, RN, is staff nurse at St. Charles Immediate Care and deputy medical examiner and law enforcement death investigator for Deschutes County in Oregon. He has been an emergency nurse since 1998. Durham started as an EMT in 1985 and then spent 10 years as a medical lab technician before finishing nursing school. He also spent 2 years as an ICU nurse for both adult and pediatric patients with a specialty in trauma. He has held positions in emergency departments as a staff nurse, trauma nurse, charge nurse, emergency department manager, and director of emergency and mental health services. Outside of the emergency department, Durham volunteers for several organizations. He provides emergency first aid for school and local sporting events; lectures to high school driver's education classes; and teaches classes to EMTs, paramedics, nursing students, firefighters, and police officers.

Laurel Grisbach, BSN, RN, CPHRM, is director of risk management and patient safety at Beta Healthcare Group, where she provides risk and patient-safety consultation and education for more than 100 healthcare facilities and medical groups throughout California. She is a certified professional in healthcare risk management and a registered nurse with expertise in emergency nursing and ED operations. Grisbach completed her patient safety leadership fellowship through the American Hospital Association and serves on the association's CPHRM Certification Committee. In addition to her work in the professional liability arena, she was a legal nurse consultant for civil and criminal cases in local and federal jurisdictions. Grisbach was an expert witness for emergency nursing, operations, and EMTALA and served as a facility-based risk manager for a region of hospitals, with responsibilities for risk management, compliance, privacy, and patient safety. She is a published author and speaks nationally on topics involving clinical risk management and risk reduction.

Linda Laskowski-Jones, MS, APRN, ACNS-BC, CEN, FAWM, FAAN, vice president of emergency and trauma services at Christiana Care Health System in Wilmington, Delaware, is a nationally recognized nurse leader and educator in emergency and trauma care. She has authored more than 100 journal articles and book chapters. She is editor-in-chief of *Nursing, the Journal of Clinical Excellence,* and is an editorial board member for the *International Journal of Emergency Nursing.* She has served on the editorial boards of the *Journal of Emergency Nursing* and the *Journal of Trauma Nursing.* Laskowski-Jones is a nurse reviewer for the American College of Surgeons Committee on Trauma Consultation and Verification Program. She has served as national course faculty for the Emergency Nurses Association Key Concepts in Emergency Department Management Course. She is a governor-appointed past president of the Delaware Board of Nursing. She serves on the Delaware Trauma System and Trauma Quality committees. She is a member of the board of directors for the Appalachian Center for Wilderness Medicine and a fellow of the Academy of Wilderness Medicine.

Rebecca S. McNair, RN, CEN, founder and president of Triage First Inc., has a 28-year history in emergency nursing. For the last 17 years, she has been an educator and consultant specializing in emergency-department triage and patient-throughput systems, customer satisfaction, teamwork, and leadership skills. Her company has received accreditation with distinction as an accredited provider of continuing nursing education. She has been published in the *Journal of Emergency Nursing* and *Physicians Weekly*, addressing triage and point-of-entry processes as well as a range of clinical topics. She co-authored the triage chapter in *Emergency Nursing Secrets* and authored eight chapters in *Triage Secrets*. Recently, she authored the foreword and the documentation chapter in *Fast Facts for Triage*. She was a member of the ENA/ACEP Joint Triage Task Force regarding the adoption of a valid and reliable five-level triage acuity scale. She has been a featured faculty member at various professional organization conferences, including an Emergency Department Practice Management Association meeting.

Fred Neis, MS, RN, CEN, FACHE, FAEN, managing director at The Advisory Board Company, obtained his BSN in 1993 and an MS in nursing administration in 1997 from the University of Kansas. He served in a variety of clinical and leadership roles in hospitals and emergency medical services until joining The Advisory Board Company in 2006. Currently, Neis leads complex partnerships aimed at transforming care delivery at large health systems. Additionally, he has been a contributor to several publications, including the Institute of Medicine (IOM) reports on *The Future of Emergency Care in the U.S. Health System* (2006) and Strauss and Mayer's *Emergency Department Management* (2013). Continuing to participate in emergency nursing, he is a conference speaker and peer reviewer for *Journal of Emergency Nursing, Advanced Emergency Nursing Journal,* and *Journal of Healthcare Management.* Outside of his role at The Advisory Board Company, he has served on several medical mission trips to Africa through Project Helping Hands (PHH), has been president of the PHH board, and volunteers for a fire department.

Nicholas A. Nelson, MS, RN, CEN, CPEN, CCRN, CPN, TNS, NRP, is an ECRN EMS instructor for emergency medical services and a per diem staff nurse for the emergency department. In his current role, he coordinates 300 emergency communications RNs at the eight hospitals of the Loyola EMS System. Besides educating emergency nurses, he instructs EMT and paramedic students, EMS and critical care transport providers, school nurses, and graduate nursing students. Nelson is also a pediatric quality coordinator in a suburban emergency department/Level I Trauma Center, a critical care transport nurse, and a state surveyor of pediatric EDs. He holds board certifications in emergency nursing, pediatric emergency nursing, adult acute and critical care nursing, and pediatric nursing. He volunteers as event medical personnel and embarked on his first international medical mission trip in 2015. Aside from nursing, he is a licensed and nationally certified paramedic, certified emergency medical dispatcher, and certified child passenger safety technician. Nelson is the 2013 recipient of the national Emergency Nurses Association's Rising Star Award.

William Schueler, MSN, RN, CEN, an emergency staff nurse and clinical nurse educator, has been an emergency nurse since 2000. In 1997, he became an EMT, which led to positions as a transport nurse and travel nurse. Through understanding and research of the pervasive problem of violence in healthcare, Schueler has been teaching violence prevention since 2012. His experience as a weight loss nurse enables him to identify with the stressors of life and how they holistically affect body weight and health. Schueler has been president of the Oregon Emergency Nurses Association and has been active in pursuing legislation to increase penalties for assaults to hospital staff. He continues to be an active martial artist and advocate for the profession of emergency nursing.

Brian Selig, DNP, RN, CEN, NEA-BC, is assistant director of perioperative and procedural services at the University of Kansas Hospital in Kansas City, Kansas. He has been a nurse since 1998 and has worked extensively in emergency nursing throughout his career. He has held positions as an ER staff RN, flight nurse, and nursing administrator. Selig has been a leader in several emergency departments, including teaching facilities, ACS Level I Trauma Centers, and a comprehensive stroke center. He has expertise in emergency nursing at mass gatherings and has established healthcare operations for teams in Major League Baseball and NASCAR. Selig has served as a commissioner for the ANCC Commission on Magnet Recognition since 2009 and is currently serving on the ANCC Magnet Commission Executive Committee. He was a 2008 AONE Nurse Manager Fellow and was the 2011 Kansas Emergency Nurses Association president. He is a 2012–2014 National Jonas Scholar.

Renee Semonin Holleran, PhD, FNP-BC, CEN, CCRN (emeritus), CFRN, CTRN (retired), FAEN, a family nurse practitioner at Alta View Senior Clinic and Hope Free Clinic, began her career in the ED in 1977 as a staff nurse. Since then, she has worked as an emergency nursing clinical nurse specialist, a transport nurse, a chief flight nurse, and now a family nurse practitioner. She has written and edited two *AJN* "Book of the Year" books: *Prehospital Nursing: A Collaborative Approach* (1994) and *Air and Surface Transport Nursing: Principles and Practice* (2011). She was editor of *Air Medical Journal* from 1996 to 2006 and editor-in-chief of *Journal of Emergency Nursing* from 2006 to 2013.

Melanie Stoutenburg, BSN, RN, CEN, clinical educator for emergency services and emergency services nurse residency program coordinator, has been an emergency room nurse since 1996. Over the years, she has served in numerous roles including staff nurse, charge nurse, clinical coordinator, and educator. Her most recent role has focused on the development and implementation of a nurse residency program that facilitates the transition of the new graduate nurse into a well-rounded professional emergency department nurse. Stoutenburg also teaches a variety of educational courses, including preparation courses for the

Certified Emergency Nursing Exam. She is an active member of both her local and state Emergency Nurses Association, serving in the positions of chapter president, state president-elect, and past chapter and state secretary.

Christi Thornhill, MSN, RN, ENP, ACNP-BC, CPNP-AC, CEN, CA-SANE, CP-SANE, has been a nurse since 1990 and a nurse practitioner since 2000. Her nursing career started in the emergency department, and she has worked as an emergency nurse in urban, suburban, and rural emergency departments as well as a flight nurse. She worked as an emergency nurse practitioner in rural emergency departments until 2008, when she obtained her post-master's degree as an acute care pediatric nurse practitioner. Thornhill worked as the lead nurse practitioner in trauma services for 6 years at Cook Children's Medical Center in Fort Worth, Texas. In 2014, she transitioned to the Child Advocacy and Resource Evaluation (C.A.R.E.) team caring for physically and sexually abused children. She is a certified sexual assault nurse examiner, a certified emergency nurse, and a certified emergency pediatric nurse. She speaks frequently on topics that include emergency and trauma care, child abuse, and human trafficking

Gayle Walker-Cillo, MSN/Ed, RN, CEN, CPEN, FAEN, stroke program clinical specialist at Morristown Medical Center in Morristown, New Jersey, has been an emergency nurse for more than 20 years, with 15 of those years as a full-time emergency clinical specialist and bedside educator. She is currently applying her emergency skills in working across the continuum to improve care of patients who experience strokes. Walker-Cillo has consulted, presented, collaborated, and authored on both state and national levels on topics that include emergency nursing, education, remediation, competence, and research. She has been on the editorial board for the *Advanced Emergency Nursing Journal,* has written and edited for Gannett and Mosby, and has been published in more than 20 peer-reviewed journals. In 2009, she was lead author of the sentinel clinical practice guideline (CPG) process for emergency nurses. She also collaborated on and co-authored *Emergency Nursing Scope and Standards of Practice 2011* and *A Framework for Creating and Evaluating Competencies for Emergency Nurses.*

Aaron Wolff, BSN, RN, CEN, director of performance excellence at Dignity Health, is an accomplished leader in professional nursing. In addition to leadership roles within the hospital, he has lectured across the nation on topics of adult, pediatric, and trauma nursing as well as nursing and hospital leadership since 2004. He has been a contributing author to many textbooks while also partnering with some of the most accomplished industry leaders to develop nursing education programs for trauma. While his interest for hospital operations and business performance improvement was born in the emergency department, his focus has expanded to include all aspects of clinical and operational efficiency in both acute and outpatient settings. Since 2008, Wolff has used tools such as LEAN, Six Sigma, and human-based design, and his passion for engineering outcomes in healthcare, to express his commitment to professional nursing.

Table of Contents

Foreword

As I was reading through the chapters of this book, I couldn't help but reminisce about the beginning of my personal journey as an emergency nurse. As a very young Army nurse, I was assigned head nurse of the emergency room of a small military hospital in what was then West Germany. Not only was I the head nurse, I was the only nurse. Our entire ER team consisted of 10 young Army medics, three foreign physicians—from Turkey, Iran, and Egypt—and me. The ER was one large room with three stretchers separated by curtains and a small, one-stretcher room. We had no clinical policies, protocols, or practice guidelines to help us. On occasion, I was designated "flight nurse," accompanying a critically ill or injured patient to a larger facility about an hour's flight north. Our aircraft was a Huey—a noisy, rattly, drafty, but very reliable helicopter, minimally equipped with an O2 E-cylinder, a BP cuff and stethoscope (which were not very useful during flight), and glass bottles of IV solutions suspended from the ceiling by strips of gauze.

Fast-forward more than four decades and witness the phenomenal growth and development of emergency nursing as a specialty. The advent of this book, which is a very thorough archive and compendium of all things emergency nursing, chronicles the history of emergency nursing, its maturation, its complexity, and key components that validate its variety and uniqueness.

For those of you who are exploring nursing specialties, whether this is your first or last stop, buckle your seat belts and get ready for a whirlwind ride into the universe of emergency nursing. Extraordinary, visionary, dedicated pioneer nursing leaders identified the need for designated practice areas, knowledgeable nurses, lifelong learning, a scope and standards of practice, and a code of ethics unique to the practice of emergency nursing. This foundational work was the beginning of a journey that continues to this day as emergency nurses work side by side with emergency physicians and emergency medical services men and women to continuously improve the specialty of emergency care.

To say that this book is carefully detailed and extremely timely would be an understatement. It captures the essence and breadth of emergency nursing. Its chapters offer you an opportunity to look into the vast universe of emergency nursing, from our rich history to the present and into the future. You can focus on a particular component of the specialty or absorb a broad range of topics.

The three sections of this book logically span the many aspects that make up emergency nursing, types of emergency care, educational preparation, certifications, and the importance of the team. It presents the practice of emergency nursing, with its challenges, regulations, populations, legal aspects, and variety of practice settings. Of particular importance to all emergency nurses, regardless of the length of time or types of experiences encountered, is the chapter on self-care. Dealing with births, deaths, and every human condition in between on any given day is an extreme challenge to one's life-balance. Self-awareness, self-care, and attentiveness to fellow emergency nurses form the bonds that help us get through the challenging times and celebrate the good times.

Led by contemporary visionary and emergency nurse extraordinaire, book editor, and author Jeff Solheim, the 17 authors are staff nurses, charge nurses, nurse managers, directors, educators, journalists, administrators, consultants, editors, nurse practitioners, medical examiners, sexual assault nurse examiners, clinical nurse specialists, ship nurses, pre-hospital nurses, flight nurses, humanitarian caregivers, and entrepreneurs—and all are emergency nurses. Their significant contributions have made this book a true atlas of emergency nursing.

As I reflect on how my own emergency nursing career began, quite by accident (or was it fate?), I will be forever grateful to the U.S. Army Nurse Corps for that fortuitous duty assignment that changed my life forever. My sincere hope is that this very thoughtful, well-written book about all things emergency nursing might inspire you to choose or continue your career in emergency nursing. Enjoy this book—absorb, ponder, deliberate, and commit. I can think of no greater, more challenging, more satisfying career than emergency nursing and no finer colleagues than emergency nurses.

–Susan Budassi Sheehy, PhD, RN, FAEN, FAAN
Adjunct Associate Professor
Daniel K. Inouye Graduate School of Nursing
Uniformed Services University of the Health Sciences, Bethesda, Maryland
Past President, Emergency Nurses Association

Introduction

A colleague of mine who works as a registered nurse on an inpatient surgical unit made an interesting observation one evening while we were enjoying dinner together. She pointed out that when you ask many nurses what they do for a living, they will respond by saying that they are an "RN" or a "nurse." She went on to comment that when you ask nurses who work in the emergency department what they do for a living, they are much more likely to identify themselves as an "emergency nurse." She asked me why it is that emergency nurses seem to feel the need to identify the area of nursing they are employed in rather than simply their career choice as a nurse.

This was not something I had given serious thought to before this conversation, but I began to pay more careful attention and found there to be some truth to this statement. While emergency nurses remain an integral part of the nursing field as a whole, they seem to have a certain sense of pride about working in the emergency department. Emergency nurses frequently identify themselves as a "nurse," along with their place of employment—the emergency department.

I will have to admit that I fall into this category myself. There has never been a day that I have regretted entering into nursing as a career. It has met and then far exceeded my expectations. I have had opportunities that I cannot imagine in any other career I might have chosen. Yet if you ask me what I do for a living, I will most likely reply that I am an "emergency nurse." There is a rush of adrenaline that comes with my work in the emergency department. There are many more moments of satisfaction than there are moments of disappointment, and for that reason, I am proud to be called an "emergency nurse."

It was this very thought that resonated with me when I was approached about editing a book about emergency nursing. Why not produce a book about the profession of emergency nursing? What is it about this particular field of nursing that makes nurses want to identify themselves as "emergency nurses" instead of simply referring to themselves as a "nurse"? It is my sincere hope as you pore through the pages that follow, you will better understand the profession of emergency nursing and what makes it so special.

The book has been divided into three distinct sections. The first section is "Emergency Nursing as a Profession and Career." The chapters in this section are designed to introduce the reader to the profession of emergency nursing. What is it about this segment of the profession that drives nurses to want to be identified with it? What is the history of emergency nursing? What career opportunities exist within emergency nursing, and what educational as well as life experiences will help nurses access those opportunities? What are the professional responsibilities that accompany being identified as an emergency nurse? What are the challenges that face the emergency nurse, and how can emergency nurses take care of themselves to ensure mental and physical health?

The second section focuses on the place emergency nurses call "home"—the emergency department. This section, "The Emergency Nurse in the Hospital Setting," introduces nurses to the emergency department. What types of emergency departments are there? How does one emergency department differ from another? When seeking a job in an emergency department, what should the emergency nurse seek out to ensure compatibility? What are the different areas in the emergency department, and who are the key players, aside from emergency nurses, who work there? There is also a chapter on triage in this section, an area of the emergency department that is unique to the emergency nurse.

The third section of the book, "Emergency Nursing Practice," is all about the practice of emergency nursing. What challenges do emergency nurses face when they go to work each day? How can nurses face those challenges? What are the laws, regulations, and pitfalls that accompany our practice? One of the challenges emergency nurses face is the fact that they care for patients across the spectrum of life from all socioeconomic and ethnic backgrounds. The final chapters of the book will focus on the varied patient populations that emergency nurses regularly encounter.

For those of you who are already emergency nurses, it is my sincere hope that this book will give you a deeper understanding of the career path you have chosen and what makes emergency nursing so unique and such a source of pride. For those of you who are considering joining the ranks of emergency nurses, I hope the contents of this book will help you decide if this is the career path for you and how best to maneuver the field to ensure you meet your personal goals. And for all other readers, I trust the contents of the pages to follow will give you insight into what drives the passion of all of us "emergency nurses."

–Jeff Solheim, MSN, RN-BC, CEN, CFRN, FAEN (and an "emergency nurse")

1

EMERGENCY NURSING DEFINED

–Renee Semonin Holleran, PhD, FNP-BC, CEN, CCRN (emeritus), CFRN, CTRN (retired), FAEN

The American Nurses Association (ANA) defines *nursing* in the following way: "Nursing is the protection, promotion, and optimization of health and abilities, prevention of illness and injury, alleviation of suffering through the diagnosis and treatment of human response, and advocacy in the care of individuals, families, communities, and populations" (ANA, 2015).

An *emergency* is defined as "a serious and unexpected situation involving an illness or an injury" (Medical Emergency, 2015). Just as there are multiple types of patients who require specific care, multiple nursing specialties have evolved to care for these populations. One of these is emergency nursing.

The focus of this chapter is to discuss the history of emergency nursing, the role of the emergency department (ED), the definition of emergency nursing and its role in emergency care, and some of the elements that constitute the practice of emergency nursing.

History of Emergency Nursing

Emergency medicine and emergency nursing are modern concepts. Historically, patient care was generally provided where the illness or injury occurred. There were no hospitals and certainly no EDs. Some patients were lucky to find a place such as a monastery or church that may have offered additional care. The early foundations of emergency care came out of war dating back to the Middle Ages (Sefrin & Weidringer, 1991).

Although emergency care is commonplace in some of the world, many parts of the globe still do not have any emergency care systems including departments staffed by nurses and physicians. In 2012, the World Health Assembly adopted Resolution 60.22 titled *Health Systems: Emergency Care Systems,* establishing a policy tool for improving emergency care access and providing emergency care globally (Anderson et al., 2012). The continued lack of a global emergency system has been brought to an uncomfortable light in global events such as the Ebola outbreak in Africa that gained national attention in 2014 and natural disasters such as the Nepal earthquake in 2015.

In 2012, there were 5,004 emergency departments in the United States (Emergency Medicine Network, 2012). The total number of emergency departments around the world is unknown.

The Role of Florence Nightingale in Emergency Nursing

Florence Nightingale has long been associated with the origins of emergency nursing; she took nurses out to the field to provide care to wounded soldiers during the Crimean War in 1854. Nightingale and her colleagues began by identifying the most injured or sickest requiring care, even on the battlefield. The care she and the nurses she trained demonstrated the value of rapid management of acute patients (Gebbie & Qureshi, 2006; Shell & Dunlap, 2008). Nightingale implemented specific interventions that affected patient care, including reducing overcrowding of patients by keeping beds 3 feet apart, providing ventilation in the care area, preventing horses from being stabled in the patient care area, and flushing latrines daily with peat charcoal (Sheingold & Hahn, 2014).

Florence Nightingale was also responsible for laying the foundation of the nursing profession and women's suffrage. She established the Nightingale Training School at the St. Thomas Hospital in London in 1865. She recognized that nurses played a significant role in the social care of patients and that this could not be separated from the patient's healthcare needs. This is never more evident than in the practice of emergency nurses who experience this today on a daily basis (MacMillan, 2012). Nightingale was operating within the circumstances that were available to her. If getting something done for a patient required collaboration and/or compromise, she was willing to do this. She worked hard, for example, to ensure that patients with mental illness were not only admitted to hospitals but could stay in the hospital for as long as was needed. Prior to her intervention, patients with mental health issues were often ignored and denied access to medical care. She demonstrated the role of advocacy, an important part of patient care in emergency nursing practice (Ayers, 2014).

 Florence Nightingale was born in Florence, Italy, on May 12, 1820, and died in the United Kingdom on August 13, 1910.

Nightingale pressed for the welfare of her nurses. She demanded better working and living conditions by promoting time off, the use of labor-saving devices, and opportunities for nurses to advance within their profession. She also monitored nursing mortality and reported these statistics (McDonald, 2013). Safety in the work environment continues to be a significant problem in emergency nursing practice today, especially the exposure to and consequences of violence in the ED.

Emergency Nursing in the 20th Century

At the beginning of the 20th century, the Henry Street Settlement in New York City created the "First Aid Room." Under the direction of nurse Lillian Wald, impoverished immigrants received care for minor emergencies such as cuts, local infections, rashes, and some accidents (Snyder, Keeling, & Razionale, 2006). Because the majority of the time nurses were mostly seeing patients without the presence of a physician, standing orders were developed. The medical community that existed at the time approved these orders, and nurses who staffed the First Aid Rooms saw between 10,000 and 23,000 patients annually for 15 years (Snyder et al., 2006).

As hospitals grew during the 20th century, emergency "rooms," later recognized as emergency departments, became a place of access for healthcare to many patients. A 1956 survey on the use of emergency rooms in the Midwest and Atlantic Seaboard found a 400% increase in the use of the emergency room by patients with many complaints (Coleman & Errera, 1963). Several reasons given for this increase included patients' inability to reach their doctors at night, weekends, or holidays. The survey also found that doctors were increasingly referring patients to the emergency room for evaluations that could not be done in an office.

As the patient census in the emergency room increased, so did questions as to whether these patients needed to be there at all. It was found that patients were defining what qualified as an emergency for themselves. It was noted early that a bad experience in the emergency room could affect the entire hospital's reputation (Kennedy, 1957). As a result, hospitals began to pay specific attention to their emergency rooms and the care provided there.

However, the areas in hospitals dedicated to the emergent care of patients were limited. Often, the ED was one room and didn't have a dedicated staff; generally, a nurse was called down from an inpatient unit or the nursing supervisor cared for the patient.

Emergency nursing and emergency medicine continued to develop into specialties during the 20th century. The medical and nursing care provided to soldiers during World War II and the Korean and Vietnam wars demonstrated that rapid and acute care could make a difference in patient outcomes. It also confirmed the value of collaborative practice among nurses, physicians, and paramedical personnel. When emergency medicine was recognized as a specialty in the late 1970s, it quickly became one of the fastest growing medical fields (Zinc, 2006). Emergency medical services (EMS) also became an integral part of emergency care.

The role of the nurse in World War II and the Korean and Vietnam wars demonstrated the importance of nursing in the triage process and the acute care of the ill and injured patient. During this time, the American Nurses Association (ANA) began to gain more members and political power to represent the profession and the work of nursing. Societal changes, including the evolving role of women, laid the foundation for nursing specialties to develop their own status.

? Fifty-nine thousand American nurses served in the Army Nurse Corps during World War II (U.S. Army Center of Military History, 2003). More than 700 nurses served in mobile army surgical units (MASH units), and 4,000 navy nurses served on hospital ships during the Korean War (Department of Defense, 2010). About 6,250 nurses served in the Vietnam War (United States Navy and Army, n.d.).

Initially, most nurses who were either assigned to an "emergency" room or were called to see a patient when one presented had to provide and perform any needed immediate care and then wait for the physician to arrive. In 1965, the ANA didn't support this role. Nurses were not to diagnosis and prescribe (Snyder et al., 2006). The specialization of nursing assisted in identifying the unique functions, responsibilities, and education needed to provide care in the ED or intensive care unit.

The concern about the lack of enough physicians in the emergency room led to the suggestion of training nurses to perform specific interventions for emergency care. Examples of some of these interventions included obtaining a pertinent medical history, instituting cardiopulmonary resuscitation, stopping hemorrhage, obtaining an EKG, inserting a naso-gastric tube, performing wound and fracture care including splinting, assisting the physician in critiquing patient care, and remaining well-informed in new methods of utilizing emergency communications (Owens, 1970).

Owens (1970) notes:

> "Every nurse involved in emergency care should serve a period of training and indoctrination in what is necessary for emergency care of the patient at the site, en route to the hospital via emergency transportation, in the emergency department, operating room, recovery room, intensive care, and coronary care units." (p. 48)

The Emergency Nurses Association (ENA)

Two visionary nurses, Anita Dorr and Judith Kelleher, took on the challenge of creating a way for emergency nursing to be recognized as a specialty. Anita Dorr formed the Emergency Room Nurses Organization. She also put together the first "Resuscitation Cart" that sits now in the Emergency Nurses Association's national office in Des Plaines, Illinois. Judith Kelleher called her association the Emergency Department Nurses Association (EDNA).

On December 1, 1970, these two nurses combined their organizations into the Emergency Department Nurses Association (EDNA). Judith Kelleher has also been credited with remarking that it is an "emergency department, not an emergency room" (Snyder et al., 2006, p. 202). The roadrunner became the symbol of the emergency room nurse based on the quick speed at which emergency nurses work. Many of us still proudly wear that pin.

Initially, EDNA and the American College of Emergency Physicians (ACEP) shared the same offices. As both associations grew, so did issues between the two groups (Patrick, 2010; Schriver, Talmadge, Chuong, & Hedges, 2003). Yet, both associations still continue to this day to work collaboratively toward ensuring that the quality of care provided in the ED is evidence-based and the needs of all emergency patients are recognized and met.

The Emergency Department Nurses Association changed its name in 1985 to the Emergency Nurses Association (ENA). The ENA board and membership felt that this better mirrored where emergency nurses were practicing and the many facets of emergency care.

Today, the ENA reports a membership of over 40,000 members. The ENA has been responsible for the development and implementation of position statements, educational products, and several publications. Table 1.1 shows the educational resources that the ENA provides.

Table 1.1 ENA Educational Resources for Emergency Nurses

Resource	Description
Trauma Nursing Core Course (TNCC)	Trauma Nursing Core Course (TNCC) is a national and international course that identifies a standardized body of trauma nursing knowledge. The TNCC (Provider) is a 2-day course designed to provide the learner with cognitive knowledge and psychomotor skills. The purpose of TNCC is to present core-level knowledge, refine skills, and build a firm foundation in trauma nursing.
Emergency Nursing Pediatric Course (ENPC)	Emergency Nursing Pediatric Course (ENPC) was developed to improve the care of the pediatric patient by increasing the knowledge, skill, and confidence of the emergency nurse. This 2-day course provides core-level pediatric knowledge and psychomotor skills needed to care for pediatric patients in the emergency care setting.
Course on Advanced Trauma Nursing (CATN)	CATN is an online advanced course in trauma care for experienced emergency nurses. The course involves critical thinking and clinical decision-making beyond the primary survey. It includes tools to anticipate complications early in the trauma continuum, resulting in better patient outcomes. CATN courses offer: Pathophysiologic concepts Long-term perspective of trauma care Evidence-based curriculum 7.3 contact hours, six interactive learning modules Individual or group study
Geriatric Emergency Nursing Education (GENE)	GENE is a comprehensive eLearning program designed to provide the best evidence-based care for older adults. This extensive course gives nurses the tools to assess special needs in older adults, to recognize atypical presentations, and to coordinate care that will help improve patient outcomes.

Source: ENA, 2015.

Examples of ENA publications include (ENA, 2015):

- *Journal of Emergency Nursing*

- *ENA Connection*

- *Core Curriculum for Pediatric Emergency Nursing*

- *Emergency Nursing Scope and Standards of Practice*

The ENA current position statements are (ENA, 2015):

- Access to Health Care (12/2010)

- Advanced Practice in Emergency Nursing (2/2012)

- Appropriate Credential Use/Title Protection for Nurses with Advanced Degrees (5/2013)

- Care of Patients with Chronic/Persistent Pain in the Emergency Setting (1/2014)

- Chemical Impairment of Emergency Nurses (7/2010)

- Collaborative and Interdisciplinary Research (12/2010)

- Communicable Diseases in the Emergency Department (5/2010)

- Cultural Diversity in the Emergency Setting (5/2012)

- Deceased Patients for Procedural Practice (7/2010)

- Disaster and Emergency Preparedness for All Hazards (1/2014)

- Education Recommendations: Trauma Nursing (7/2010)

- Emergency Nursing Certification (10/2014)

- Emergency Registered Nurse Orientation (7/2011)

- Firearm Safety and Injury Prevention (1/2013)

- Forensic Evidence Collection (7/2010)

- Healthy Work Environment (3/2013)

- Holding, Crowding, and Patient Flow (7/2014)

- Human Trafficking Patient Awareness in the Emergency Setting (2/2015)

- Injury Prevention (10/2014)

- Interfacility Transfer (9/2010)

- Mobile Electronic Device Use in the Emergency Setting (9/2013)

- Nurse Leaders in Emergency Care (10/2012)

- Nurse Practitioners and Retail Health Care Clinics (2/2012)

- Observation Units (5/2011)

- Obstetrical Patient in the Emergency Department (5/2011)

- Palliative and End of Life Care in the Emergency Setting (9/2013)

- Patient Experience/Satisfaction in the Emergency Care Setting (10/2014)

- Patient Handoff/Transfer (1/2013)

- Patient Safety (12/2010)

- Pediatric Procedural Pain Management (12/2010)

- Prevention, Wellness, and Disease Management (1/2014)

- Professional Liability and Risk Management (9/2012)

- Protection of Human Subjects' Rights (9/2003)

- Registered Nurse Delegation in the Emergency Setting (9/2013)

- Resuscitative Decisions (7/2014)

- Safe Discharge from the Emergency Setting (12/2013)

- Sexual Assault and Rape Victims (9/2010)

- Social Networking by Emergency Nurses (2/2012)

- Specialty Certification in Emergency Nursing (9/2012)

- Staffing and Productivity (2/2011)

- Substance Abuse (7/2010)

- Telephone Triage (7/2010)

- Triage Qualifications (2/2011)

- Use of Protocols in the Emergency Setting (1/2014)

- Utilization of Paid Reservations for Emergency Department Services (5/2012)

- Violence in the Emergency Care Setting (10/2014)

- Weighing Patients in Kilograms (9/2012)

- Weighing Pediatric Patients in Kilograms (3/2012)

It's important to note that emergency nursing, medicine, and emergency medical services (EMS), including emergency transport, are all historically intertwined. As emergency patient care has evolved into a specialty that now provides non-urgent, urgent, and emergent care from birth to death, emergency nursing continues to play a key role in this process.

Advanced Practice Nursing in the Emergency Department

In 1965, Loretta Ford opened a 4-month-long pediatric nurse practitioner program at the University of Colorado. Her vision was to increase access to pediatric care by using nurses in an expanded role that would make care more affordable in underserved areas (Snyder et al., 2006). The success of this program set the foundation for the expansion of the role of nursing in patient care.

In the 1970s, funding became more available for advanced practice nursing in other areas, including emergency nursing. Initially, these were certificate programs that lasted from 16 to 68 weeks. Curriculum and length of training varied, depending on the programs.

Through these programs, the emergency nurse practitioner can learn how to (Hardy, 1978):

■ Take a medical history

■ Perform a physical examination

■ Assess clinical information

■ Develop a health-maintenance program that includes prevention

■ Perform laboratory tests

■ Initiate resuscitation, including CPR

■ Perform wound care

■ Immobilize injured limbs

■ Determine the management of diagnosed injuries and illnesses

■ Counsel patients on psychosocial issues

■ Counsel patients on medications

In 1976, the University of Virginia offered the Emergency Nurse Practitioner Program. Nurses needed to have 2 years of experience and a committed ED physician preceptor. Upon completion of the program, graduates were able to apply in Virginia for emergency nurse practitioner licensure and were approved emergency medical technicians and CPR instructors (Snyder et al., 2006). The opportunity to obtain a master's degree was also offered to graduates of the program.

The University of Texas School of Nursing admitted its first ENP students in 1994. As of 2008, a survey completed by Davis-Moon and Storer found that there are five nurse practitioner programs and four that have post-master's certificates in emergency care (Davis-Moon & Storer, 2008). For more information on educational requirements for the nurse practitioner, see Chapter 4, "Education of the Emergency Nurse."

In 1999, the ENA adopted the *Scope of Practice for the Practitioner in the Emergency Setting* (Cole, Ramirez, & Luna-Gonzales, 1999). This document outlines the role, educational preparation, and practice arrangements for ENPs. In 2010, the ENA NP Validation Team published the results of a Delphi Study designed to identify the competencies for practice in emergency care for nurse practitioners (Hoyt et al., 2010).

The advanced practice nurse is a role not only in the United States but in many other parts of the world, including Europe and Australia. The advanced practice role of the nurse in the ED continues to develop as they become an integral part of the staff in many EDs, especially in underserved and rural parts of the world.

Role of the Emergency Department

In 2011, more than 136 million visits were made to EDs in the United States (Centers for Disease Control and Prevention [CDC], 2015). Emergency department visits continue to grow, yet EDs are closing, initiating ambulance diversions, increasing waiting times, and boarding patients who are critically ill and injured. This overcrowding in EDs is occurring because of decreasing numbers of doctors and nurses and limited hospital beds (Castillo et al., 2011; Hoot & Aronsky, 2008; Institute of Medicine [IOM], 2006).

 Boarding patients—When ED patients are admitted to an inpatient unit but the inpatient unit cannot accept the patient due to staffing or other constraints and the patient must wait in the ED.

Since the 1950s, hospitals, nurses, and physicians have expressed concern about the use of the emergency room for non-emergencies (Coleman & Errera, 1963; Zinc, 2006). In 1974, Rosen, Segal, Coppleson, and Fauman wrote that there was an increasing need to implement a method of triage in the ED to help recognize who required immediate care. They noted that nurses were the most experienced and competent at performing triage (Rosen, Segal, Coppleson, & Fauman, 1974).

Emergency departments have become the source of care for many types of patients, but particularly for patients who are poor and uninsured. Many societal changes have had an impact on the ED. The establishment of Medicare and Medicaid in 1965 increased the ED census. Patients who did not have medical insurance coverage could now have care they did not have access to in the past (Zinc, 2006).

In 1966, the Committee on Trauma and the Committee on Shock published a landmark paper entitled "Accidental Death and Disability: The Neglected Disease of Modern Society," which focused attention on the unnecessary mortality and morbidity of injured patients. From this paper came the drive and, most importantly, the funding for the development of emergency services throughout the United States. The ED became one of the focal points for this care (Zinc, 2006).

The Emergency Medical Treatment and Active Labor Act (EMTALA), which became a federal law in 1986, created a right to emergency care whether the patient is or is not a United States citizen. EMTALA ensures that EDs cannot refuse to provide a medical screening examination and stabilizing care when patients present for care. For more information on EMTALA and how it affects the ED, see Chapter 12, "Risk Management and Quality Issues Affecting the Emergency Nurse."

 Another piece of legislation that has the potential to affect the ED is the Affordable Care Act. According to the American College of Emergency Physicians ([ACEP], 2014), visits to the ED increased in the 6 months after the passage of this law, and the increased availability of health insurance for many individuals through this law is expected to cause the census in the ED to continue to climb.

Lee (2015) poses the question as to whether social media, including television shows that glamorize the ED, has played a recent role in the continued increase in the ED census. Major illnesses and injuries are common features of social media and television shows. Reality television also uses cameras to film resuscitations and evaluations with multiple modes of technology that save a patient's life daily (Lee, 2015). Who would not want to be cared for in this manner?

The increase in uninsured patients, open access, and the ability to provide 24-hour-a-day care have stressed the capacity of EDs. Patients' perception of what the ED can provide and why they may choose to come to the ED continues to challenge all who work within this environment (Soremekun, Takayesu, & Bohan, 2011). The ED plays an important role in patient care, and emergency nurses continue to be an essential part of the collaborative teams who work in EDs.

Emergency Nursing as a Specialty

In 2011, the ANA recognized emergency nursing as a nursing specialty and described emergency nursing as "the care of individuals across the lifespan with perceived or actual physical or emotional alterations of health that are undiagnosed or require further interventions. Emergency nursing care is episodic, primary, typically short-term, and occurs in a variety of settings" (ANA, 2011, p. 1; Bonalumi & King, 2007; Fazio, 2010; Patrick, 2010).

The ENA states that emergency nurses provide care across the lifespan in a variety of patient care settings, including the pre-hospital, transport, and hospital environments. Emergency nursing interventions may be minimal to life-saving. An integral part of emergency nursing is prevention. Unique to emergency nursing practice is the application of the nursing process to patients of all ages who require stabilization and/or resuscitation for a variety of illnesses and injuries (ENA, 2011).

In 2011, the ENA published *Emergency Nursing Scope and Standards of Practice*. Incorporated within the *Scope and Standards* is ENA's *Code of Ethics*. The ENA *Code of Ethics,* updated in 2015, is the framework for providing competent, holistic, safe, and ethical patient care, as well as ensuring that all individuals have access to care.

Per the ENA *Code of Ethics,* the emergency nurse (ENA, 2015, p. 1–3):

- Collaborates with multidisciplinary teams across the spectrum to ensure safe practice and safe care

- Acts with compassion, integrity, and respect for human dignity while recognizing and safeguarding the autonomy of the individual

- Maintains competence within, and accountability for, emergency nursing practice

- Acts to protect the individual when healthcare and safety are threatened by incompetent, unethical, or illegal practice

- Exercises sound judgment in exercising responsibility, reporting, delegating, and seeking consultation

- Respects the individual's right to privacy and confidentiality

- Advocates for and works to improve public health and secure access to healthcare for all

- Embraces the role of advocate for patients, families, all healthcare workers, and communities in discussion of healthcare policy

- Supports and participates in research needed to close the gap in knowledge, practice, and education

- Promotes and fosters a healthy work environment and a Just Culture

 Just Culture—An atmosphere or culture where frontline care providers feel comfortable disclosing errors (including their own) without fear of reprisal.

The *Emergency Nursing Scope and Standards of Practice* includes Standards of Practice and Standards of Professional Performance. Standards 1 to 6 are grounded in the nursing process, which contains Assessment including Triage, Diagnosis, and Outcomes Identification; Planning including Coordination of Care, Health Teaching, and Health Promotion; Consultation; Prescription Authority; and Treatment and Evaluation.

Triage and collaboration are important components in emergency nursing practice. Because emergency nursing care is generally episodic, emergency nurses must quickly assess and identify who is sick, sicker, or the sickest so care can rapidly be initiated. Collaboration is mandatory because many patients have multiple issues that demand a transition of care. For an in-depth look at the triage process, see Chapter 10, "The Emergency Nurse in the Role of Triage."

Standards 7 to 16 designate the behaviors of professional nurses, including advanced practice nurses, who work in the specialty of emergency nursing (ENA, 2011). Standard 7 describes ethical emergency nursing practice, which has now been incorporated into the ENA *Code of Ethics*. Table 1.2 contains a summary of standards 8–16 for professional practice (ENA, 2011, p. 17).

Table 1.2 Emergency Nursing Standards of Professional Practice 8–16

Standard	Description
Standard 8 Education	Education for emergency nursing for competence and current nursing practice
Standard 9 Evidence-Based Practice and Research	Use of evidence-based practice and research in emergency nursing practice
Standard 10 Quality of Practice	The emergency registered nurse contributes to quality nursing practice
Standard 11 Communication	Need for effective communication

continues

Table 1.2 Emergency Nursing Standards of Professional Practice 8–16   (continued)

Standard	Description
Standard 12 Leadership	Emergency nurse demonstrates leadership in profession and practice of emergency nursing
Standard 13 Collaboration	Collaboration with patients, families, communities, and all who interact in providing emergency care
Standard 14 Professional Practice Evaluation	Evaluation of emergency nursing practice using current practice guidelines, rules, and regulations
Standard 15 Resource Utilization	Use of appropriate resources to plan and provide safe patient care
Standard 16 Environmental Health	Safe practice, safe care within the emergency care environment

The first *Emergency Nursing Core Curriculum* was released in 1987 (though there was a core curriculum developed in 1975 by EDNA to help guide the education and training of the emergency nurse). The 6th edition was published in 2007, and a 7th edition is slated for release in 2016. This curriculum outlines the practice of emergency nursing based on the nursing process. This core provides the foundation of the knowledge base for the practice of emergency nursing. It's also a part of the framework for the Certified Emergency Nurse exam (CEN).

The first CEN exam was offered in July of 1980. The exam is managed by the Board of Certification for Emergency Nursing (BCEN). The CEN exam measures the attainment of a defined body of nursing knowledge pertinent to the specialty of emergency nursing. Currently, about 30,000 nurses hold the CEN certification. There are CENs throughout the world, but the CEN exam is based on emergency nursing practice in the United States (BCEN, 2015).

In 2005, the Pediatric Nursing Certification Board and the BCEN began working together to develop a certification for pediatric emergency care. The Certified Pediatric Emergency Nurse exam (CPEN) was first offered in 2009 (BCEN, 2015).

The BCEN also offers certification for transport nursing, including the Certified Flight Registered Nurse (CFRN) and the Certified Transport Registered Nurse (CTRN). Another certification, Trauma Certified Registered Nurse, will be made available beginning in 2016 (BCEN, 2015). For more information on obtaining certification, see Chapter 4. For more information on certification as it relates to the professionalism of nursing and how to prepare for certification exams, see Chapter 5, "The Emergency Nurse as a Professional."

Emergency Nursing Competencies

Who are emergency nurses and what skills are needed to be a part of this nursing specialty? Kennedy, Curtis, and Waters (2014) conducted a study that described the personality of an emergency nurse. A standardized personality test instrument was completed by 72 emergency nurses. Five personality domains were evaluated: neuroticism, extraversion, openness to experience, agreeableness, and conscientiousness. Emergency nurses were found to score significantly higher than the population norm on extraversion, openness to experience, and agreeableness (Kennedy et al., 2014). Emergency nurses are generally a different group of nurses who enjoy the challenges of patient care in a chaotic, rapidly changing work environment.

 Extraversion—This variation on the word "extrovert" indicates an individual satisfied by activities or thoughts outside of one's own self.

In order to practice and function safely in this environment, the practice of emergency nursing requires specific competencies. A primary competency in emergency nursing practice is the ability to *triage* (sort out who is the sickest) and coordinate care of all patients who present to the ED (ENA, 2011).

Several published papers have attempted to describe the competencies related to the practice of emergency nursing and how to evaluate nurses' ability to perform them. The BCEN has also performed role delineation studies over the years to identify the elements of emergency and transport nursing practices.

McCarthy, Cornally, O'Mahoney, White, & Weathers (2013) used a quantitative description design to evaluate how frequently 199 nursing procedures were performed by emergency nurses. The study was conducted across 11 EDs in Ireland. Even though this research was conducted in Ireland, the tool was based on Campo, McNulty, Sabitini, and Fitzpatrick's (2008) assessment of nurse practitioners' competencies. The authors identified specific competencies and organized them using Benner's five domain categories of practice: diagnostic function, administering and monitoring therapeutic interventions, effective management of rapidly changing situations, organizational and workload competencies, and the helping role. Table 1.3 contains some examples of the identified competencies in each of these categories (McCarthy et al., 2013, p. 53–54).

Table 1.3 Examples of Procedures in Emergency Nursing

Category	Competencies
Diagnostic Functioning	Attaching ECG monitoring Administering pain medication and assessing patient response Assessing airway, breathing, and circulation and the patient's response to interventions
Administering and Monitoring Therapeutic Interventions	Applying cervical immobilization Performing venipuncture; inserting peripheral venous catheters Female urethral catheterization
Effective Management of Rapidly Changing Situations	Seeking assistance with care of patient who is deteriorating rapidly
Organizational and Workload Competencies	Working as part of an interdisciplinary team Communicating effectively with multidisciplinary team
The Helping Role	Planning patient care Conducting holistic assessment

Harding, Walker-Cillo, Duke, Campos, and Stapleton (2013) developed a framework for creating and evaluating competencies for emergency nurses. Using the *Emergency Nursing Scope and Standards of Practice,* these authors present an ED triage competency validation form that can be used to evaluate the emergency nurse's triage abilities. A good evaluation of an emergency nurse's triage competency needs to include the type of triage stratification system used, method of communication, the interventions required and allowed for critically ill or deteriorating patients, employer resources, and the type of communication modalities that are used in the ED in which the nurse practices (Harding et al., 2013, p. 256–261).

Summary

Emergency nursing is a specialty that provides care to individuals across the lifespan with perceived or actual physical or emotional alterations of health that are undiagnosed or require further interventions. Emergency nursing care is episodic, primary, typically short-term, and occurs in a variety of settings (ANA, 2011; Bonalumi & King, 2007; Fazio, 2010; Patrick, 2010).

Two visionary nurses, Anita Dorr and Judith Kelleher, took on the challenge of creating a way for emergency nursing to be recognized as the specialty it is. Their vision and work have continued to be realized through the Emergency Nurses Association. Emergency nursing is practiced all over the world.

EDs provide care for all patients, whether they present in full cardiopulmonary arrest or just have a stubbed toe. Emergency nurses are an integral part of the ED, and the practice of emergency nursing requires specific competencies and experiences. Just as there are new societal and disease challenges, emergency nursing continues to develop to meet patients' needs. Emergency nurses are the heart and soul of emergency care.

References

American College of Emergency Physicians (ACEP). (2014, May 21). *ER visits up since implementation of the Affordable Care Act* [news release]. Retrieved from http://newsroom.acep.org/2014-05-21-ER-Visits-Up-Since-Implementation-of-Affordable-Care-Act#Closed

American Nurses Association (ANA). (2015). *What is nursing?* Retrieved from http://www.nursingworld.org/EspeciallyForYou/What-is-Nursing

American Nurses Association (ANA). (2011, August 23). *ANA recognizes emergency nursing as a specialty* [Press release]. Retrieved from http://www.nursingworld.org/FunctionalMenuCategories/MediaResources/PressReleases/2011-PR/ANA-Recognizes-Emergency-Nursing-Specialty-Practice.pdf

Anderson, P. D., Suter, R. E., Mulligan, T., Bodiwala, G., Razzak, J. A., & Mock, C. (2012). World Health Assembly Resolution 60.22 and its importance as a health care policy tool for improving emergency access and availability globally. *Annals of Emergency Medicine, 60*(1), 35–44. doi: 10.1016/j.annemergmed.2011.10.018

Ayers, K. (2014). How did Florence Nightingale survive being a trauma coordinator? *Journal of Trauma Nursing, 9*(4), 89–92.

Board of Certification for Emergency Nursing (BCEN). (2015). *Certified Emergency Nurse (CEN)* and *Certified Pediatric Emergency Nurse (CPEN)*. Retrieved from http://www.bcencertifications.org/Get-Certified.aspx

Bonalumi, N., & King, D. (2007). Professionalism and leadership. In S. Hoyt & J. Selfridge-Thomas (Eds.), *Emergency nursing core curriculum* (6th ed., pp. 1046–1056). Philadelphia, PA: W. B. Saunders.

Campo, T., McNulty, R., Sabatini, M., & Fitpatrick, J. (2008). Nurse practitioners performing procedures with confidence and independence in emergency care setting. *Advanced Emergency Nursing Journal, 30*(2), 153–170.

Castillo, E., Vilke, G., Williams, M., Turner, P., Boyle, J., & Chan, T. (2011). Collaborative to decrease ambulance diversion: The California emergency department diversion project. *Journal of Emergency Medicine, 40*(3), 300–307.

Centers for Disease Control and Prevention (CDC). (2015). National Hospital Ambulatory Medical Care Survey: 2011 emergency department summary tables 1, 4, 14. 24. Retrieved from http://www.cdc.gov/nchs/fastats/emergency-department.htm

Cole, F. L., Ramirez, E., & Luna-Gonzales, H. (1999). *Scope of practice for the nurse practitioner in the emergency setting*. Des Plaines, IL: Emergency Nurses Association.

Coleman, J. V., & Errera, P. (1963). The general hospital emergency room and its psychiatric problems. *American Journal of Public Health, 53*(8), 1294–1301.

Davis-Moon, L., & Storer, A. (2008). *A survey of emergency nurse practitioner programs in the United States*. Retrieved from http://www.nursinglibrary.org/vhl/handle/10755/162689

Department of Defense. (2010). *Nurses in the Korean War: New roles for a traditional profession.* Retrieved from http://www.koreanwar60.com/nurses-korean-war-new-roles-traditional-profession

Emergency Medicine Network. (2012). *National Emergency Department Inventory.* Retrieved from http://www.emnet-usa.org/nedi/nedi_usa.htm

Emergency Nurses Association (ENA). (2011). *Emergency nursing scope and standards of practice.* Des Plaines, IL: Emergency Nurses Association.

Emergency Nurses Association (ENA). (2015). Retrieved from https://www.ena.org/publications/Pages/Default.aspx

Fazio, J. (2010). Emergency nursing practice. In P. Kunz Howard & R. Steinmann (Eds.), *Sheehy's emergency nursing: Principles and practice* (6th ed., pp. 8–15). St. Louis, MO: Mosby Elsevier.

Gebbie, K., & Qureshi, K. (2006). A historical challenge: Nurses and emergencies. *Online Journal of Issues in Nursing, 11*(3), 2. doi: 10.3912/OJIN.Vol11No03Man01

Harding, D., Walker-Cillo, G., Duke, A., Campos, G., & Stapleton, S. (2013). A framework for creating and evaluating competencies for emergency nurses. *Journal of Emergency Nursing, 39*(3), 252–264.

Hardy, V. G. (1978). The emergency nurse practitioner: The role and training of an emergency health professional. *Journal of the American College of Emergency Physicians, 7*(10), 372–376.

Hoot, N. R., & Aronsky, D. (2008). Systematic review of emergency department crowding: Causes, effects, and solutions. *Annals of Emergency Medicine, 52*(2), 126–136. doi: 10.1016/j.annemergmed.2008.03.014

Hoyt, S., Coyne, E. A., Ramirez, E. G., Peard, A., Gisness, C., & Gacki-Smith, J. (2010). Nurse practitioner Delphi Study: Competence for practice in emergency care. *Journal of Emergency Nursing, 36*(5), 439–449.

Institute of Medicine (IOM). (2006). *Hospital-based emergency care at the breaking point.* Washington, DC: National Academy of Sciences.

Kennedy, B., Curtis, K., & Waters, S. (2014). The personality of emergency nurses: Is it unique? *Australasian Emergency Nursing Journal, 17,* 139–145.

Kennedy, R. H. (1957). Give the emergency room the status it deserves. *Hospitals, 31,* 35–36.

Lee, G. (2015), Emergency departments: A victim of our own success? *International Emergency Nursing, 23*(2), 45–46.

MacMillan, K. M. (2012). The challenge of achieving interprofessional collaboration: Should we blame Nightingale? *Journal of Interprofessional Care, 26*(5), 410–415. doi: 10.3109/13561820.2012.699480

McCarthy, G., Cornally, N., O'Mahoney, C., White, G., & Weathers, E. (2013). Emergency nurses: Procedures performed and competence in practice. *Journal of Emergency Nursing, 21,* 50–57.

McDonald, L. (2013). What would Florence Nightingale say? *British Journal of Nursing, 22*(9), 542.

Medical emergency. (2015). In *Oxford English Dictionary* online. Retrieved from www.oxforddictionaries.com/definition/english/medical-emergency

Owens, J. C. (1970). Operating room nursing and emergency. *AORN, 12*(5), 46–49.

Patrick, V. (2010). Emergency nursing: A historical perspective. In P. Kunz Howard & R. A. Steinmann (Eds.), *Sheehy's emergency nursing: Principles and practice* (6th ed., pp. 3–7). St. Louis, MO: Mosby Elsevier.

Rosen, P., Segal, M., Coppleson, L., & Fauman, B. (1974). A method of triage within an emergency department. *Journal of the American College of Emergency Physicians, Mar/Apr,* 85–86.

Schriver, J., Talmadge, R., Chuong, R., & Hedges, J. (2003). Emergency nursing. *Journal of Emergency Nursing, 29*(5), 431–439.

Sefrin, P., & Weidringer, J. W. (1991). History of emergency medicine in Germany. *Journal of Clinical Anesthesia, 3*(3), 245–248.

Sheingold, B. H., & Hahn, J. A. (2014). The history of health care quality. *International Journal of African Nursing Sciences, 1,* 18–22.

Shell, C. M., & Dunlap, K. D. (2008). Florence Nightingale, Dr. Ernest Codman, American College of Surgeons Hospital Standardization Committee, and the Joint Commission: Four pillars in the foundation of patient safety. *Perioperative Nursing Clinics, 3*(1), 19–26.

Snyder, A., Keeling, A., & Razionale, C. (2006). From "First Aid Rooms" to advanced practice nursing: A glimpse into the history of emergency nursing. *Advanced Emergency Nursing Journal, 3,* 198–209.

Soremekun, O. A., Takayesu, J. K., & Bohan, S. J. (2011). Framework for analyzing wait times and other factors that impact patient satisfaction in the emergency department. *Journal of Emergency Medicine, 41*(6), 686–692.

United States Navy and Army. (n.d.). *Personnel.* Retrieved from www.mrfa.org/vnstats.htm

U.S. Army Center of Military History. (2003). *The Army Nurse Corps.* Washington, DC: Government Printing Office.

Zinc, B. (2006). *Anyone, anywhere, anytime: A history of emergency medicine.* Philadelphia, PA: Mosby Elsevier.

THE TRADITIONAL ROLE OF THE EMERGENCY NURSE

–Darin L. Durham, BSN, RN; and Jeff Solheim, MSN, RN-BC, CEN, CFRN, FAEN

Many images may come to mind when the words "emergency nurse" are spoken. For some people, it might be a memory of a person who took care of them or a loved one during a past visit to the emergency department (ED). Others may envision a character from a popular television show. For many people, an emergency nurse conjures up visions of delivering care in a high-adrenaline environment—perhaps performing cardiopulmonary resuscitation, stemming the flow of blood from a traumatic wound, or administering a life-saving bolus of medication. Although these activities may make up part of the day for an emergency nurse, they are not representative of the full range and responsibility of this role. Emergency nursing is a complex profession that encompasses many duties, some of which include the standard vision of the emergency nurse, but many that do not. This chapter explores some of the traditional functions of the emergency nurse.

Direct Patient-Care Roles

Although the role of the emergency nurse can be varied, the majority of emergency nurses provide direct patient care. Yet even in the area of direct patient care, there are wide variations in how that role is applied. Examples of patient-care roles include staff nurse, travel nurse, transport nurse, nurse practitioner, and clinical nurse leader.

Staff Nurse

Registered nurses who provide direct patient care in an institution are often referred to as "staff nurses." Another common title is a "clinical nurse." As this chapter and the chapter that follows demonstrate, emergency nurses can take on many roles, but the traditional role of the staff nurse remains the backbone of institutional nursing. Staff nurses either provide direct patient care to ED patients or delegate and oversee that care to other personnel within the department.

Staff nurses are often referred to as "generalists" and perform a wide variety of duties. The most obvious role of the emergency nurse is to apply the nursing process to the care of patients who present to the ED. The emergency nurse performs patient assessments and makes a judgment about the actual or potential health problem the patient has. Armed with this information, the nurse develops a plan of care, implements that plan, and then evaluates the effectiveness of the care.

The application of the nursing process is not unique to being a staff nurse in the ED; nurses in every clinical area utilize the nursing process to deliver care to patients. But several factors create a unique environment that differentiates emergency nursing from other areas of nursing.

The first is the episodic nature of the ED. The arrival of patients and the acuity of those patients is unpredictable. The workload of the emergency nurse can change dramatically from literally one minute to the next. It's possible that several patients may arrive in a short period of time with high acuity problems requiring intensive nursing care. A major event such as a multi-casualty trauma can result in the influx of numerous patients simultaneously, or the lack of inpatient beds can result in the accumulation of many high-acuity patients requiring significant nursing care. Potentially, all of these events could occur simultaneously, and the emergency nurse must be able to prioritize and adapt to ensure high-quality and safe care. Because of this unpredictable workload, some of the qualities listed by the Emergency Nurses Association (ENA, n.d.) as advantageous for staff nurses include:

- The ability to shift gears and accelerate the pace of work as needed

- Multi-tasking ability

- The ability to maintain calm amid chaos

- The capability to think fast and on your feet

- Good observation, assessment, and prioritization skills

- Good interpersonal and customer service skills

- Stamina

- Good personal coping skills

- Being an assertive patient advocate

- Having a good sense of humor

Another factor that makes staff nursing in the ED unique from other areas of nursing is the collaborative yet independent nature of practice created by the ED environment. In most EDs, physicians are physically present in the unit 24 hours a day, giving the emergency nurse immediate access for collaboration on patient care issues. Ironically, despite physical availability of physicians for collaboration, emergency nurses frequently state that one thing that draws them to emergency nursing is the independence in practice that the ED allows. When nurses work in triage for example, they are usually physically isolated from the rest of the department and must make independent decisions directly affecting patient care. Many EDs have implemented standing orders or protocols that allow nurses to initiate radiology and other diagnostic tests to expedite patient movement through the ED. Multiple studies have shown that when protocols are appropriately implemented, length of stay decreases and patient care is improved (Robinson, 2013). It's essential to remember that although protocols may give the impression of independent practice, they are approved by medical staff, and they should be carefully followed and only implemented when the patient fits the criteria outline in the protocol (Patrizzi, Gurney, Baxter, Bush, & Crook, 2013).

 Standing Order or Protocol—"An agreed framework outlining the care that will be provided to patients in a designated area of practice. They do not describe how a procedure is performed, but why, where, when, and by whom the care is given" (Ebling Library, 2015).

Another thing that makes emergency nursing unique is the varied population served by emergency nurses. Unlike other nursing specialties that may focus on a specific age range (e.g., pediatric or adult patients) or a specific body system (e.g., orthopedics or obstetrics), emergency nurses serve all ages experiencing disorders to every body system. In fact, the very definition of emergency nursing outlined by the American Nurses Association (2011) highlights this uniqueness:

> "Emergency Nursing is the care of individuals across the lifespan with perceived or actual physical or emotional alterations of health that are undiagnosed or require further interventions. Emergency nursing care is episodic, primary, typically short-term, and occurs in a variety of settings." (p. 1)

For this reason, emergency nurses have to have a broad knowledge base and skill set.

Common Educational Preparation

The minimum educational requirement for a staff nurse is an associate's degree or diploma in nursing. As the profession of nursing has become increasingly complex, a push for a minimum of a baccalaureate degree to practice as a staff nurse has gained momentum. Some hospitals require nurses to have a baccalaureate degree as a condition of hire, especially in critical care units such as the ED. Individuals interested in emergency nursing are strongly advised to seek a baccalaureate degree to increase their chance of hire into the ED. For additional information on nursing education and the baccalaureate degree as an entry to practice, see Chapter 4, "Education of the Emergency Nurse."

Suggested Career Path

There are no national standards regarding the education and experience required to be a staff nurse except that the individual holds a license to practice as a registered nurse. Therefore, the suggested career path to being a staff nurse in the ED may be as varied as the number of EDs.

Although new graduate nurses sometimes get hired into the ED, this usually involves a lengthy and expensive internship or orientation program. For that reason, many EDs seek nurses with prior experience, even from different clinical areas such as the intensive care unit or cardiology. Even if the clinical area is vastly different from the ED, the nurse may have developed assessment and organizational skills that transfer nicely to the ED setting.

Nurses interested in becoming emergency nurses may consider the following suggestions:

- **Take numerous courses to improve skills in the emergency setting.** Although these courses are rarely required as conditions of employment, taking these courses prior to applying for an emergency nurse position demonstrates the applicant's dedication to the position and may make the applicant stand out from other nurses interested in the position. Courses that are required in many EDs include the Advanced Cardiovascular Life

Support Course (ACLS), the Pediatric Advanced Life Support (PALS) Course, the Trauma Nursing Core Course (TNCC), and the Emergency Nursing Pediatric Course (ENPC).

■ **Gain experience and skills in other positions that translate into the skills required to be a staff nurse in the ED.** Applicants who bring past experience as unlicensed assistive personnel in an ED (e.g., emergency department technician), pre-hospital experience such as an emergency medical technician (EMT) or paramedic, and experience as a registered nurse in a different clinical area, especially one with a critical-care focus such as the intensive care unit, may make the applicant more marketable when seeking a position within the ED.

Specialty Areas Within the ED

In a smaller ED, the staff nurse may receive orientation to care for all ages and types of patients. In larger hospitals, the department may be divided into various sections, and the emergency nurse may be assigned to one section for a shift or part of a shift caring for a specialized subset of patients (e.g., trauma patients or patients with psychiatric illnesses). Sometimes the staff nurse may permanently work with a specialized subset of patients (e.g., permanently assigned to work in the triage or pediatric area of the ED). In EDs with specialized areas, it's not uncommon for the emergency nurse to be trained in one area at a time until the nurse demonstrates competency in all areas. Some common "specialty areas" contained in the ED include:

■ Resuscitation rooms (Advanced Cardiac Life Support training is usually required to work in this area.)

■ Critical care area (Advanced Cardiac Life Support training is usually required to work in this area.)

■ Trauma rooms (A course in trauma nursing such as the Trauma Nursing Core Course is usually required to work in this area.)

■ Acute care area (This area may be further subdivided into areas such as obstetrics, gynecology, isolation rooms, etc.)

■ Low acuity area (sometimes called "fast track")

■ Pediatric area (A course in pediatric care such as the Pediatric Advanced Life Support Course or the Emergency Nursing Pediatric Course is usually required to work in this area.)

■ Psychiatric area

■ Observation unit (an area designed for patients who do not meet criteria for hospital admission but require ongoing care and assessment)

■ Triage area (For more information on requirements to work in triage and the process of triage, see Chapter 10, "The Emergency Nurse in the Role of Triage.")

Travel Nurse

A travel nurse is a staff nurse who chooses to work on a temporary contract rather than be permanently employed at a particular institution. There are multiple companies that coordinate travel nurse assignments. Each company is unique, with different benefits and conditions of employment; therefore, you need to thoroughly research the field before choosing a company. Contracts for 13-week assignments at one hospital are very common in the industry (although contracts may be as short as 8 weeks or as long as 23 weeks). At the end of the 13-week assignment, you may be able to extend the contract if you're enjoying the experience or may choose to accept a new 13-week assignment at a different institution.

The pay for travel nurses is often slightly higher than for nurses permanently employed at the institution. Travel companies frequently provide furnished housing or a housing stipend to the travel nurse. Benefits differ greatly among companies, with some companies offering competitive health, dental, retirement, and continuing-education benefits, while others offer less-competitive benefits.

The advantages of travel nursing include the ability to experience a variety of geographical areas of the country as well as experience different ways of doing things in a variety of healthcare settings. Many travel nurses find the financial rewards of travel nursing to be greater than if they were permanently employed at a particular institution.

Travel nurses experience disadvantages as well:

■ Less influence on choosing the shifts that they work and often less flexibility in setting their work schedule.

■ Rarely have the opportunity to become involved in unit committees and decisions regarding how the unit functions. Although this may be an advantage for nurses who aren't interested in this type of involvement, it can be frustrating for others who may desire greater input. Involvement at this level helps develop leadership skills that can be advantageous for future career advancement; therefore, travel nursing may be seen as an impediment to advancing to alternate jobs in nursing.

■ While travel lets the nurse experience new places and make new friends, it also takes the travel nurse away from home and family. It can make the maintenance of personal and community relationships difficult.

The National Association of Travel Healthcare Organizations has lots of great information on travel nursing. You can access its website at http://www.natho.org/about.php.

There are many variations on travel nursing aside from the traditional 13-week temporary assignment. Many communities have *registries,* companies that place nurses in local institutions for single shifts. Nurses may work at a different hospital every day. Unlike a travel nurse, nurses who work with registries can live at home and maintain family and community ties. The pay is often higher when working with a registry, and nurses may have more flexibility in their schedules, choosing what shifts and days they are available to work. The work, however, may be more sporadic and less likely to have benefits and assistance with housing.

There are also occasional opportunities for nurses to pick up travel assignments in foreign countries. These assignments are usually longer than 13 weeks but may offer very competitive wages and benefits. Companies also exist for nursing leaders to do travel assignments as "temporary management," which can be financially lucrative but may involve contracts of lengths much greater than 13 weeks.

Common Educational Preparation

The educational requirements for working as a travel nurse are identical to those of a staff nurse.

Suggested Career Path

Travel nurses usually receive much less orientation when starting a temporary assignment than a new staff nurse would receive if they were accepting a job at the same hospital. This is because travel nurses are expected to arrive at the job with the knowledge and experience to begin working with minimal training. Most travel companies will expect travel nurses to have between 12 and 24 months experience in the clinical area in which they will be working. If you're interested in becoming a travel nurse, first seek permanent employment at a facility that provides you with as much clinical experience as possible before seeking a travel assignment. Most hospitals expect you to come with basic courses like Advanced Cardiovascular Life Support (ACLS) up-to-date; therefore, find as many opportunities as possible to complete courses and gain skills before looking for a travel assignment.

Transport Nurse

A variation on staff nursing is transport nursing. Transport nurses also provide direct patient care, but they do so outside of the traditional hospital setting. Transport nursing may be considered a specialty distinct from emergency nursing; however, many of the skills needed to be an effective emergency nurse translate well to transport nursing.

Transport nurses may work in a variety of settings:

- **Flight nursing**

    - Rotor wing (helicopter), which often involves short flights transporting patients from their point of origin to a hospital or transporting patients from one hospital to another.

    - Fixed wing (airplane), which involves longer flights, most often to transport a patient from one state or country to another.

- **Ground transport nursing:** These nurses transport patients via ambulance from one location to another. Although most people envision pre-hospital personnel such as paramedics providing ground transport services, some companies hire nurses to work in the ambulance providing the complex care required to transport critically ill patients. Many ground transport nurses may be involved with a specialty ground transportation company that transports critically ill or injured pediatric patients or patients requiring complex intensive care en route.

Transport nurses typically work very independently, utilizing pre-established protocols. Because of the autonomous nature of this work, transport nurses frequently learn advanced skills that are not considered part of the normal competencies of an emergency nurse, such as intubation and advanced airway maintenance. Requirements unique to transport nursing (especially transport nurses who work on a helicopter) are physical requirements, such as height and weight limitations.

 Interested in more information about flight nursing? *The Air Medical Crew National Standard Curriculum* provides an in-depth look at flight nursing. Other books include *Flight Nursing Principles and Practice* and *Fundamentals of Aerospace Medicine.*

Common Educational Preparation

Transport nurses must be RNs. Exact requirements differ from one employer to another, but a bachelor's degree is frequently required for most transport companies, and some may even require a master's degree. Some employers may also require that transport nurses have education as a pre-hospital provider in an emergency medical technician or paramedic position (Air and Surface Transport Nurses Association [ASTNA], n.d.).

Suggested Career Path

Employers may require between 1 and 5 years of experience in the ICU, ED, or other critical care area before being considered for a transport job. Applicants with pre-hospital experience often have an advantage when being considered for a job as a transport nurse. You should complete courses such as Advanced Cardiovascular Life Support (ACLS), the Trauma Nursing Core Course (TNCC), Pediatric Advanced Life Support (PALS), and a Neonatal Resuscitation Program (NRP). Completion of national certifications such as the Certified Emergency Nurse (CEN), Critical Care Registered Nurse (CCRN), Certified Transport Registered Nurse (CTRN), and Certified Flight Registered Nurse (CFRN) would also give you an advantage when seeking a transport nursing position (ASTNA, n.d.).

Nurse Practitioner

Many emergency nurses are drawn to emergency nursing because of the sense of autonomy that they feel. That autonomy is probably most fully realized as a nurse practitioner. Nurse practitioners "provide nursing and medical services to individuals, families, and groups … diagnosing and managing acute episodic and chronic illnesses" (American Association of Nurse Practitioners [AANP], 2013). The scope of practice for a nurse practitioner expands beyond the registered nurse in many areas, including the ability to diagnose, interpret diagnostic tests, and prescribe medications and treatments (AANP, 2013). To learn more about the history of nurse practitioners in the United States, see Chapter 1, "Emergency Nursing Defined."

Common Educational Preparation

The minimum educational requirement to practice as a nurse practitioner is a master's degree; in the future, a doctorate may be required. For an in-depth discussion of the educational and certification requirements of a nurse practitioner, see Chapter 4.

Suggested Career Path

There is no specific career path that leads to becoming a nurse practitioner. This job requires educational preparation. Some nurses work for many years in a variety of different roles before going back to school to become a nurse practitioner; other nurses seek this designation early in their career.

Clinical Nurse Leader

Many emergency nurses find fulfillment working directly with patients at the stretcherside. They have no desire to seek an administrative role or even to work as an advanced practitioner. With this in mind, the American Association of Colleges of Nursing (AACN) developed a new educational track to provide advanced education for nurses wanting to take a leadership role in providing direct patient care called a *clinical nurse leader* (CNL). This individual oversees the integration of care and is usually directly involved in providing care to patients in complex situations. "The CNL collects and evaluates patient outcomes, assesses cohort risk and has decision-making authority to change care plans when necessary" (AACN, 2012). It's important to note that the clinical nurse leader position is neither administrative nor considered an advanced practice role. However, like an advanced practice registered nurse, CNLs must take a certification exam to practice in this role.

Common Educational Preparation

A CNL must complete a master's degree with a focus on being a CNL.

Suggested Career Path

An emergency nurse becomes a CNL by completing his or her master's degree. Although experience as an RN before obtaining this degree is preferable, there is no specific career path that will assist in obtaining this role.

Administrative Roles

Some emergency nurses may choose to apply their skills in roles that don't involve direct patient care. One of these roles is leadership or administration. It's important to note that many emergency nurses who choose the administrative track continue to provide patient care in addition to their leadership duties.

Charge Nurse

A natural progression in career advancement within nursing is to move from staff nurse to charge nurse. In some hospitals, the charge nurse assignment is rotated among staff with experience in the department. In other departments, it may be an identified position that is carried out by a select group of individuals. The charge nurse is to a department what the conductor is to an orchestra. The charge nurse directs the daily operations of the department, making adjustments when needed. Generally, the charge nurse is viewed as the shift manager and handles the administrative as well as operational functioning of the department during the shift. The charge nurse is usually responsible for human resource issues on shift, ensuring adequate staffing, making work assignments, and dealing with personnel issues as they arise. The charge nurse liaises with pre-hospital staff and other departments to ensure patient flow is maintained. A charge nurse is often tasked with the responsibility of completing reports required by the institution or accrediting agencies.

A good charge nurse knows the resources available to handle issues as they arise and knows how to access those resources. Good charge nurses also display exceptional organizational skills, have superior communication skills, know how to handle conflict effectively, and can multitask without difficulty.

Common Educational Preparation

Because staff nurses are frequently assigned to the charge nurse role, the educational preparation may be identical. A bachelor's degree in nursing, however, generally includes leadership training beneficial in the charge nurse role. In some institutions, the charge nurse role is considered a stepping stone to other management positions, which almost always require a minimum of a baccalaureate degree in nursing. Therefore, emergency nurses contemplating career advancement should seriously consider education at a bachelor's degree or higher.

Suggested Career Path

Frequently, charge nurses are assigned from among the staff nurses working each shift, although in some departments, the position may be a permanent designation. Therefore, excelling at the staff nurse role is often used as one of the decisive factors in assigning the charge nurse role. Being a charge nurse, however, requires more than exceptional clinical skills. Leadership, communication, and people skills, as well as a thorough knowledge of the department, are also foundational to being a charge nurse. Taking additional training in these skills will help position you for the charge nurse role. Because intimate knowledge of the workings of the department and the hospital as a whole are also important, consider taking on additional responsibilities, such as volunteering for unit or hospital-wide committees or improvement projects within the department. These activities not only demonstrate commitment to the department but also allow you to stand out when it comes time to assign or select a charge nurse.

Manager

Although the charge nurse is responsible for the functioning of the unit during the shift on which he or she is working, the manager has 24-hour responsibility for the unit, even when he or she is not physically present. Being the manager of a nursing unit requires a different skill set than being a staff nurse (see Table 2.1).

Table 2.1 Differences Between Staff Nurses and Managers	
Staff Nurse	*Manager*
Doer	Planner, Designer
One-on-one interactions	One-to-many interactions
Reactive personality	Proactive personality
Require immediate gratification	Accept delayed gratification
Deciders	Delegators
Value autonomy	Value collaboration
Independent	Participative
Patient advocate	Organizational advocate
Identify with profession	Identify with organization

Source: Mayer, Kaplan, & Kelly, 2014, p. 36.

Although managers should possess the same skills as the charge nurse, the nurse manager must also have knowledge and skills in (Turner, Stone-Griffith, & Kopka, 2014):

- Human resource management (including hiring, termination, evaluations, training, disciplinary action, scheduling, payroll, and adjusting staffing to budget and staff satisfaction)

- Staffing (including scheduling, adjusting staffing to budget and census, payroll)

- Patient care (patient satisfaction, ensuring quality care, patient flow)

- Quality and risk (including core measure, risk audits, EMTALA, dashboards, data collection, survey readiness, policy development and review, Hospital Consumer Assessment of Healthcare Providers and Systems [HCAHPS])

- Interpersonal relationships (with physicians, pre-hospital personnel, other departments in the hospital, staff, peers, nursing students)

- Finance (budgeting, variance reports, supplies, billing, coding)

- Facility (committees, facility initiatives, community meetings)

Common Educational Preparation

The skill set required to be a manager demands the education offered at the baccalaureate level, and most nurse managers would be best served to have a master's degree in either nursing leadership or business administration. Although the exact educational requirements will be established by each institution, the American Nurses Credentialing Center (ANCC) requires nursing leaders to have a bachelor's degree or higher for Magnet certification (ANCC, 2014). Even though many hospitals have not sought Magnet designation, they have adopted many of the recommendations for Magnet status, including the education recommendations for nursing leaders.

Suggested Career Path

Nurses seeking leadership roles should pursue every opportunity to gain leadership experience. This may involve embracing the charge nurse role when it is available. Staff nurses may also accept additional assignments within the unit or institution to gain a deeper understanding of healthcare from a different perspective than a staff nurse. Sitting on the hospital-wide disaster committee, for example, allows you to meet other key players from around the hospital and learn how each one contributes to the institution. Similarly, seizing the opportunity to be involved with a performance improvement activity at the unit level gives you a broader scope not only of quality improvement but also how multiple factors contribute to outcomes. These types of experiences not only develop leadership competencies but may also be viewed during the interview process as an indication of commitment to personal development.

To develop leadership competencies, look outside of the hospital for experiences that develop these skills. Assuming leadership at a community level such as the local parent-teacher association, or leadership within a professional organization such as the Emergency Nurses Association, also helps develop skills in leadership and may also help to establish relationships that can be beneficial for career advancement into leadership in the future.

Director

In some hospitals, nurse managers report to a nursing director (in other hospitals, the nurse manager performs the role of both the manager and director). A nursing director shares the leadership responsibilities of the unit with the nurse manager but usually takes on most of the administrative duties, leaving managerial duties to the nurse manager. Table 2.2 takes the duties of the nurse manager listed earlier in this chapter and demonstrates how these duties are frequently divided between the nurse manager and a nurse director. It's not uncommon for a nursing director to be responsible for multiple units and have multiple nurse managers reporting to him or her.

Table 2.2 Common Division of Duties Between the Nurse Manager and the Nurse Director

Category	Tasks	Who's Responsible
Human resource management	Termination Evaluations Training Disciplinary action Scheduling Payroll Adjusting staffing to budget Staff satisfaction	Nurse manager
Quality and risk	Core measure Risk audits EMTALA Dashboards Data collection Survey readiness Policy development and review Hospital Consumer Assessment of Healthcare Providers and Systems [HCAHPS]	Nurse director
Staffing	Scheduling Adjusting staffing to budget and census Payroll	Nurse manager
Finance	Budgeting Variance reports Supplies Billing Coding	Collaborative between the nurse manager and nursing director
Facility	Committees Facility initiatives Community meetings	Collaborative between the nurse manager and nursing director
Patient care	Patient satisfaction Ensuring quality care Patient flow	Collaborative between the nurse manager and nursing director

Common Educational Preparation

Although specific educational requirements for a nursing director are unique to each institution, the administrative requirements of this job nearly always necessitate a master's degree in nursing or business administration. Some nursing directors have doctorate degrees.

Suggested Career Path

A common career path toward an administrative role such as a nursing director involves gaining experience as a staff nurse, then advancing leadership experience as a charge nurse. Most nursing directors also work as nurse managers prior to becoming a director, although this is not a mandatory prerequisite in most cases. Emergency nurses interested in nursing administration should actively seek leadership experiences and advanced degrees in nursing.

Trauma Coordinator (Trauma Program Managers)

Although trauma is often erroneously thought of as being part of the ED, effective care of the trauma patient extends beyond the ED throughout the hospital. While trauma patients are initially seen in the ED, they will likely pass through surgical services, critical care areas, medical-surgical units, and finally the rehabilitation department. Trauma patients frequently require utilization of nearly every ancillary department in the hospital. Therefore, trauma coordinators are usually not employees of the ED but work for the trauma department. Although a registered nurse from any area of the hospital with experience and knowledge in trauma care may serve as trauma coordinator, the skills that an emergency nurse brings to the job make them well suited for this position.

Trauma coordinators work in conjunction with the trauma medical director to coordinate trauma care throughout the entire patient's stay, not just in the ED. Trauma coordinators must have intimate knowledge of trauma designation or verification requirements, ensure adherence to those requirements, and generally take the lead during trauma designation or verification surveys (for more information on trauma designation and verification, see Chapter 7, "Types of Emergency Departments"). Trauma coordinators are usually intimately involved in trauma performance improvement, collecting data regarding care of the trauma patient, and trauma-patient outcomes. When care or outcomes are substandard, the trauma coordinator assists with the planning, implementation, and evaluation of interventions to improve care (Curtis & Ramsden, 2011). One of the biggest challenges a trauma coordinator faces is coordinating services from a variety of different spectrums including physicians, pre-hospital personnel, nursing units, and ancillary departments, many of which may spend little time caring for trauma patients and therefore have less motivation to be involved in the process.

Common Educational Preparation

The educational preparation required for this role is dependent heavily on the individual institution. The leadership qualities required of a trauma coordinator in a large hospital that sees thousands of trauma patients every year may be different from a small rural hospital that sees fewer than 100 trauma patients each year. However, the trauma-coordinator role is an administrative role for which preparation at a bachelor's degree or above will benefit the position.

Suggested Career Path

Trauma coordinators must see trauma from a trauma system perspective, being able to understand the entire process from prevention of trauma through rehabilitation. Therefore, nurses interested in being a trauma coordinator are best served by selecting a career path that exposes them to as many facets of trauma care as possible. Serving on committees that help plan trauma care, attending trauma educational events, and taking courses focused on care of the trauma patient will all help to make the nurse more marketable for this position.

 The American Trauma Society has an educational offering entitled "Trauma Program Manager Course," which is designed for nurses already in the role of trauma coordinator but is also helpful for nurses wanting to learn more about the position (American Trauma Society, n.d.).

Other Hospital Roles for Emergency Nurses

One advantage of being an emergency nurse is the plethora of opportunities that this role prepares you for. Emergency nurses may leave the traditional patient care role or augment it with a variety of other duties for which their experiences uniquely prepare them for. Examples of other roles that emergency nurses are well suited for include clinical educators—especially in the emergency department—safety coordinators, and telephone triage nurses.

Clinical Educators

Healthcare is a dynamic field, especially as the focus shifts to providing evidence-based care. (For more information on evidence-based care and research, see Chapter 5, "The Emergency Nurse as a Professional.") Although emergency nurses have a professional responsibility to ensure that their practice is current, clinical educators help in this process by recognizing deficits in knowledge and providing educational opportunities for nurses in the ED. Clinical educators also frequently oversee the orientation of new employees and coordinate education on new equipment, policies, procedures, and processes within the department.

It's not uncommon for a unit educator to play a leading role in preparing the unit for various accreditation surveys such as The Joint Commission or a Magnet survey. Nurse educators are usually responsible for measuring individual nursing competencies and working with nurses who may lack competency in a particular skill or clinical area.

Although many nurse educators are not clinical nurse specialists (CNS), the educational preparation of the CNS makes them ideal candidates to be involved in the role of clinical education. A CNS has either a master's degree or a doctorate and has successfully completed a certification exam. A CNS, like a nurse practitioner, is an advanced practitioner, although they have different roles. According to the National Association of Clinical Nurse Specialists (n.d., p. 1), a CNS provides direct patient care and "improves patient outcomes through expert consultation, care coordination, monitoring quality improvement indicators and expert communication between the health care team and the family."

Common Educational Preparation

Although educational requirements for the position of nurse educator are unique to each institution, most employers will prefer that the unit educator have a minimum of a bachelor's degree and most will prefer a master's degree with specialization in education. If the role is to be filled by a CNS, then a minimum of a master's degree is required, but a CNS can also be prepared at the doctoral level.

Suggested Career Path

If you're interested in becoming an educator, focus heavily on being an educational leader on the nursing unit. Offering to help with competency measurement, becoming a unit preceptor, or training as an instructor in a course such as the Trauma Nursing Core Course (TNCC) may demonstrate to the institution your dedication to educating others. These types of activities also help develop skills that are useful in the educator role.

Safety Coordinators

Emergency nurses may have a sole position as a safety coordinator in the department or have this duty assigned to them as part of a regular staff position in the department. The safety coordinator typically reports to a safety committee in the hospital and represents his or her department. The coordinator is responsible for making sure safety issues are addressed with staff and monitors events that occur in the department. Their goal is to prevent these events from occurring through education, monitoring, and reporting.

The goal of a safety coordinator is to provide a safe working environment for the staff and a safe environment for the patient.

Common Educational Preparation

There is no special educational preparation to serve as a safety coordinator.

Suggested Career Path

Nurses interested in becoming a safety coordinator should seek continuing education in safety requirements.

Telephone Triage Nurse

Emergency nurses perform triage regularly, so adapting to the role of a telephone triage nurse or telehealth nurse seems like a natural progression. Telehealth nurses perform assessments via phone instead of in person. They utilize specific scripts and protocols to answer health questions and determine whether additional healthcare is necessary and, if so, where the patient should seek that healthcare. Although nurses who work for poison control centers have a very specific knowledge base regarding toxicology, they also practice telehealth nursing.

Common Educational Preparation

The educational preparation for a telehealth nurse is similar to that of a staff nurse; however, there are numerous additional courses available to provide you additional competencies needed to be successful in this role.

Suggested Career Path

Experience as a staff nurse in the ED is an asset to the telehealth nurse, especially in the area of triage. Additional courses in pharmacology and toxicology as well as crisis management will also be helpful (Johnson & Johnson, n.d.).

Summary

The visions created by "emergency nurse" are likely as varied as the role itself. Some people may envision a scene from a television show of a chaotic environment in a resuscitation room. Others may remember a visit to the emergency department where a nurse provided much-needed pain medication. Some may think of that comforting hug provided by an individual in scrubs when they learned of the death of a loved one. Emergency nurses have numerous opportunities to practice including direct as well as indirect patient care roles. It's essential for the emergency nurse to know about the different roles to understand how they interact with one another and how to prepare for each role to ensure success within a career path.

References

Air and Surface Transport Nurses Association (ASTNA). (n.d.). *Frequently asked questions.* Retrieved from http://www.astna.org/faq.html

American Association of Colleges of Nursing (AACN). (2012, May 29). *Clinical nurse leader: Frequently asked questions.* Retrieved from www.aacn.nche.edu/cnl/frequently-asked-questions

American Association of Nurse Practitioners (AANP). (2013). *Scope of practice for nurse practitioners.* Retrieved from www.aanp.org/images/documents/publications/scopeofpractice.pdf

American Nurses Association (ANA). (2011). *ANA recognizes emergency nursing as a specialty practice.* Silver Spring, MD: American Nurses Association.

American Nurses Credentialing Center (ANCC). (2014). *Organization eligibility requirements.* Retrieved from http://www.nursecredentialing.org/OrgEligibilityRequirements

American Trauma Society. (n.d.). *Professional development for the trauma program manager.* Retrieved from http://www.amtrauma.org/?page=TPMCourse

Curtis, K., & Ramsden, C. (2011). *Emergency and trauma care for nurses and paramedics.* Philadelphia, PA: Elsevier.

Ebling Library. (2015, May 28). *Standard, guidelines, protocol, policy.* Retrieved from http://researchguides.ebling.library.wisc.edu/content.php?pid=325126&sid=3267902

Emergency Nurses Association (ENA). (n.d.). *Why emergency nursing?* Retrieved from www.ena.org/membership/Pages/WhyEmergencyNursing.aspx

Johnson & Johnson. (n.d.). *Telephone triage nurse.* Retrieved from www.discovernursing.com/specialty/telephone-triage-nurse

Mayer, T. A., Kaplan, J., & Kelly, C. (2014). Managing professionals in organizations: The role of physician and nurse leaders. In R. W. Strauss & T. A. Mayer (Eds.), *Strauss and Mayer's emergency department management* (pp. 36–38). New York, NY: McGraw-Hill.

National Association of Clinical Nurse Specialists. (n.d). *Advanced practice registered nurses.* Retrieved from http://www.nacns.org/docs/APRN-Factsheet.pdf

Patrizzi, K., Gurney, D., Baxter, T., Bush, K., & Crook, J. (2013). *Use of protocols in the emergency setting.* Des Plaines, IL: Emergency Nurses Association.

Robinson, D. J. (2013). An integrative review: Triage protocols and the effect on ED length of stay. *Journal of Emergency Nursing, 39*(4), 398–408.

Turner, P., Stone-Griffith, S., & Kopka, K. (2014). Leadership, nursing director. In R. W. Strauss & T. A. Mayer (Eds.), *Strauss and Mayer's emergency department management* (pp. 117–121). New York, NY: McGraw-Hill.

3

UNIQUE ROLES OF THE EMERGENCY NURSE

–Patricia L. Clutter, MEd, RN, CEN, FAEN

Experienced emergency nurses are uniquely positioned to enter into an array of additional nursing opportunities. Multiple career paths or additional roles are available in which the background, education, and experiences of the emergency nurse merge together to provide for prospective "outside the box" adventures. While some emergency nurses may choose to simply change specialty fields within the confines of the hospital structure, others desire to step outside of the normal boundaries and take "the road less traveled."

Some nurses choose to completely leave the traditional job of caring for patients at the bedside in the emergency department (ED) or flight nursing for new and distinctive career prospects, while others may find themselves combining their love for conventional patient care and stability within the hospital walls with a part-time or casual role in another, less recognized type of nursing. There are many novel approaches to nursing care in which emergency nursing credentials and qualifications may open doors that might not be available to others.

The spectrum of nursing contains a never-ending list of potential job openings, and each nursing specialty creates possibilities for future employment. This chapter explores positions in which emergency nursing experience can prepare emergency nurses who crave a change of pace, routine, and environment for success in a new journey. Taking on new and different challenges can be a conduit to personal and professional satisfaction.

Entrepreneurship/Intrapreneurship

One of the more common roads for nurses to take is that of an entrepreneur. This usually involves starting a company, requiring insight into the marketplace, ingenuity, business acumen, financial backing, and the ability and fortitude to work long hours. There are endless opportunities to take the emergency nurse into the world of entrepreneurship. Consider your passions and determine which route is the best one for you. It could be a company that specializes in education or a product that holds a special interest for both yourself and either the general public or a specific audience of healthcare professionals. Other potential businesses include new and innovative strategies to successfully administer EDs, the invention and patenting of novel products to assist other emergency nurses in their everyday work, creating discharge instructions for patients, publishing books and literature, or perhaps helping busy professionals care for themselves through fun products or vacation-planning strategies. The only limiting factor is your imagination and dedication to the idea.

If entrepreneurship is not attractive or not possible at this particular point in your career, consider intrapreneurship. This is a situation in which you look at established companies and/or organizations and determine whether there is a place for you within that structure. For instance, lecturing independently through a reputable educational company or becoming an instructor or coordinator for recognized curricula such as the Trauma Nursing Core Course (TNCC) or the Emergency Nursing Pediatric Course (ENPC). Other options might include looking within your own department and taking on new responsibilities that provide for an outlet for your interests and fuel your inner self. Perhaps you are detail-oriented, and helping to write policies within your department appeals to you. Or maybe there are committees that pique your interest and would help you to feel more fulfilled while still allowing you to continue that all-important bedside nursing that is such an important piece of yourself. Working through organizations such as the Emergency Nurses Association (ENA) or Sigma Theta Tau International can also help you to accomplish other goals that are not fulfilled through bedside care. Various committees, work groups, or special projects through an association can help to provide for an increased sense of self and worth.

Remember that you're in control of your own future no matter which route you take. Look around and determine whether you would like to pursue other options in the nursing field that appear attractive to you, whether it be a full-time or an "on the side" type of situation.

The first nurse entrepreneur/intrapreneur was one of the most famous nurses of all time—Florence Nightingale. She was a clinical nurse, a military nurse, a researcher, a nurse educator, an international nurse, a nurse consultant, and a nurse author, and she was also very active in the political arena.

Forensic Nursing

Forensic nursing aligns readily with the world of emergency care. Many nurses think that forensic nursing employs only the sexual assault nurse examiner (SANE). Although the SANE is an important facet of forensic nursing, it's not the only feature. The following sections discuss the spectrum of forensic nursing.

Sexual Assault Nurse Examiner (SANE)

The sexual assault nurse examiner (SANE) provides care to victims of sexual assault, acquires and preserves forensic evidence, offers outpatient resources, and may function in the role of an expert witness during court trials (All Nursing Schools, 2015; American Forensic Nurses, Inc., 2010).

Nurses seeking a SANE position should seek continuing education courses, certification programs, and university-based elected courses or formal programs. There are SANE-A (adult) and SANE-P (pediatric) certifications available. For more information on sexual assault and the emergency department patient, see Chapter 15, "The Emergency Nurse and the Abused Patient."

For more information about becoming a SANE, see:

- International Association of Forensic Nurses (IAFN): http://www.forensicnurses.org/

- American Forensic Nurses, Inc.: http://amrn.com/about_us.html

- All Nursing Schools: http://www.allnursingschools.com/nursing-careers/article/forensic-nursing

Correctional Nurse

The correctional nurse functions in local or federal incarceration and detention institutions, including juvenile facilities. They may care for individuals held in detention or incarcerated for periods of time. This may include caring for ill persons of this population on initial entry or during their time of detainment. This may occur at the bedside or as situations occur within the jail environment.

Education for this role may include learning regulations and guidelines relative to security issues, legal aspects, and health considerations for residents of these facilities. The nurse may also need to learn to utilize firearms (All Nursing Schools, 2015; American Nurses Credentialing Center [ANCC], 2014b; National Commission on Correctional Health Care [NCCHC], 2015; Nursing School Degrees, 2012a).

Nurses can find specialty conferences, continuing education classes, and peer-reviewed journals to find out more about being a correctional nurse. Certifications for this position include CCHP (Certified Correctional Health Professional), CCHP-A (Advanced), CCHP-MH (Mental Health), and CCHP-RN (Registered Nurse).

Interested in becoming a correctional nurse? See these websites for more information:

■ National Commission on Correctional Health Care: http://www.ncchc.org/

■ All Nursing Schools: http://www.allnursingschools.com/nursing-careers/article/forensic-nursing/

■ American Nurses Credentialing Center: http://www.nursecredentialing.org/PsychiatricMentalHealthNursing

Forensic Clinical Nurse Specialist

Forensic clinical nurse specialists may function in many areas including the clinical arena, educator, administrative roles, research initiatives, and as consultants. They may subspecialize in areas such as geriatrics or psychiatry. The psychiatric specialist may work with offenders providing guidance and treatment during their incarceration and after release. The geriatric expert can work with the aspect of abuse and neglect within this expanding group of citizens (All Nursing Schools, 2015; ANCC, 2014a; ANCC, 2014b; American Psychiatric Nurses Association [APNA], 2015; Nursing School Degrees, 2012a).

Forensic clinical nurse specialists are expected to complete a master's or doctoral program; there is also an AFN-BC (Advanced Forensic Nursing-Board Certified) certification program available. A specialist can also be certified in gerontology and psychiatry.

If you're interested in becoming a forensic clinical nurse specialist, see:

■ American Psychiatric Nurses Association (APNA): http://www.apna.org/i4a/pages/index.cfm?pageid=3737

■ All Nursing Schools: http://www.allnursingschools.com/nursing-careers/article/forensic-nursing/

- American Psychiatric Nurses Graduate Programs by State: http://www.apna.org/i4a/pages/index.cfm?pageid=3311

- American Nurses Credentialing Center/Advanced Forensic Nursing: http://www.nursecredentialing.org/ForensicNursing-Advanced

Nurse Coroner/Death Investigator

A nurse coroner or death investigator deals with suspicious and violent deaths and the events surrounding those deaths. They may be involved in the morgue with autopsy responsibilities and at the crime scene itself. They may work with families to help determine cause of death and become expert witnesses in the courtroom. They may also work with victims of assault or violent situations (ANCC, 2014a; IAFN, Forensic Nurse Death Investigator Education Guidelines, 2013; Nursing School Degrees, 2012b; Study.com, 2015).

Education for this position includes master's and doctoral programs as well as an FNDI Program (Forensic Nurse Death Investigator) degree. Certifications include AFN-BC (Advanced Forensic Nurse-Board Certified).

Find out more about being a nurse coroner at:

- Forensic Nurse Death Investigator Education Program: https://c.ymcdn.com/sites/iafn.site-ym.com/resource/resmgr/Education/Nurse_Death_Investigator_Edu.pdf

- Forensic Nursing Programs: http://www.nursing-school-degrees.com/Nursing-Schools/Forensic-Nursing.html#context/api/listings/prefilter

- Nursing School Degrees: http://www.nursing-school-degrees.com/Nursing-Careers/nurse-coroner.html

- American Nurses Credentialing Center (ANCC): http://www.nursecredentialing.org/ForensicNursing-Advanced

- Study.com: http://study.com/articles/Nurse_Coroner_Job_Description_Duties_and_Requirements.html

Legal Nurse Consultant

The role of the legal nurse consultant is usually seen as one who works within an attorney's office, but a legal nurse consultant may also be a registered nurse who works independently and subcontracts with law offices. This nurse may also work for insurance companies, in business or industrial settings, or in government agencies. A legal nurse consultant may assist with legal proceedings as an analyst of medical records in malpractice suits or as an expert witness in the courtroom. Other areas to be considered are in product liability cases (medical and nonmedical), medication-related instances, risk management situations (in hospital or as an independent entity), criminal cases, regulatory circumstances, worker's compensation cases, environmental cases, or in determining healthcare fraud (American Association of Legal Nurse Consultants [AALNC], 2015; Milazzo, n.d.).

Nurses can seek consulting education in colleges and universities as well as paralegal programs. Certifications to be considered for this position are LLNC (Legal Nurse Consultant Certification) and CLNC (Certified Legal Nurse).

For more information about becoming a legal nurse consultant, see:

- American Association of Legal Nurse Consultants (AALNC): www.aalnc.org

- Legal Nurse Consulting: www.legalnurse.com

Nurse Attorney

Nurses who choose to continue their education and become attorneys may find themselves in the courtroom in a variety of circumstances, including malpractice situations, insurance-related disagreements, product litigation, or personal-injury legal actions. They may also lobby legislators for changes in healthcare-related practices, or work with nursing organizations on issues of importance to the practice of nursing and the care of patients. These nurses decipher and analyze medical legal cases and make an impact on malpractice questions. They may become authors, editors, or subject-matter experts for nursing and legal journals, or they may work within a healthcare-policy research institute. In addition to an undergraduate degree, nurse attorneys need a JD (Juris Doctor) degree (American Association of Nurse Attorneys, 2015). This group of nurses has an association known as the American Association of Nurse Attorneys (TAANA); its website is www.taana.org.

Nursing Jobs With the Federal Government

Have a penchant for excitement and unusual job situations? The federal government may be a good place to start. The following sections describe a few of the jobs in which your nursing knowledge can be an asset.

Federal Bureau of Investigation

The Federal Bureau of Investigation (FBI) hires nurses as forensic experts. The nurse in this position deals with evidence collection and handling, serves as witnesses in the courtroom, and works in various areas dealing with forensic situations. The FBI also hires nurses in various other positions such as in domestic and international field offices where they may provide care for staff or those in custody of law enforcement. FBI nurses can become special agents and may be present in arrest situations in order to provide immediate care to injured parties. The application process is long and has many requirements, including being a U.S. citizen and not having any felony arrests in the past. Substance abuse can also prevent you from being hired for these positions. Written exams and oral interviews are given, and a background check and security clearance must be passed (Blum, 2009; Rossheim, 2015).

 To read about the life of an FBI nurse, read *Special Agent: My Life on the Front Lines as a Woman in the FBI* by Candice DeLong.

Central Intelligence Agency

The Central Intelligence Agency (CIA) also has openings for nurses who are interested in joining forces with one of the most secretive agencies in the United States. This may require that your family and friends not be aware of your occupational choice. Duties may include working with OSHA requirements, health education for employees, caring for acute health issues, dealing with medical screenings, or working within the travel medicine genre. One of the requirements is relocation to the Washington, DC area. Other minimum prerequisites include a bachelor of science degree (healthcare area) and at least 5 years working as a registered nurse in the specialty fields of emergency nursing, critical care, or occupational health. Again, U.S. citizenship is required, and successful completion of both medical and psychological examinations as well as polygraph interviews and a thorough background investigation are mandated. Nurse practitioners are also utilized in this field (CIA, 2015). You can search for and apply for these positions at https://www.cia.gov/careers/opportunities/support-professional/occupational-health-nurse.html.

National Aeronautics and Space Administration

Did you ever wonder what it might be like to work in a place where concerns might center on the biochemical problems with rocket fuel? Or maybe strong radiation exposure? Consider a career with NASA! This role encompasses caring for the hundreds of employees that comprise the NASA family. Not only do NASA nurses work at Spaceport at Kennedy Space Center in Florida, but there are other facilities such as a railroad, airports, fire and police departments, the numerous institutions that house either military or private individuals, and an EMS service. While a lot of what they do entails aspects of occupational nursing, nurses at the Spaceport facility are present during launches and landings (NASA, n.d.; Rothwell, 2001b).

An interesting counterpart to this is a group called the Space Nursing Society, which deals with the topic of nursing in space itself. Some of the members of this group work for NASA, and they plan to write textbooks and provide educational programs dealing with the special problems of caring for patients in space. They deal with such questions as bone loss in astronauts at the international space station, the gravitational pull on Mars, and exposure to different types of toxic gases that might be emitted from soils on different planets, as well as psychological issues (Dryden, 2005; Space Nursing Society, n.d.; Wood, 2006).

 Connect with like-minded individuals on the Facebook page for the Space Nursing Society.

Secret Service

Some nurses might find themselves providing medical care to those who are in positions of power in the United States' highest office. The White House must employ nurses who can work within the clinic areas offering healthcare services either to the employees who work within the confines of the White House or to the many visitors that tour the nation's most prestigious home. There is also a registered nurse and physician present at all times in the office next to the Oval Office. In addition to these duties, a Secret Service nurse may also travel with White House dignitaries within the United States or on overseas trips. They may accompany the president, the first lady, or vice-president and their families or be a part of the advance team that determines the best hospital to utilize in the areas visited and prepare it for the upcoming visit (NurseZone, 2001; White House Medical Unit, n.d.).

Emergency nurses are exceptionally suited for these roles because they must be able to respond to any of the multiple types of emergency issues that might arise. Nurses with backgrounds in trauma, general emergency, and intensive care will find their skills put to the test in this arena. The job may require long periods of travel, and flexibility within their current environment is a must. Critical thinking can help Secret Service nurses determine proper care provisions in foreign countries. The WHMU (White House Medical Unit) nurse most often has military experience, but it is not mandatory, and a few have been hired from within the non-military professional sector. Political astuteness is not a factor in the hiring process; however, the hiring process is long and requires the proper credentials, qualifications, and personality to competently cope with all that this position offers (NurseZone, 2001; White House Medical Unit, n.d.).

Department of State

As a member of the Foreign Service, a nurse provides care and promotes health services to those individuals and their families who work around the world representing the United States. This can include healthcare and prevention services for all age ranges, functioning as the medical liaison with local hospitals and workers, dealing with the myriad of administrative responsibilities that accompany a health unit, directing emergency-response preparedness, and supervising other health department personnel which may be local. To apply for this position, the nurse must be between the ages of 21 and 60 (may be age 20 to apply) and be a citizen of the United States. This person obtains top secret security clearance and must be medically cleared for Foreign Service work. A "suitability clearance" must also be achieved. A nurse practitioner or physician's assistant from an accredited university in the family practice area is considered for this position after the person has 5 years of direct patient care in the clinical area. Some of the attributes sought after for this position include (U.S. Department of State, 2015):

- Emergency, occupational, or urgent care experience

- Expertise in public/community health

- Clinical expertise, including an understanding of infectious disease processes

- Management/supervisory knowledge and skills

- An understanding of the intricacies of working with people of different lifestyles or cultures

- Ability to respond to medical crises

- Capability to work in high-stress conditions

- Aptitude to work with limited resources

- Objective and logical judgment skills

- Excellent written and oral communication talents

- Proficiency in preparing and implementing healthcare-related programs

- Adaptable to work in difficult, possibly isolated areas

- Firm convictions

- Allegiance to country

- Self-confidence

- Firm ethical convictions

- Organizational skills

 Want to apply for a position in the State Department? Go to http://careers.state.gov/.

Cruise Ship Nurse

Traveling the seas while caring for patients can be exciting and rewarding. Passengers on these vacation venues are scared and unsure when medical crises occur away from home. They depend on the knowledge and skills of the nurse and other medical crew onboard. As a cruise ship nurse, you may care for seasickness, dehydration, an acute myocardial infarction, a stroke, a ruptured spleen, fractures, or a traumatically injured passenger/crew member. Experience obtained during bedside emergency nursing on land correlates directly to the ship, except for the fact that the usual ancillary personnel who help during each shift are not present, nor are many of the tools that are taken for granted each day. There are no CT scanners, no ultrasound machines, and no sophisticated ventilators (though there is a ventilator on most ships). There are also no X-ray technicians, lab personnel, or respiratory therapy staff to take care of their respective areas. The nurse assumes all roles.

The usual complement onboard a large cruise ship is two to three registered nurses and a physician. Some cruise lines have a passenger physician and a crew physician. The crew physician is onboard for several months at a time, and his or her role involves the day-to-day care of the 600 to 800 crew members as well as taking on roles within the infirmary, such as first call nurse. Nurses may be on call 24 hours a day. On the cruise line for which this author works, each day carries a different position. The first call nurse is responsible for the clinic all day except for 2 hours in the afternoon, when the second call nurse takes over. The first call nurse takes all calls for medical assistance until 8am the next morning. The second call nurse helps in the infirmary as needed and runs the clinic for the 2 afternoon hours when the first call nurse rests. Third call is the day off. This may be in port, when the nurse can go ashore if there are no required fire, boat, man-overboard, or abandon-ship drills or high patient loads/acuities that require the nurse to remain onboard. If at sea, you can take this day to rest or catch up on behind-the-scenes tasks. You can take the time to do your paperwork responsibilities that may include counting inventory; checking expiration dates in the alternate infirmary; performing wheelchair, face masks, and AED checks; cleaning the sterilizer; or putting the voyage journal together. These functions are performed at pre-designed intervals and usually are weekly or monthly duties.

A history of emergency or critical care nursing is important in the hiring process for this role. Anything that can walk through the doors of an ED can walk through the doors of the ship infirmary. Learning to take X-rays, perform laboratory testing, and deal with the disembarkation of a passenger or crew member with an acute, life-threatening illness or injury are just a few of the many items to check off the orientation list.

Do not expect the pay to be exceptional. Many nurses take full-time contracts and do this for their full-time employment. Others may work part time, which for some cruise lines is 2 weeks at a time. You can't take this job thinking it'll be a vacation. If you enter this vocation with that thought in mind, your contract will not be pleasant.

For employment in the cruise ship industry, go to the individual cruise ship website and look for the employment section.

Questions that should be considered when choosing a cruise line to work with:

- What is the complement of medical officers onboard?

- What kind of intensive care area is onboard?

- What medications are available?

- What equipment is used?

- Do all the medical officers onboard speak the same language?

- Does the cruise line provide thrombolytics onboard?

- What kind of backup assistance is available via phone?

- What kind of training should I expect?

- Do they allow me to bring my spouse or other person onboard with me?

 WARNING: Cruise ship nursing is *not* like the old television show *The Love Boat* or the movie *Out to Sea*! But it is fun and interesting.

Humanitarian Nursing

Performing humanitarian work in either the domestic or international field is a dream of many healthcare professionals. An emergency nursing background lays a firm foundation for this rewarding career choice. This may be chosen as a part-time job or a once-a-year event, or you may choose to seek out a full-time position that lasts from 6 months to several years. Many organizations await your application to fill a needed role.

When considering work in the developing world, consider the impact it will make on not only yourself, but on your family as well. Having a loved one gone for a considerable amount of time, without being able to contact home, can take a toll on those left behind. Make sure that both sides of your personal relationship can handle the absence.

Some trips are physically challenging, while others can be more fixed (in that although you are in a developing country and working in harsh conditions, one-stop unpacking is available, and a bed and a shower are available each night). On some teams, constant movement from village to village may be the norm, requiring constant packing, unpacking, and carrying your personal backpack each day. There may be long hikes while transporting supplies or rivers to ford. You may be transported in tightly packed trucks, in the back of a pickup, in a ramshackle bus, in a long boat, or on a crude raft. Days may pass with no real beds or showers; when showers are present, they may be a cold trickle of water. Other trips may be held in one location, thus not requiring the constant travel. You may reside in a hotel or compound and be transported each day to the location of the clinic.

The clinics can be a challenge all on their own. You may find yourself struggling to determine how to teach people to mix rehydration fluid, but unsure as to how they are going to acquire clean water to use with it. There are often few or no hospitals nearby, and it can become a quandary as to how to deal with an individual with potential appendicitis, a severe burn, or acute cholecystitis in remote areas of the world. There are also issues with diagnosing some of the endemic infectious processes such as leishmaniosis, dengue fever, or leprosy. It is always helpful to have local physicians or nurses as part of the medical team. Critical thinking is the most important skill needed for this type of nursing.

Make sure before you leave that you have a clear image of what the mission is for the particular group that you choose. Emergency nurses usually want to provide medical care. Not all groups do this. Make sure you ask and are provided with an unmistakable answer as to the vision and purpose of the trip. Is there a religious affiliation with the group? Some groups require attendance at church services or, at the least, prayer before medications are provided. Just make sure that you fit in with the group that you choose to join.

Be aware that when on a mission trip, again either domestic or international, you may not see "the big things." Most patients that come to the clinics are there for simple processes such as upper respiratory infections, urinary tract infections, yeast infections, and the occasional abdominal pain. Some trips have their share of more acute illnesses and injuries, but the norm is to care for the less acute and more chronic issues. However, for the people who come to the clinic for care, the medical team is seen as a gift to them. Simple interventions such as Tylenol or ibuprofen for constant back pain, antacids for chronic reflux, or an antibiotic for a UTI are welcome relief from long-standing problems. Of course, you must be prepared for catastrophic events such as extensive burns or patients in need of surgical intervention. The rewards are seen in the smiles you receive when you take the time to listen and treat patients like they count. Because, of course, they do.

Education should be a large part of the process of caring for individuals who do not have regular access to care. Talk to the team leader to determine what percentage of time should be devoted to educating the patients and their families. Whether formal or more informal, education will guide them in the future, because the clinic will not always be there, and it is difficult for them to find even the minimal type of medications that are provided by the medical team. Teaching proper lifting techniques, hand washing, brushing teeth, access to clean water, and simple first-aid techniques can be the best thing that is left behind. See Table 3.1 for a list of some organizations that organize humanitarian trips that nurses may participate in.

Table 3.1 Organizations Whose Humanitarian Missions Include Nurses

Organization	Website
Doctors Without Borders	www.doctorswithoutborders.org
Project Helping Hands	www.projecthelpinghands.org
Convoy of Hope	www.convoyofhope.com
Big Creek Missions	www.bigcreekmissions.com
Samaritan's Purse	www.samaritanspurse.org
Project Hope	www.projecthope.org
International Medical Relief	www.internationalmedicalrelief.org
AmeriCares	www.americares.org

Go to www.missionfinder.org/medical-dental-doctor-relief to see a listing of multiple organizations that offer medical care in both domestic and international venues. Another website that deals with this type of nursing is www.onenurseatatime.org. This site not only provides a directory of organizations but also offers financial scholarships to help nurses to participate in mission trips, networking, and educational opportunities.

Disaster Nursing

Disaster nursing is another aspect of humanitarian work, but it carries with it a different set of tools and needs. For those interested in this venue of nursing, you must be ready to leave within a very short time period; disasters don't happen on a schedule. This is a very intense type of nursing and requires someone who can handle harsh conditions and severe situations. When approaching a disaster site, no words can totally prepare you. The area may be strewn with bodies of injured individuals. There may not be a true "medical clinic," and making the most of what is available is a quintessential characteristic for these nurses.

When faced with disasters, the impact of the surrounding devastation, loss of family connections for those injured, and the fact that severely injured people must be cared for with a minimum of supplies, diagnostics, and treatment options prevail. It may be difficult to adjust your mentality if your usual environment is a hospital ED setting where you're used to resuscitating everyone; you may have to get used to leaving the most injured who require intensive resuscitation to concentrate on those you can quickly help. It's a nursing role that provides deep satisfaction and fills a demanding need, but the reality of the destruction may take a toll on you physically, psychologically, emotionally, and spiritually.

For those interested, contact organizations such as the Red Cross and DMAT (Disaster Medical Assistance Team) teams in your area. DMAT teams are deployed by the federal government to crisis situations and have required meetings and education throughout the year. A stipend is provided for those who respond to these team deployments (Public Health Emergency, 2014, 2015).

To join a DMAT team, search for the DMAT in your state. Each state has its own website and should provide information regarding how to join. Be prepared to be deployed on short notice to disaster areas.

Camp Nursing

Who wouldn't want to spend time in a lovely setting, waking up every morning to beautiful landscapes and the trill of a robin in the nearby trees? Camp nursing can be an enjoyable respite from the daily grind of the ED. There are numerous camps throughout the United States seeking emergency nurses to work through the summer or for shorter periods of time. Caring for campers and camp employees can run the gamut of simple insect bites to full-fledged anaphylactic shock. Ask questions before accepting this job, such as how many medical staff members are present, the location of the closest hospital or emergency support, the expected responsibilities, what supplies/medications are available for your use, and other duties you might be expected to perform. Some camps may be day camps close to your primary location or overnight camps that encompass longer contracts.

You must be able to multitask, have the ability to critically think through demanding situations, have managerial aptitudes, have flexibility and adaptability, and be skilled in autonomous nursing. You may be the only medical professional in the camp, or you may be a part of a larger team that includes an onsite physician.

Look for advertisements in nursing journals or simply browse the Internet for these positions. Some allow you to bring your children for free, which is a bonus. The pay varies, so make sure that this is something that you can tolerate financially. Be aware that you may be the only medical professional present and therefore must be able to act independently and utilize your critical thinking and astute assessment skills. The website www.acn.org is a repository of camp nurse jobs both U.S. and international. This is the national Association of Camp Nurses and includes many features including educational offerings, a magazine called *Compass Point,* annual meeting information, and practice guidelines (Association of Camp Nurses, 2015). Other websites that may be helpful for those who are interested in this type of fascinating nursing are www.campnursejobs.com and www.campnurse.info.

 Remember that with compact licensure, many states have reciprocity, and it will not be necessary to obtain a license in each individual state if the camp you decide to work in is not in the state in which you are licensed.

On-Set Nursing

Some nurses can find themselves on the set of a movie or television show. These jobs are a bit harder to find, but are reachable. The nature of this occupation requires potentially long hours and the ability to care for patients of all ages in a variety of locations and lengths of contracts. An emergency nurse background is an incomparable piece on your resume that can help you to find employment in this lesser-known arena. Nurses are utilized on movie sets, in television series, and in advertisements. They may be the healthcare provider on the set or an on-set medical advisor. It's not all glamour and glitz though. You might be needed when the set is under construction, for any behind-the-scenes duties that occur during pre- and post-production. But you might also find yourself on the set with movie stars (Nursing Entrepreneurs, 2015; Rothwell, 2001a).

 Information about on-set nursing is harder to find. Try looking up Casala, Ltd. in Los Angeles or Kathy's Medical Production Company in Long Island, NY.

Finding Other Nursing Options

There are many ways that nurses can find other exciting endeavors. Consider some of the following thoughts that can help you to be successful in these new ventures:

- Believe in yourself. If you don't, no one else will.

- Surround yourself with others who believe in you, too.

- Don't be afraid to try new things. Keep the fear and anxiety that's usual for a new or unknown project in check.

- Stick to the project through to the end. It may take several tries to get things right, and you might find that you have a passion for it by the end.

- Learn from your failures. Everything may not turn out exactly as you would like. You may need to go on to the next adventure or adjust to a learning curve.

- Take a break every once in a while to regroup. It's fine to kick back and not take on new projects for a bit. Give yourself room to breathe and to relight the fire within yourself.

- Keep your eyes and ears open and read the fine print. You never know when a small advertisement in the back of the journal that you normally read will be the door that opens a new opportunity.

- Subscribe to magazines that foster your non-professional interests. You just might be able to carve out a niche for yourself.

- Attend conferences, network, and visit the vendor area. There is no better way to discover new options than to visit with others and find out what is available.

- Use your professional organization. This cannot be stressed enough. There are a myriad of things that you can do beyond what is expected of you in your workplace. And yet, the workplace is not always the place where your talents might be put to work. Look outside the workplace to find such an avenue.

- Search the Internet. This is the most common method to find new opportunities.

- Further your education. It is important to obtain higher degrees; just make sure they are in the proper field of interest for yourself. (Refer to Chapter 4 for additional information on nursing education and the opportunities opened to you via various nursing degrees.) Not everyone needs a master's degree in nursing. Not everyone wants to be a nurse practitioner. A master's degree in education can open many doors and provide for new and exciting prospects. For others, a business degree might be the best option. Determine where your talents lie and map out any education you need.

- Help each other out. Be a source of contagious excitement for your colleagues! Everyone needs a cheerleader.

- Taking risks is important. Everyone is scared of new environments and tasks. But nothing risked is nothing gained.

- If you take on multiple projects, prioritize them to keep them going. This can be overwhelming at times, so be sure to think things through well before accepting new projects.

- Don't burn bridges. You never know when you might need someone's expertise or a reference from an old place of business (if you choose to leave). Be careful about burning bridges that cannot be rebuilt.

Summary

This chapter provided an overview of a variety of nursing options for emergency nurses that offer an exciting and fun change of pace. Emergency nursing is wonderful because it allows the nurse to hone her or his assessment, intervention, evaluation, and psychomotor skills, which can then be transposed into some of these "out of the box" careers. Others that were not delved into with depth include school nurse, researcher, consultant, educator/lecturer, and author. Keep your eyes and ears open and remember that the only thing keeping you from your dream job is fear of the unknown. Let your imagination take you to new worlds and then search out the details and make progress into the known. Career options that seem too "out there" are truly within your grasp and require only that first step.

References

All Nursing Schools. (2015). *Eight great forensic nurse specialties*. Retrieved from http://www.allnursingschools.com/nursing-careers/article/forensic-nursing/

American Nurses Credentialing Center (ANCC). (2014a). *Advanced forensic nursing*. Retrieved from http://www.nursecredentialing.org/ForensicNursing-Advanced

American Nurses Credentialing Center (ANCC). (2014b). *Psychiatric–mental health nursing*. Retrieved from http://www.nursecredentialing.org/PsychiatricMentalHealthNursing

Blum, A. (2009, November 26). On the front lines: FBI profiler had high-stakes career. *The News-Herald*. Retrieved from http://www.thenewsherald.com/articles/2009/11/26/entertainment/doc4b056de01eead169537334.txt

Central Intelligence Agency (CIA). (2015). *Occupational health nurse* [job description]. Retrieved from https://www.cia.gov/careers/opportunities/support-professional/occupational-health-nurse.html

DeLong, C. (2001). *Special agent: My life on the front lines as a woman in the FBI*. New York, NY: Hyperion. Retrieved from http://www.amazon.com/Special-Agent-Front-Lines-Woman/dp/0786867078

Dryden, P. W. (2005, August). Preparing for space travel: Nursing at NASA. *Medscape*. Retrieved from http://www.medscape.com/viewarticle/508554

International Association of Forensic Nurses. (2013). *Forensic nurse death investigator education guidelines.* Elkridge, MD: International Association of Forensic Nurses.

Milazzo, V. (n.d.). *Types of services.* Retrieved from http://www.legalnurse.com/legal-nurse-consulting/types-of-legal-services

NASA. (n.d.). Retrieved from http://quest.arc.nasa.gov/space/frontiers/ohara.html

NurseZone. (2001). *Nurses a heartbeat away from the president.* Retrieved from www.nursezone.com/nursing-news-events/more-features/Nurses-a-Heartbeat-Away-from-the-President_21294.aspx

Nursing Entrepreneurs. (2015). *Nurse-owned businesses movie set first aid nurses (motion pictures).* Retrieved from http://www.nursingentrepreneurs.com/directory.entrepreneurs.category.movie.set.first.aid.nurses.htm

Nursing School Degrees. (2012a). *Forensic nursing programs.* Retrieved from http://www.nursing-school-degrees.com/Nursing-Schools/Forensic-Nursing.html#context/api/listings/prefilter

Nursing School Degrees. (2012b). *Nurse coroner.* Retrieved from http://www.nursing-school-degrees.com/Nursing-Careers/nurse-coroner.html

Public Health Emergency. (2014). *National Disaster Medical System.* Retrieved from http://www.phe.gov/Preparedness/responders/ndms/Pages/default.aspx

Public Health Emergency. (2015). *National Preparedness Month 2015.* Retrieved from http://www.phe.gov/Preparedness/news/events/NPM2015/Pages/default.aspx

Rossheim, J. (2015). *The FBI is hiring, and not just special agents.* Retrieved from http://career-advice.monster.com/job-search/company-industry-research/fbi-jobs/article.aspx

Rothwell, K. (2001a). *Making movie magic: Nurses work behind the scenes in Hollywood.* Retrieved from http://www.nursezone.com/nursing-news-events/more-features/Making-Movie-Magic-Nurses-Work-Behind-the-Scenes-in-Hollywood_20932.aspx

Rothwell, K. (2001b). *Nurses at NASA—Mission control: Occupational safety.* Retrieved from: http://www.nursezone.com/Nursing-News-Events/more-features/Nurses-at-NASA%E2%80%94Mission-Control-Occupational-Safety_21310.aspx

Space Nursing Society. (n.d.). In *Wikipedia.* Retrieved March 13, 2014, from http://en.wikipedia.org/wiki/Space_Nursing_Society

Study.com (2015). *Nurse coroner: Job description, duties and requirements.* Retrieved from http://study.com/articles/Nurse_Coroner_Job_Description_Duties_and_Requirements.html

U.S. Department of State. (2015). Retrieved from http://careers.state.gov

White House Medical Unit. (n.d.). In *Wikipedia.* Retrieved May 3, 2015, from http://en.wikipedia.org/wiki/White_House_Medical_Unit

Wood, D. (2006). *Space Nursing Society prepares for future flights.* Retrieved from http://www.nursezone.com/nursing-news-events/more-features.aspx?ID=15458

EDUCATION OF THE EMERGENCY NURSE

–*Nicholas A. Nelson, MS, RN, CEN, CPEN, CCRN, CPN, TNS, NRP*

Nurses have not always been formally educated. Prior to the 20th century, individuals simply declared themselves as nurses when providing patient care. This resulted in varied levels of care, and the need for formalized education was recognized in the 1800s. Since that time, nursing education has evolved from hospital-based diploma programs to a variety of different nursing doctoral programs. This chapter reviews the educational preparation of the emergency nurse and provides an overview of opportunities that exist with each type of educational preparation.

Nursing Education Today

Modern nursing education has a long and varied history, often influenced by external factors. Basic nursing education has transitioned from the hospital-based apprentice model to formalized educational programs in colleges and universities. These programs prepare graduates for a wide range of settings and care of complex patients.

As nursing has continued to evolve into a profession and academic discipline (McEwen & Wills, 2014), much controversy exists regarding entry-level education of the registered nurse (RN). Today, several points of entry into professional nursing practice remain and will likely continue for the foreseeable future. New nurses seeking to become emergency nurses should weigh the routes of entry into what is best for their personal circumstances but realize that ultimately the emergency nurse is a lifelong learner. As such, you must be committed to furthering your education. Clinical nursing experience is fundamental to any RN and builds a strong foundation in becoming a competent emergency nurse.

Basic nursing education prepares you for entry into nursing practice as a generalist. The specialty of emergency nursing is unique compared to all other areas of nursing practice; patients of every age, with virtually every type of condition, present to the ED. Emergency nursing practice includes patients with medical and surgical conditions, including traumatic injuries. You must be knowledgeable and skilled to assess, identify, and intervene quickly and efficiently. Therefore, an essential component of emergency nursing practice extends well beyond the entry-level nursing program and into the clinical practice environment via continuing education courses and clinical orientation.

Advanced nursing education is at the graduate level and prepares nurses for specialist practice. Nursing education has a tiered approach that is cumulative, in which specialty education is built upon entry-level educational programs. As a result, formal nursing education specific to emergency nursing is available at the graduate level.

The Future of Nursing Education

In 2010, the Institute of Medicine (IOM) released its landmark report on nursing, *The Future of Nursing: Leading Change, Advancing Health,* which outlined significant changes to the nursing profession and overall health in the United States (IOM, 2011). The report listed four key messages (IOM, 2011, p. 29):

- Nurses should practice to the full extent of their education and training.

- Nurses should achieve higher levels of education and training through an improved education system that promotes seamless academic progression.

- Nurses should be full partners, with physicians and other health professionals, in redesigning healthcare in the United States.

- Effective workforce planning and policy-making require better data collection and improved information infrastructure.

Eight recommendations were identified by the IOM. The following recommendations pertain directly to nursing education (IOM, 2011, p. 35–37):

- **Recommendation 2:** Expand opportunities for nurses to lead and diffuse collaborative improvement efforts, in part by nursing education programs providing entrepreneurial professional development that will enable nurses to initiate programs and businesses that will continue to improve health and healthcare.

- **Recommendation 3:** Implement nurse residency programs that facilitate transition-to-practice after completion of pre-licensure or advanced practice programs or when transitioning into new clinical practice areas.

- **Recommendation 4:** Increase the proportion of nurses with a baccalaureate degree to 80% by 2020 by ensuring nursing schools offer defined academic pathways that promote seamless transition to higher levels of education beyond articulation agreements; encourage diploma and associate degree nurses to enter RN to bachelor of science in nursing (BSN) programs within 5 years of graduation by offering tuition reimbursement, creating a supportive environment, and through salary differential and promotion; expansion of baccalaureate programs; expansion of loans and grants for second-degree nursing students; institute interprofessional learning; and recruit and advance diverse students.

- **Recommendation 5:** Double the number of nurses with a doctorate by 2020 to increase nurse faculty and researchers (including increasing diversity) by ensuring the Commission on Collegiate Nursing Education (CCNE) and National League for Nursing Accrediting Commission (NLNAC) monitor for progress that at least 10% of BSN graduates matriculate into master's or doctoral programs within 5 years of graduation; expansion of funding for graduate degree nurses; and make academic and clinical nurse faculty salaries and benefits competitive.

- **Recommendation 6:** Ensure that nurses engage in lifelong learning by continually updating curricula; ensuring clinical competency and the knowledge and skill to provide care across settings and the lifespan by nursing students; requiring faculty to participate in continuing professional development; and implementing interprofessional continuing competency programs.

Five years later, substantial progress has been made toward these goals. However, significant work remains to ensure that the nursing profession is a leader of redesigning the U.S. healthcare delivery system and meeting the needs of the population. Nursing education remains a fundamental underpinning toward these goals.

Accreditation

Accreditation in nursing education is two-fold. In addition to accreditation of the educational institution, such as the college or university, nursing programs may be accredited by specialty agencies. Origins of nursing accreditation in the U.S. date back to 1893, with formal accrediting activities beginning in 1920 by multiple organizations (Accreditation Commission for Education in Nursing [ACEN], 2013a).

 Accreditation—"[T]he recognition that an institution maintains standards requisite for its graduates to gain admission to other reputable institutions of higher learning or to achieve credentials for professional practice. The goal of accreditation is to ensure that education provided by institutions of higher education meets acceptable levels of quality" (U.S. Department of Education, Office of Postsecondary Education, n.d.).

The United States Department of Education currently recognizes two specialty-accrediting organizations for nursing education in the U.S.: The Accreditation Commission for Education in Nursing (ACEN) (formerly NLNAC, National League for Nursing Accrediting Commission, Inc.) and the Commission on Collegiate Nursing Education (CCNE, 2013).

The ACEN formal nursing educational programs are (ACEN, 2013a):

Practical Nursing	Certificate
Diploma	Associate
Baccalaureate	Master's
Post-Master's Certificate	Clinical (Practice) Doctorate

The CCNE formal nursing education programs are (CCNE, 2013):

Baccalaureate	Master's
Post-Graduate APRN Certificates	Doctor of Nursing Practice

The CCNE also offers post-baccalaureate nurse residency programs.

Specialty education accreditation serves the public interest and the educational community by setting standards for nursing programs. The standards ensure that nursing educational programs are effective and strive for improvement (ACEN, 2013b; CCNE, 2013).

It's in the interest of the nursing profession and the public at large that every nurse pursues education that is appropriately accredited. Institutions of higher learning are more likely to accept transfer of academic credits from accredited programs, and applicants to degree completion (e.g., RN to BSN) or advanced nursing programs (e.g., doctorate of nursing practice [DNP]) may be required to have graduated from an accredited entry-level nursing program for acceptance. A list of accredited nursing programs is available from the U.S. Department of Education, ACEN, and CCNE.

Nursing Degree Titles: What's the Difference?

Prospective students may wonder, what is the difference between a BSN and a BS with a major in nursing or an MSN and an MS in nursing? For all intents and purposes, these different degrees meet the same competencies for specialty education accreditation and are considered equivalent. So why the difference? Largely, the title of the degree rests with the institution's academic structure, the governing body approving the nursing program, and the focus of the institution.

Although there are exceptions, programs that offer a BS in nursing or a BS with a major in nursing may be housed in an academic department of nursing within a multidisciplinary college or school, such as a college of health sciences or school of nursing and health studies. Other times, the governing body overseeing the nursing program may not be specific to the nursing college or school. The focus of the college or university may also influence the degree title. For example, institutions with a liberal arts focus may award the bachelor of arts in nursing (BAN) or bachelor of arts (BA) with a major in nursing (Augustana College Department of Nursing, 2012; St. Olaf College, n.d.). For master's programs that award an MS in nursing or MS with a major in nursing (instead of an MSN), the institution's graduate college may oversee the graduate nursing program. The graduate college's governing structure may be composed of multidisciplinary faculty (University of Illinois at Chicago, n.d.), and therefore, they have chosen to award an alternative to the MSN. Students in nursing programs leading to an MS may be admitted to the college of nursing and the graduate college (University of Illinois at Chicago, n.d.).

Although these degrees are almost always interchangeable, they are different degrees (Northwest Nazarene University, n.d.). Nursing program graduates should use the appropriate post-nominal credentials for the degree in which they were awarded, because that is the degree that was approved by the institution's governing body.

Entry Into Practice

There are four main routes of entry into nursing practice at the professional nursing (registered nurse) level in the United States: diploma, associate degree, bachelor's degree, and master's degree. Each varies in length and the setting in which they are administered. Bridge programs also exist for licensed practical or vocational nurses (LPN/LVN) or other healthcare providers. Regardless of the type of initial nursing educational preparation, all pre-licensure programs prepare the graduate to sit for the National Council Licensure Examination Registered Nurse (NCLEX-RN) exam. Successful completion of the NCLEX-RN exam is a prerequisite for professional nursing licensure in the states and territories of the United States. It is important to note that legally, no state authorizes an expanded scope of practice for RNs prepared at various levels of entry into practice (i.e., diploma, associate, baccalaureate, or master's degree). In other words, an RN graduating with a diploma in nursing practices equally in the eyes of the law as an RN who graduates with a master's degree.

Regardless of the type of initial nursing educational preparation, all pre-licensure programs prepare the graduate to sit for the NCLEX-RN exam.

Entry Into Practice Debate

In 1965, the American Nurses Association (ANA) published a paper advocating for the baccalaureate degree–prepared nurse as the standard for professional nursing education (ANA, 2013). Since that time, the ANA and other organizations, such as the American Association of Colleges of Nursing (AACN) have held fast to their position that nurses should complete bachelor of science in nursing (BSN) programs before entry into the profession (American Association of Colleges of Nursing [AACN], 2014) and that associate degree and diploma programs prepare graduates for "technical" nursing practice—that is, task-based nursing interventions. This debate of professional versus technical nursing practice persists today, but proponents of all levels of entry nursing programs agree that all nurses must commit to lifelong professional learning, including advancement of formal nursing education (AACN, 2012).

Though the disagreement over basic educational preparation of RNs will likely not be resolved soon, some trends have emerged. Today, hospital employers may require or give preference to nurses prepared with a minimum of a BSN more than in the past. Similarly, employers may require as a condition of employment that RNs complete a BSN within a certain time period for continued employment. Healthcare organizations are increasingly partnering with schools of nursing for BSN degree completion programs that are subsidized or reimbursed by the employer. Several states have debated mandating BSN degree completion within 10 years after entry into practice (Future of Nursing Campaign for Action,

2014); yet, no state has initiated this requirement due to strong opposition. What is clear is that nursing, like all other healthcare professions, is becoming increasingly challenging and more demanding. Therefore, all nurses must be committed to learning.

Diploma Programs

Diploma nursing programs are hospital-based and prepare the graduate for entry into nursing practice and to assume direct-care nursing roles.

Overview

Diploma programs were once the dominant entry into nursing practice. In the mid-1960s, 75% of nursing programs graduated diploma-prepared nurses (Catalano, 2015, p. 82). As of 2011, only about 10% of entry-level nursing programs in the U.S. award a diploma in nursing (AACN, 2011a). These programs are hospital-based and focus more on practical and clinical experiences through an apprentice approach. Diploma programs today continue to serve local communities and educate nurses who may not have other options for entry into professional nursing (Association of Diploma Schools of Professional Nursing [ADSPN], 2015).

Length

Programs leading to a diploma in nursing are 3 years in length. Diploma programs typically offer pre- and co-requisite courses within the nursing program or through partnerships and collaborations with institutions of higher learning.

Jobs

With a diploma, you can become a direct-care emergency staff nurse, and with appropriate clinical experience, you can be a(n):

- ED charge nurse

- ED clinical preceptor

- Flight or ground transport nurse

Among other factors, the shift of entry-level nursing education into the college and university system means that diploma nurses may have to seek formal education for career advancement.

Positives

Unlike other types of nursing programs, diploma programs often incorporate hands-on clinical training early in the program. Hospital-based diploma programs may be financially cost-effective compared to BSN programs. Some hospitals may even sponsor students through the program (ADSPN, 2015). Admission requirements may be as minimal as a high school diploma or GED, which may better suit students who don't thrive in the typical academic setting.

Negatives

Hospitals seeking a designation from the American Nurses Credentialing Center's (ANCC) Magnet Recognition Program® may only hire BSN-prepared nurses (AACN, 2015b). However, only 7% of U.S. hospitals to date have received this designation (ANCC, 2015). Diploma-prepared RNs likely have to return to school for a nursing degree to assume positions in nursing leadership or education roles. Because diploma programs are not housed in institutions of higher learning, transfer of credits may be a challenge. Diploma nursing programs may have articulation agreements with colleges or universities, thereby facilitating the transition.

Associate Degree Programs

Similar to the diploma nursing program, the focus of the associate degree nursing program is to prepare the graduate for entry into nursing practice, primarily in direct-care roles.

Overview

Unlike diploma programs, associate degree in nursing programs are most commonly based in community colleges. Some 4-year colleges and universities have associate degree nursing (ADN) programs as well (Mason, Isaacs, & Colby, 2011).

 Multiple associate degrees in nursing are awarded in the United States, including the associate of science in nursing (ASN), associate of applied science in nursing (AAS), and the associate degree in nursing (ADN). Each is equivalent to one another; ADN is the collective term.

The concept of the ADN-prepared nurse came about in the 1950s in response to a critical nursing shortage (National Organization for Associate Degree Nursing [NOADN], 2006). In order to increase the number of nurses, the length of the nursing program was shortened to 2 years but placed into the community college to maintain academic standards (NOADN, 2006). In 1958, the ADN program was piloted at seven sites in four states (NOADN, 2006).

Today, associate degree nursing programs remain one of the most popular routes for entry into professional nursing practice. As of 2006, there were more than 940 ADN programs in the United States, of which community colleges accounted for over 600 (NOADN, 2006). Such programs account for more than half of the pre-licensure preparation of RNs in the U.S. (American Association of Community Colleges Health Professions Education Center [AACCHPEC], 2011).

Length

Although associate degrees in general are considered to be 2-year degrees, most ADN programs require a total of 3 years. Most of these programs require a total of 70-plus semester credits for completion.

Jobs

Nurses with an associate degree can be direct-care emergency staff nurses. With appropriate clinical experience, these opportunities are available:

- ED charge nurse

- ED clinical preceptor

- Flight or ground transport nurse

Those seeking to practice as emergency nurses may find some challenges at Magnet hospitals requiring or highly preferring a BSN or higher degree (AACN, 2015b). Alternatively, graduates of ADN programs may have to commit to BSN degree completion for continued employment. Nurses seeking to advance to leadership or education positions in emergency nursing will likely have to return to school for a baccalaureate degree or higher in nursing.

Positives

Associate degree nursing programs are significantly less costly than most 4-year college and university BSN programs (Fulcher & Mullin, 2011). As tuition costs continue to skyrocket across the United States, community college tuition remains significantly lower and more realistic for students with limited financial means or those wanting to minimize student loans. Many hospitals offer a tuition benefit or have partnered with colleges or universities to offer cohort RN to BSN programs at reduced or even no cost to the RN seeking to complete his or her baccalaureate degree.

Negatives

Emergency nurses with an associate degree will most likely have to return to school for a baccalaureate degree (or higher) in nursing to assume other roles. Critics may view ADN-prepared nurses as "technical" nurses who focus on the technical aspects of nursing care, are not prepared for leadership or administrative roles, or lack critical thinking.

Baccalaureate Degree Programs

Nursing programs awarding a bachelor's degree prepare graduates for entry-level nursing practice and to assume direct-care nursing roles in various healthcare settings. In addition, these programs prepare the graduate for additional roles and set the foundation for advanced graduate-level nursing education.

Overview

Baccalaureate nursing programs incorporate additional components of professional practice, such as leadership and introduction to nursing theory and research. Baccalaureate programs are based on *The Essentials of Baccalaureate Education for Professional Nursing Practice* (AACN, 2008), which serve as the fundamental underpinnings of baccalaureate generalist nursing practice. These essentials include liberal education, leadership, evidence-based practice, information management and use of technology, the healthcare delivery system, interprofessional collaboration, population health, and professionalism (AACN, 2008).

 The most common baccalaureate degree in nursing awarded in the United States is the Bachelor of Science in Nursing (BSN). The Bachelor of Science in nursing (BS) and Bachelor of Arts in Nursing (BAN) are alternatives awarded by some institutions of higher learning and are equivalent to the BSN.

Although 4-year colleges and universities issue the vast majority of bachelor degree nursing programs, 23 community colleges in six states award a baccalaureate degree in nursing as of September 2014 (Community College Baccalaureate Association, 2014; Mason et al., 2011).

Length

Bachelor degree nursing programs are generally 4 years in length: 1 year of prerequisite courses and 3 years of nursing courses. In addition to the content of ADN programs, BSN programs include additional studies in nursing leadership and management, nursing research, public health and community nursing, physical and social sciences, and humanities. BSN programs may offer an advantage over other entries into practice programs, providing an in-depth clinical or leadership experience to facilitate transition into practice. Prospective nurses interested in emergency care may be able to take advantage of such experiences and better position themselves for employment in the ED.

Jobs

A bachelor's degree gives a nurse the opportunity to work as a direct-care emergency staff nurse. With the appropriate clinical experience, these opportunities are also available:

- ED charge nurse

- ED clinical preceptor

- ED assistant/nurse manager

- ED clinical staff educator

- Transport nurse

- ED nurse case manager

These graduates are prepared for the broadest range of entry-level nursing positions across healthcare settings and patient populations. Those hospitals pursuing Magnet designation may prefer or require new hires to hold a BSN (AACN, 2015b).

Positives

The BSN-prepared nurse is largely considered to be the standard for entry into nursing practice. With some practical experience, the BSN nurse can assume a variety of leadership and educational roles. The BSN nurse has a wide degree of job latitude in nursing practice, including emergency nursing. The nurse prepared at this level is also ready to seamlessly step into graduate level nursing study.

Negatives

Advocates of associate degree nursing programs argue that BSN programs lack adequate practical, hands-on experience. Baccalaureate degree programs tend to be significantly more costly than ADN or diploma programs (Fulcher & Mullin, 2011). Additionally, 4-year colleges and universities may not be geographically accessible for prospective students in rural or remote areas. The program length may also be prohibitive or a deterrent for some prospective students, instead opting to enter into practice via the ADN route and completing the undergraduate degree at a later time.

RN Completion Programs

There are unique programs that exist to prepare those with previous education and training as an LPN or allied health providers for graduation to professional nursing practice (Mason et al., 2011). Also known as RN completion programs or bridge programs, these programs prepare the graduate to sit for the NCLEX-RN exam like traditional educational programs.

Overview

Bridge nursing programs most frequently award an associate degree in nursing, though some do award a BSN. These programs take advantage of the healthcare provider's previous training and clinical experience that may overlap with basic nursing education that is often found in the first semester or year of a professional nursing program. It's important to note that each program's criteria and requirements vary greatly. In general, the applicant must be a licensed healthcare provider in the appropriate related field, have graduated from an accredited program, and generally have practiced for about 1,000 hours.

Length

LPN to RN (ADN) or LPN to BSN programs are generally the most standardized and may reduce the professional nursing program completion by up to an academic year by transferring previous academic credits. Licensed practical nurses entering ADN or BSN programs typically complete a specifically designed transition course at the beginning of the program and then progress with the traditional students.

Bridge programs for paramedics, respiratory therapists, and other allied health providers are more limited, and requirements tend to vary. In general, however, these students may be required to complete an assessment examination, complete bridge courses, and then enter the program at an advanced placement.

Jobs

Graduates of bridge nursing programs are prepared for the same roles as graduates of traditional nursing programs. The type of program (ADN or BSN) may affect additional roles aside from the direct-care emergency staff nurse.

Positives

Emergency nursing is challenging and unique from all other nursing specialties. New graduate nurses entering into ED staff positions may encounter various challenges, in which previous clinical experience may be beneficial. Namely, skills like interaction with patients, physical assessment and history, and some technical procedures in which LPNs and other allied healthcare providers are experienced may increase the likelihood of standing out from other applicants, and will likely prove beneficial in their novice practice as emergency nurses.

Negatives

Some graduates of nursing degree completion programs may have difficulty transitioning from their previous role and experiences into that of an emergency nurse. Unlike practical nursing, which is largely built around medically stable patients, and the narrow focus of the pre-hospital environment to which paramedics are accustomed, novice emergency nurses may need additional time or resources to acclimate to their new role in the ED.

Accelerated Bachelor Degree Programs

Accelerated BSN (ABSN) programs are designed for the adult learner seeking to change careers, to enter professional nursing practice, and to assume direct-care nursing roles across the healthcare spectrum.

Overview

ABSN programs feature a condensed and fast-paced curriculum that builds upon the adult student's previous education and life experience. As of 2013, there were 293 such programs throughout the U.S. and Puerto Rico, and 13 more in the planning phase (AACN, 2015a).

Length

Accelerated baccalaureate nursing programs vary in length between 11 and 18 months of full-time study, often including prerequisites (AACN, 2015a). Students complete the same type and number of clinical hours as traditional, first-degree nursing students.

Jobs

Like the traditional BSN program, graduates of accelerated programs are prepared for a wide variety of roles in emergency nursing, especially with clinical experience. Some colleges have found that their accelerated program graduates move into leadership positions more quickly and tend to be more successful in their positions (AACN, 2015a).

Positives

ABSN programs offer the fastest route into professional nursing practice (Mason et al., 2011). As adult learners, second-degree nursing students tend to be older, more motivated, and have higher academic standards compared to the high school graduate in a traditional BSN program (AACN, 2015a). All of these characteristics translate positively into motivated students and then RNs. According to the American Association of Colleges of Nursing (2015a, p.2), "Employers report that these graduates are more mature, possess strong clinical skills, and are quick studies on the job."

Negatives

Admission requirements generally include a minimum GPA of 3.0, greater than many traditional BSN programs (AACN, 2015a). Many students seeking a second degree in nursing will be prepared to complete prerequisite courses in the natural sciences. However, ABSN programs may have special courses to meet these requirements (AACN, 2015a). Financial aid is very limited for ABSN students, so the cost of a second bachelor's degree may be prohibitive for some (AACN, 2013). Due to the intense nature of these programs, an interview with faculty may be part of the application process to ensure that applicants understand and can commit the necessary resources to be successful (AACN, 2013). Students who may have years of experience and competence in one setting may experience difficulty returning to the undergraduate setting (AACN, 2013). The rigors of this program may not afford the time for outside employment and place additional demands on the student's personal life. For those who need to work or find that the demands are too great on their personal lives, they may have the option to transfer into the traditional BSN program as a part-time student (AACN, 2013).

Master's Entry Programs

Master's entry into nursing practice (MENP) programs, also known as graduate or generic entry master's programs, are designed for the adult learner seeking to change careers, to enter professional nursing practice, and to assume a variety of nursing roles across the healthcare spectrum.

Overview

Master's degree entry programs are an alternative to accelerated BSN programs and are a natural academic progression for the student with a previous bachelor's degree. All MENP programs include entry-level nursing education, thereby qualifying the graduate to sit for the NCLEX-RN exam and become licensed as a registered nurse. These programs include additional graduate-level content in anatomy and physiology, health assessment, pharmacology, leadership, and research.

An increasing number of master's entry programs also prepare the graduate as an advanced generalist (clinical nurse leader or CNL). For more information on the CNL role, see Chapter 2, "The Traditional Role of the Emergency Nurse." These programs are consistent with the AACN's call for advanced generalist registered nurses who are better prepared for complex healthcare needs (AACN, 2012). Graduates of master's entry CNL programs complete additional coursework and clinical hours beyond the basic nursing preparation and are eligible to sit for the CNL examination.

Some entry-level master's degree nursing programs first prepare the graduate in entry-level nursing education (thereby qualifying to sit for the NCLEX-RN exam and become a licensed RN), and then students complete the graduate coursework by focusing on an advanced practice nursing role, such as a clinical nurse specialist or nurse practitioner. Upon the completion of the MSN degree, graduates of these programs would be eligible to sit for the chosen APRN role's certification examination and then seek APRN licensure. An increasing number of these programs are transitioning to the CNL role and moving the APRN role into a doctor of nursing practice (DNP) program.

Length

Graduate entry master's degree nursing programs vary in length between 2 and 3 years. Programs that incorporate education in an APRN role may be longer, but the basic nursing education is completed within 12 to 18 months of intense study. These programs also vary based on part- or full-time study.

Jobs

A master's degree gives nurses the opportunity to be a direct-care emergency staff nurse or clinical nurse leader. And with appropriate clinical experience, a nurse with a master's degree could be a(n):

- ED charge nurse

- ED clinical preceptor

- ED assistant/nurse manager

- ED clinical staff educator

- Flight or ground transport nurse

- ED nurse case manager

Graduates of master's entry programs are prepared for a wide variety of roles across healthcare settings. Most graduates will initially practice in direct-care roles, but they may find themselves in leadership, education, or other non-clinical roles with adequate clinical experience. Like graduates of ABSN programs, MENP graduates tend to be highly valued by employers and generally transition well into practice.

For graduates of graduate-level entry programs that include an advanced practice track, most students seek employment as direct-care staff nurses while completing the advanced practice portion of the program. After, most graduates transition into an APRN role related to the focus of their program.

Positives

Graduate entry programs into nursing are quicker than the traditional BSN and offer the graduate an alternative to a second undergraduate degree. These programs often include in-depth education and additional clinical hours and experiences beyond what most undergraduate entry-level nursing programs offer. Additionally, they tend to provide opportunities that are not available to other nursing students, such as a cumulative research project or thesis. The new CNL role has yet to be clearly demonstrated in terms of outcomes and effects in the ED, but it is likely that graduates of these programs will have additional opportunities in their careers. If you're seeking to ultimately become an APRN, the master's entry route is the most efficient.

Negatives

Similar to ABSN programs, the admission requirements are rigorous and stricter than other entry points into professional nursing education. Students may need to complete additional prerequisite coursework (often in the natural sciences), have a minimum GPA of 3.0, and hold a bachelor's degree from an accredited college or university. An interview may also be a part of this program due to its intense nature. Like ABSN programs, master's entry programs require a great deal of coursework, studying, and clinical time, and may leave little time for a personal life or the ability to work outside of the program. As with any other graduate program, tuition is more expensive. Unlike second-degree BSN programs, however, financial support in the form of student loans, grants, and scholarships is more available. Some graduates of programs that include basic and advanced practice nursing education may not obtain significant practice experience (or any experience) as an RN prior to becoming an APRN. Some employers or nursing colleagues may view this negatively.

Bridge Programs

There is significant overlap between the educational requirements for the various degrees in nursing. Bridge programs exist to capitalize on this overlap. A bridge program allows a nurse with one degree to apply the educational credits from that degree to another one, decreasing the amount of schooling required to advance education. For example, a baccalaureate degree in nursing normally takes 4 years of full-time schooling to complete. A nurse with a diploma in nursing may be able to enter a bridge program, utilizing credits from the diploma program to reduce the time required to complete a baccalaureate degree to half the time.

RN to BSN Bridge Programs

RN to BSN programs allow for the completion of the baccalaureate degree for ADN- and diploma-prepared RNs.

Overview

Also known as BSN completion programs, RN to BSN programs build upon the nurse's entry-level education utilizing *The Essentials of Baccalaureate Education for Professional Nursing Practice* (AACN, 2008), which also serve as the foundation for traditional BSN programs. Students complete practical experiences, as well as coursework in nursing and the liberal arts and sciences. Employers may partner with nursing programs to offer cohorts of their employees seeking to complete the BSN.

Between 2013 and 2014, RN to BSN program enrollment increased more than 10% for the 12th straight year (AACN, 2015b). Nearly all RN to BSN programs exist in the U.S., with more than half of those offering a portion of the program online (AACN, 2015b).

Length

Based on the program's requirements, the student's previous academic preparation, and type of program, RN to BSN programs are 1 to 2 years in length and may be completed on a full- or part-time basis.

Jobs

Graduates of bridge, traditional, and accelerated BSN programs have many career options. An advantage of graduates of RN to BSN programs is that they already have clinical experience and may be prepared to immediately assume leadership or education roles in emergency nursing.

Positives

Nurses completing BSN education may be eligible for clinical ladder promotion or an increase in salary. Additionally, BSN-prepared nurses may have increased levels of job security.

Negatives

RN to BSN programs that are not covered by employment benefits may quickly add up financially for students. However, federal loans and grants are available for many students completing a baccalaureate degree.

RN to MSN Bridge Programs

RN to MSN bridge programs are an alternative to RN to BSN programs for RNs who hold a nursing diploma or associate degree or a baccalaureate degree in a non-nursing discipline. Such programs are designed for an efficient transition to graduate nursing education that is quicker than the traditional academic progression.

Overview

In accordance with the IOM's *Future of Nursing* report, RN to MSN programs are an attractive alternative for RNs without a bachelor's degree in nursing who want to pursue graduate-level nursing education (IOM, 2011). These programs incorporate both *The Essentials of Baccalaureate Education for Professional Nursing Practice* (AACN, 2008) and *The Essentials of Master's Education in Nursing* (AACN, 2011b) and may award a BSN after completion of the undergraduate requirements.

RN to MSN programs are structured for initial completion of the baccalaureate content absent from the student's diploma or associate degree nursing program (AACN, 2015b; Mason et al., 2011). Completion of upper-level undergraduate liberal arts and sciences courses will vary based on the student's previous education and the program's requirements (Mason et al., 2011). The student then moves into the graduate-level portion of the program. Some students with non-nursing bachelor's degrees may be required to complete as few as two or three undergraduate nursing courses before matriculating into the graduate nursing curriculum.

Like traditional master's degree programs, most RN to MSN programs offer a variety of tracks or specialties, leading to an advanced generalist (CNL) role, advanced nursing practice role, or advanced practice nursing (APRN) role.

Length

RN to MSN programs take about 3 years to complete full-time. Program length is dependent upon the type of advanced nursing education. For example, a focus as a nurse educator generally requires fewer courses and clinical hours than that of an emergency nurse practitioner program. Students enrolling in programs with articulation agreements that facilitate transfer of academic credit between programs will generally have less coursework to complete (AACN, 2015b).

The number of RN to MSN programs has tripled since the early 1990s, when there were 70 (AACN, 2015b). As of March 2015, there were 214 RN to MSN programs in the U.S. (AACN, 2015b).

Jobs

Upon completion of the program, graduates are positioned for a wide variety of positions and jobs, based on the focus of their graduate program. The MSN-prepared registered nurse is ready for many positions and roles, including emergency nursing. The upcoming Table 4.1 lists master's degree program foci.

Positives

RN to MSN programs are less expensive and quicker than separately completing a BSN and MSN. If you're lacking a bachelor's degree in nursing and want graduate nursing education, the RN to MSN route is ideal.

Negatives

Misperceptions that RN to MSN programs do not adequately meet the baccalaureate nursing curriculum persist (AACN, 2015b). On the contrary, students must first complete baccalaureate coursework to set the foundation of the graduate studies of the program according to nursing specialty accreditation standards (AACN, 2015b).

Advanced Nursing Education

Advanced nursing education at the graduate level is specialized, building upon basic nursing education. There are three options for graduate-level nursing education: master's degree, post-master's certificate, and doctoral degree. See Table 4.1 for a summary of educational requirements for various types of advanced nursing positions. Advanced nursing educational programs may prepare the graduate as an advanced practice nurse or for advanced nursing roles. At the graduate level, nurses can pursue specialty education related to emergency nursing.

Table 4.1 Emergency Nursing-Related Graduate Programs	Master's Degree	Post-Master's Certificate	Doctor of Nursing Practice	Doctor of Philosophy in Nursing/Doctor of Nursing Science
Clinical Nurse Leader	X			
Emergency/ Trauma Clinical Nurse Specialist	X	X	X	
Emergency/ Trauma/Flight Nurse Practitioner	X	X	X	
Forensic Nursing	X	X	X	
Informatics/ Quality/Safety	X	X	X	X
Nursing Administration/ Management/ Leadership	X	X	X	X
Nursing Education	X	X	X	X
Nursing Scientist/Researcher				X

Master's Degree

Master's-level nursing education is the basis for specialized advanced nursing education and prepares graduates for additional nursing practice roles. Several emergency nursing–related programs are available through master's degree programs.

Overview

Master's nursing programs prepare the graduate for more broad nursing practice, incorporating additional scholarship in areas of the sciences and humanities, leadership, quality improvement and safety, translation and integration of scholarship into practice, informatics and healthcare technologies, health policy and advocacy, interprofessional collaboration, clinical prevention and population health, and graduate level nursing practice as outlined by *The Essentials of Master's Education in Nursing* (AACN, 2011b). In addition to didactic coursework, all master's nursing programs must include supervised clinical experiences (AACN, 2011b) and be accredited by ACEN or CCNE.

The Master of Science in Nursing (MSN) is the most common master's degree in nursing. Other equivalent degrees awarded in the United States include the Master of Science in nursing (MS), Master of Nursing (MN), Master of Arts in nursing (MA), and Master of Arts in Nursing (MAN). Despite the various (or similar) names, they are considered equivalent.

Length

Length of master's degree nursing programs varies considerably by focus. Programs preparing graduates for advanced practice roles as nurse practitioners or clinical nurse specialists are the longest and may exceed 60 credit hours. However, most MSN programs require between 36 and 40 hours for completion. MSN programs may be completed on a full- or part-time status.

Jobs

Depending on the program's focus, master's prepared nurses may assume multiple jobs in emergency nursing, including:

- Direct-care emergency staff nurse

- Clinical nurse leader

- ED charge nurse

- ED clinical preceptor

- ED assistant/nurse manager

- ED administrative nurse director

- ED clinical staff educator

- ED nurse case manager

- Flight or ground transport nurse

- Emergency, trauma, or flight APRN

- Forensic nurse

- Nurse informaticist/quality improvement

- Academic educator

Positives

The master's degree provides the graduate with in-depth study and practical experiences in a focused area. Some master's degrees can be completed in 2 years or less, and most are designed for the practicing nurse.

Negatives

The master's prepared nurse, especially APRN, may be perceived as inadequate when compared to other health professionals educated at the doctoral level. With the development of the DNP degree, some employers may prefer doctoral preparation of APRNs and advanced specialty nurses.

For the nurse pursuing graduate education, many nursing programs have developed partnerships with other colleges to award joint degrees. In addition to MSN study, these programs allow the graduate student to pursue specialized education in a relevant but non-nursing field, such as business administration (MBA), healthcare administration (MS, MHA), law (JD), public health (MPH), and public administration (MPA). Typically, joint degree programs transfer credit from one program toward the other, thereby reducing the time to completion of either degree.

Post-master's certificate programs, also known as post-graduate certificate programs, are designed for master's-prepared nurses seeking additional specialty education without completing another graduate degree. Most nurse practitioner and clinical nurse specialist programs can be completed via this route. The main advantage to this method of education is that the nurse does not have to repeat previous education, and instead must only complete the missing content, which may include supervised clinical experiences. With the increasing popularity of the DNP degree, some graduates of post-master's certificate programs may feel the need to return for doctoral education.

Doctoral Degrees

The first doctoral program for nurses was developed in 1924 at Columbia University as a doctor of education (EdD), combining nursing and education to develop nurse educators (Chism, 2010). Although the first PhD in nursing program began in 1934, the nursing PhD didn't gain traction until the 1970s (Chism, 2010). Many nurses pursued PhDs and EdDs in nursing-related fields, such as the basic sciences, education, psychology, and sociology (Chism, 2010). The doctor of nursing science (DNS) degree was developed in the 1960s as the first nursing practice degree but ultimately became a research doctorate (Chism, 2010).

The doctor of nursing (ND) degree was another attempt to create a practice doctorate, which more recently was replaced by the doctor of nursing practice (DNP) degree (Chism, 2010).

Clearly, the evolution of doctoral nursing education is diverse. Today, however, doctoral education in nursing has been streamlined and is divided into two areas: the practice doctorate (DNP) and the research doctorate (PhD/DNS) (AACN, 2008).

Doctor of Nursing Practice

The doctor of nursing practice (DNP), a practice-focused doctorate, is a newer concept in nursing education that prepares graduates for the highest level of nursing practice and is therefore a terminal degree.

Overview

Doctor of nursing practice programs are focused on preparing the nurse to assume a role as an advanced practice nurse providing direct patient care at a higher level of practice or to assume an advanced nursing practice role such as leadership. Goals of all DNP programs, regardless of focus, are to prepare the graduate to translate research into practice, conduct scholarly activities, and be a leader in the healthcare system (Chism, 2010). The DNP is a response to the call for increased numbers of doctorate-prepared nurse faculty, an alternative to the nursing research doctorate, and a way to provide care in an increasingly complex healthcare system (AACN, 2008). Components of all DNP programs are outlined in *The Essentials of Doctoral Education for Advanced Nursing Practice,* which include leadership, health policy, health advocacy, and information technology (AACN, 2006).

In 2004, the AACN (2015c) member schools voted that APRN education should transition to the DNP level by 2015. Since this statement was issued, significant debate has surrounded the concept of the DNP and the call for APRN education to occur at the doctoral level. Despite the controversy, the DNP has gained popularity, and many programs have begun or have fully transitioned. While significant progress to this end has been made, APRN education remains at various levels of graduate education. Other organizations, including the Institute of Medicine, have held fast that APRN education should remain at the graduate level via the master's degree, post-master's certificate, or doctoral degree (IOM, 2011).

Length

There are two routes of entry to the DNP: post-master's and post-baccalaureate. Post-master's DNP programs are designed for the RN or APRN holding an MSN or equivalent degree. These programs may be full- or part-time and require completion of about 45 to 50 additional credit hours. The programs may focus on advanced education of the nurse's current role or prepare the graduate for a new role. Post-baccalaureate DNP programs are designed for entry by the BSN-prepared RN for APRN or advanced nursing practice roles. Some programs also allow entry for the associate degree–prepared RN who holds a bachelor's degree in a related field, but require bridge courses as pre- or co-requisites to the advanced studies. Baccalaureate-to-DNP programs are 3 to 4 years in length and may be completed on a full- or part-time basis.

In 1979, the first doctor of nursing (ND) degree program was launched by Case Western Reserve University as an entry-level, practice-focused doctoral degree (similar to the doctor of medicine degree) and an alternative to the PhD in nursing (AACN, 2004; Chism, 2010; Fitzpatrick, 2008). Over the years, other ND programs offered entry-level and advanced practice nursing education (Chism, 2010). The ND has since been phased out, and some institutions have transitioned their ND programs to the DNP.

A clinical research doctor of nursing practice degree (DrNP), similar to the doctor of public health (DrPH) degree, had a brief existence in the U.S. in the mid-2000s. These programs were designed to be a hybrid of practice and clinical research for APRNs to engage in advanced independent practice (AACN, 2008; Chism, 2010; Dreher, Donnelly, & Naremore, 2005) and cumulated in a clinical research dissertation or a scholarly portfolio. These programs have since transitioned to the DNP degree.

Jobs

Jobs that a DNP-prepared nurse can hold are:

- ED nurse administrators and managers

- ED APRNs

- ED clinical educators

- Academic educators

Positives

The DNP provides parity with other healthcare professions that have adopted doctoral-level education (Chism, 2010). Graduates gain experience through residency requirements and complete a scholarly capstone project. The DNP is an alternative for nurses who do not seek a career in research.

Negatives

DNP programs require more time for completion than master's degrees. The DNP continues to be surrounded by controversy, even among nurses.

Doctor of Philosophy in Nursing and Doctor of Nursing Science

Doctor of philosophy in nursing programs prepare graduates at the highest level of nursing science to become researchers and advance nursing knowledge (AACN, 2010). The doctor of nursing science degree is considered equivalent to the PhD in nursing (U.S. Department of Education, International Affairs Office, 2008), as few distinguishers have been identified (AACN, 2004). For a side-by-side comparison of the doctor of nursing practice degree and other nursing doctoral degrees, see Table 4.2.

Table 4.2 Comparison of Doctoral Nursing Programs

	Doctor of Nursing Practice (DNP)	*Doctor of Philosophy (PhD) in Nursing/Doctor of Nursing Science (DNS/DNSc)*
Type of Degree	Terminal practice doctorate	Academic (research) doctorate
Program Objectives	Prepare nurses for the highest level of nursing practice as leaders and to translate research into practice	Prepare nurses for the highest level of nursing science and to advance the body of nursing knowledge
Students	Nursing practice–oriented Advanced practice nurses/students	Nursing research–oriented
Roles of Graduates	Advanced practice nurses Nurse leaders Nurse educators	Nurse scientists Nurse researchers Nurse leaders Nurse educators
Program Cumulating Activity	Scholarly capstone project that translates scientific evidence into practice	Original research that expands nursing science and successful defense of dissertation
Routes of Entry	Post-Baccalaureate Post-Master's	Post-Baccalaureate Post-Master's
Program Length	2–4 years (full-time)	4–7 years (full-time)
Program Specialty Accreditation	Accreditation Commission for Education in Nursing (ACEN) Commission on Collegiate Nursing Education (CCNE)	No specialty accreditation; oversight by institutional governing bodies and regional accreditation

Overview

As the terminal academic degree in nursing, the PhD in nursing focuses on theory, research methodology, and in some cases, pedagogy. The PhD and DNS degrees prepare nurse scholars to conduct original bodies of research, expand nursing knowledge, and disseminate research. PhD-prepared nurses are essential toward nursing advancing into a full academic discipline and for setting the foundation on which nursing practice is built. Like practice-doctorate nursing education, research-focused doctoral nursing programs are based on the *Indicators of Quality in Research-Focused Doctoral Programs in Nursing* (AACN, 2001).

Length

There are two routes of entry into the PhD/DNS: post-baccalaureate and post-master's. BSN to PhD programs are usually completed full-time. PhD programs must be completed in 7 years, with an average completion of 4 to 6 years. MSN to PhD programs are shorter in length, but students may be more likely to complete the doctoral studies on a part-time basis. The duration of the program also varies based on the progression of the dissertation. Upon successful defense of the dissertation, the PhD/DNS is awarded. Nurses with research doctorates may go on to complete optional post-doctoral programs.

Jobs

Doctorate-prepared nurses can become:

- Nurse researchers
- Nurse scientists
- Academic faculty
- Nurse executives

Positives

The PhD-prepared nurse is a scholar and expert on his or her area of study. The PhD degree is universally recognized and carries significant clout.

Negatives

Research-based doctorates require considerable devotion to study and research over many years, which may be unrealistic or unappealing to some nurses. The academic rigor of such programs can be stressful and allow little time for clinical practice (or work of any kind outside of the program).

Dual Doctorates — DNP to PhD in Nursing Programs

As unique degrees with separate foci, some highly motivated DNP-prepared nurses seek a PhD in nursing. A few programs in the U.S. are designed with this nurse in mind. Bridge DNP to PhD in nursing programs are designed for DNP graduates who seek to earn a PhD by agreeing to transfer a limited number of credits from the DNP program that apply toward the PhD curriculum. Some programs may transfer up to nearly half of the credits normally required for the PhD program, cutting the duration of the program in half.

DNP and PhD in Nursing Programs

Alternatively, dual DNP-PhD in nursing programs seek to combine the two roles and prepare the graduate for the highest level of clinical practice and to conduct research and expand nursing knowledge. Such programs may begin with the foundational PhD coursework, transition into the practice specialty courses of the DNP, and then return to complete the PhD dissertation. Often, dual doctoral programs are slightly shortened due to overlap of content but offer a unique learning experience by incorporating the features of both programs simultaneously.

The doctor of education (EdD) in nursing education is a doctoral degree that combines the disciplines and professions of nursing and education. Only a handful of higher education institutions in the U.S. offer this degree, which prepares graduates to advance the body of nursing education knowledge, apply nursing education principles to change health, become an expert in nursing pedagogy, and fully prepare for academic or clinical education (Teachers College, Columbia University, n.d.). The EdD in nursing education is sometimes considered an alternative to the PhD in nursing or nursing education. Like other research doctorates, the EdD in nursing education culminates in a dissertation and oral defense.

APRN Specialty Programs

Clinical nurse specialist (CNS) and nurse practitioner (NP) programs may be completed through the master's degree, post-master's certificate, or doctor of nursing practice degree level, and are accredited. Regardless of the level of graduate education, each program meets the same core competencies and includes graduate-level courses in advanced physiology/pathophysiology, health assessment, and pharmacology, in addition to clinical experiences.

In 2008, the *Consensus Model for APRN Regulation: Licensure, Accreditation, Certification & Education* was published and outlined the future of APRN regulation in the United States (APRN Consensus Work Group & National Council of State Boards of Nursing [NCSBN] APRN Advisory Committee). As supported by more than 48 national nursing organizations as of 2010 (APRN, 2008), this model strives to standardize and streamline APRN practice, including education and certification. As a result, the education of emergency APRNs (clinical nurse specialists and nurse practitioners) has been significantly redesigned.

Advanced practice registered nurses in each of the four roles (clinical nurse specialist, nurse anesthetist, nurse midwife, and nurse practitioner) are to be educated in at least one of the six population foci (APRN, 2008):

- Family

- Adult-gerontology

- Neonatal

- Pediatrics

- Women's health

- Psychiatric/mental health

The APRN educational program may also include specialty education of a focus within the identified population, such as emergency, trauma, or flight nursing. Specialty certification may not be used alone for state APRN licensure. For example, a family nurse practitioner (FNP) program with an emergency nurse practitioner (ENP) specialty track will prepare the graduate to practice primary care of infants to geriatrics, as well as the specialty care of patients who present to the ED. The graduate of an FNP/ENP program will be eligible for certification as a family nurse practitioner and gain state licensure as an APRN. It is only after this point, and meeting additional requirements, that the APRN may be eligible for certification as an ENP.

Clinical Nurse Specialist

Clinical nurse specialist (CNS) programs prepare graduates in at least one of the six population foci identified by the APRN Consensus Model across the health continuum, from wellness through acute care (APRN, 2008). Population foci that are best suited to the emergency care setting include adult-gerontology, family, and pediatrics. Only one self-described program specifically prepares the CNS for practice in emergency care (AAENP, 2015a).

Overview

CNS educational programs include the core graduate-level courses, as required by the APRN Consensus Model (APRN, 2008), including supervised clinical experience in emergency, critical care, and/or trauma settings.

The Emergency Nurses Association states:

> "In addition to graduate course completion, APRNs wishing to specialize in emergency care must obtain educational preparation related to emergency care and may do so through various pathways including: 1) successful academic course completion specific to emergency care; 2) continuing education course completion; and/or 3) on-the-job instruction in emergency care." (ENA, 2011, p. 5)

Additionally, the ENA has developed 25 specialty competencies for the emergency CNS (ENA, 2011).

Jobs

A CNS-educated nurse can be a(n):

- Emergency clinical nurse specialist

- Urgent care clinical nurse specialist

- Trauma clinical nurse specialist

- ED clinical educator

Nurse Practitioner

Nurse practitioner programs that prepare the graduate to practice in the emergency setting include adult-gerontology acute care or primary care, family, or pediatric acute care or primary care NP programs. Programs with emergency specialties prepare the graduate to step directly into the ED.

Overview

Although nurse practitioners have been providing care in the ED since the 1970s (Keough, Cole, Jennrich, & Ramirez, 2003), programs specific to the emergency nurse practitioner (ENP) are relatively new. Prior to the first ENP program, and even today, NPs who practice in an emergency setting may not have completed formal ENP training (AAENP, 2015c).

The first dedicated ENP program was developed at the University of Texas at Houston (Keough et al., 2003), and currently only eight self-described ENP programs exist in the United States (AAENP, 2015a).

Emergency NP programs prepare the graduate in at least one of the six population foci identified by the APRN Consensus Model and then provide additional education in the emergency specialty. Emergency NP programs have seen a recent switch toward the family NP focus because these graduates are prepared to treat all patient populations in the emergency setting. Applicants to emergency NP programs are required to have at least 1 year of emergency nursing experience.

According to the ENA (2008), nurse practitioners in emergency care demonstrate entry-level core and emergency competencies but can obtain further educational preparation through various pathways including:

- Successful academic course completion

- Continuing education course completion

- On-the-job instruction in emergency care

Additional specialties for emergency-related NP programs include trauma nurse practitioner programs and one flight nursing program for adult-gerontology acute care NPs (AAENP, 2015a). Applicants to programs that prepare graduates for certification eligibility as acute care NPs are required to have at least 1 year of acute or critical care experience in the appropriate patient population.

Jobs

A nurse practitioner can follow one of these paths:

- Emergency nurse practitioner

- Urgent care nurse practitioner

- Trauma nurse practitioner

- Flight nurse practitioner

- Convenient care nurse practitioner

See Table 4.3 for a comparison of advanced practitioner educational programs.

Table 4.3 Comparison of APRN Graduate Education

	Master's Degree	Post-Master's Certificate	Doctor of Nursing Practice
Length	18–24 months (full-time)	Varies	Post-BSN: 3–4 years (full-time) Post-MSN: 2–3 years (full-time)
Credit hours	40–60 hours (additional 5–9 hours for emergency specialty; dual population foci programs are more than 60 hours)	30–40 hours, varies by institution and previous education	70–80 hours
Clinical hours	672–750 hours (substantially more hours for dual population foci)	None	1000-plus hours (upwards of 500 additional hours for dual population foci)
Positives	Quick route into practice No practice residency required, fewer clinical hours	Builds upon previous MSN education, saving considerable time APRNs can complete an additional population focus with fewer courses	Terminal practice degree in nursing Practice residency allows for additional training in the clinical setting Completion of a scholarly capstone project
Negatives	Graduates of these programs may feel pressured to complete the DNP	Graduates of these programs may feel pressured to complete the DNP	Takes considerably longer to complete than the MSN or post-master's certificate

 Post-graduate fellowships for emergency nurse practitioners are the latest progression in ENP education. These optional programs, sometimes referred to as residencies, are designed to build upon entry-level competencies and certifications (AAENP, 2015b). Fellowship programs for emergency NPs are about a year in length and may be interdisciplinary in nature, including physician assistants (AAENP, 2015b). Post-graduate fellowships for ENPs have been gaining popularity but are not required for licensure or certification. These programs service the novice ENP and experienced NPs seeking additional training or experience.

Continuing Education

Lifelong learning is a hallmark of the emergency nurse, regardless of level of practice, role, or setting. Programs that offer continuing education (CE) are an efficient means to stay current and meet state licensing and certification body requirements. Emergency nurses complete various standardized continuing education courses, attend conferences and seminars, and read peer-reviewed journals in order to remain current with emergency nursing practice. For more information on the responsibility of the emergency nurse to seek out continuing education, see Chapter 5, "The Emergency Nurse as a Professional."

CE Courses

A standardized set of continuing education courses are commonly required or preferred by employers of emergency RNs and APRNs, depending on the type of emergency department (ED). These courses are also common in the pre-hospital and ground or flight transport settings. Experienced emergency nurses frequently become instructors in these courses:

- **Air and Surface Transport Nurses Association:** Transport Nurse Advanced Trauma Course (TNATC)

- **American Burn Association:** Advanced Burn Life Support (ABLS)

- **American Heart Association:**

    - Advanced Cardiovascular Life Support (ACLS)

    - Basic Life Support for Healthcare Providers (BLS)

    - Pediatric Advanced Life Support (PALS) (in conjunction with the American Academy of Pediatrics)

- **Emergency Nurses Association:**

    - Course in Advanced Trauma Nursing (CATN)

    - Emergency Nursing Pediatric Course (ENPC™)

    - Geriatric Emergency Nursing Education (GENE)

    - Trauma Nursing Core Course (TNCC™)

- **FEMA Emergency Management Institute:** IS-100.HCB: Introduction to the Incident Command System (ICS 100) for Healthcare/Hospitals

- **Society of Trauma Nurses:** Advanced Trauma Care for Nurses (ATCN)

Conferences and Seminars

Conferences and seminars are ideal means to earn formal CE credit, as well as engage in other aspects of professionalism within the emergency nursing specialty. National conferences attract hundreds to thousands of nursing and healthcare professionals, feature expansive exhibit halls, include opportunities for networking and professional growth, and include hands-on, round-table, lectures, and other forms of presentations.

Several national conferences are held annually and are ideal for the emergency nurse. These conferences include the following:

- Emergency Nursing (formerly the Annual Conference and Leadership Conference) (Emergency Nurses Association)

- Annual Conference (Society of Trauma Nurses)

- National Teaching Institute & Critical Care Exposition (American Association of Critical-Care Nurses)

- Air Medical Transport Conference (Air Medical Physician Association, Air and Surface Transport Nurses Association, and International Association of Flight and Critical Care Paramedics)

- Critical Care Transport Medicine Conference (Air Medical Physician Association, Air and Surface Transport Nurses Association, and International Association of Flight and Critical Care Paramedics)

Seminars focus on a particular subject or topic and may last up to 2 days. Of particular note are courses for emergency APRNs and other advanced practice providers. These workshops provide the advanced practice student or recent graduate, as well as the experienced APRN, with hands-on and lecture-style learning that is specific to emergency care. These programs can serve as an educational bridge by incorporating important emergency care information, especially for the graduate student in a non-emergency specialty program. Most programs provide the participant with CE credit.

Seminars for the emergency APRN may include:

- Suturing

- Splinting

- Advanced airway management

- Radiology diagnostic interpretation

- Focused examinations (e.g., ears/eyes, nose, throat (EENT); dental; ophthalmologic; dermatologic; orthopedic; etc.)

- 12-lead ECG interpretation

- High-risk emergency boot camp

- Pediatric emergency boot camp

Journals

Staying abreast of the most recent practice recommendations, medical science breakthroughs, and the newest products may be difficult for the emergency nurse. Peer-reviewed journals are an excellent method to keep up-to-date on the latest changes in emergency nursing. Most journals also offer opportunities for formal CE credit. The following journals represent popular publications related to emergency nursing:

- *Advanced Emergency Nursing Journal,* the official journal of the American Academy of Emergency Nurse Practitioners

- *Air Medical Journal,* official journal of the five leading air medical transport associations in the U.S.

- *Journal of Emergency Nursing,* the official journal of the Emergency Nurses Association

- *Journal of Trauma Nursing,* the official publication of the Society of Trauma Nurses

- *Prehospital Emergency Care,* the official journal of the National Association of EMS Physicians, the National Association of State EMS Officers, the National Association of EMS Educators, the National Association of EMTs, and the National Registry of Emergency Medical Technicians

Nursing Certifications

Nursing certification is the voluntary process by which nurses seek formal recognition of specialized experience, knowledge, and skills (American Board of Nursing Specialties [ABNS], 2005). Obtaining specialty nursing certification is a means to validate the emergency nurse's commitment to continual learning (ABNS, 2005). Although not mandatory for professional nursing licensure as a registered nurse, certification is recommended and highly valued by the nursing community, employers, and the public. Certification of APRNs is mandatory for licensure as an APRN.

Tables 4.4 through 4.7 list certifications ideal for the emergency registered nurse (4.4), advanced emergency nursing practice roles (4.5), emergency clinical nurse specialist (4.6), and nurse practitioner (4.7). Each certification body has unique requirements, which may include nursing practice, completion of a graduate degree, or clinical practice as an APRN. Due to the implementation of the APRN Consensus Model, some APRN certifications may be eligible only for renewal, while others will soon be phased out. Contact the certification organization for more information.

Table 4.4 Emergency Nursing Certifications

Certification Organization	Certification
AACN Certification Corporation	Certification in Acute and Critical Care Nursing (CCRN®)
Board of Certification for Emergency Nursing	Certified Emergency Nurse (CEN®)
	Certified Flight Registered Nurse (CFRN®)
	Certified Transport Registered Nurse (CTRN®)
	Trauma Certified Registered Nurse (TCRN™)*
Board of Certification for Emergency Nursing and Pediatric Nursing Certification Board	Certified Pediatric Emergency Nurse (CPEN®)

*TCRN exam is scheduled to become available in 2016.

Table 4.5 Certifications for Advanced Nursing Practice Emergency Nurses

Certification Organization	Certification
American Nurses Credentialing Center	Nurse Executive-Board Certified (NE-BC)
	Nursing Case Management (RN-BC)
AONE-Credentialing Center	Certified in Executive Nursing Practice (CENP)
AONE-Credentialing Center and ANCC Certification Corporation	Certified Nurse Manager and Leader (CNML)
Association of Air Medical Services	Certified Medical Transport Executive (CMTE)
Commission on Nurse Certification	Clinical Nurse Leader (CNL®)
National League for Nursing	Certified Nurse Educator℠ (CNE)

Table 4.6 Advanced Practice Emergency Nursing Certifications— Clinical Nurse Specialists

Certification Organization	CNS Certification
American Nurses Credentialing Center	Adult-Gerontology CNS (AGCNS-BC) Pediatric CNS (PCNS-BC)
AACN Certification Corporation	Adult-Gerontology CNS (ACCNS-AG®) Pediatric CNS (ACCNS-P®)

Table 4.7 Advanced Practice Emergency Nursing Certifications—Nurse Practitioner

Certification Organization	NP Certification
American Nurses Credentialing Center	Adult-Gerontology Acute Care NP (AGACNP-BC) Adult-Gerontology Primary Car NP (AGPCNP-BC) Family NP (FNP-BC) Pediatric Primary Care NP (PPCNP-BC) Emergency NP (ENP-BC)
AACN Certification Corporation	Adult-Gerontology Acute Care NP (ACNP-AG®)
AANP Certification Program	Adult-Gerontology Primary Care NP (NP-C®) Family NP (NP-C®)
AANP Certification Program and American Academy of Emergency Nurse Practitioners*	Emergency NP (ENP-C)*
Pediatric Nursing Certification Board	Acute Care Certified Pediatric Nurse Practitioner (CPNP®-AC) Primary Care Certified Pediatric Nurse Practitioner (CPNP®-PC)

*The ENP certification was announced in early December 2015. No further details were available as this book went to press.

Certification as an emergency nurse practitioner (ENP-BC) is available from ANCC to assess the entry-level clinical knowledge and skills of nurse practitioners in the emergency nursing specialty, after initial nurse practitioner certification and licensure. Unlike other NP certifications, the ENP certification is not intended to meet the requirements for APRN licensure, and certification is granted through portfolio assessment instead of examination (AAENP, 2015c). Eligibility to apply for portfolio assessment includes (AAENP, 2015c):

■ Certification in one of the accepted NP populations

■ A nursing graduate degree from an acute care, adult-gerontology primary care, family, pediatric acute care, or pediatric primary care nurse practitioner program

■ Meet minimum practice requirements in emergency nurse practitioner practice

The ENP-BC is currently the only advanced practice nursing credential for those practicing in the emergency environment. In December 2015, plans for an exam-based Emergency Nurse Practitioner certification (ENP-C) were announced by the American Academy of Nurse Practitioners Certification Program (AANPCP) and the American Academy of Emergency Nurse Practitioners (AAENP) (AANPCP, 2015). Although details regarding eligibility criteria, application process, and launch date have yet to be disclosed, this certification program will align with the APRN Consensus Model and meet national accreditation standards (AANPCP, 2015). For more information on preparing for a certification exam, see Chapter 5, "The Emergency Nurse as a Professional." For more information on preparing for a certification exam, see Chapter 5.

Summary

Nursing education has continued to evolve as needed to make strides toward becoming a full profession and recognized academic discipline. However, multiple points of entry into basic nursing education mean that the RN can be prepared via hospital diplomas, community college associate degrees, senior college and university baccalaureate degrees, or entry-level master's degrees. Lifelong learning, including continued formal learning, is a hallmark of nursing practice.

At the graduate level, nurses complete advanced nursing education in specialty advanced nursing or APRN roles. Nurses seeking positions in leadership, education, and clinical research can pursue master's degrees, post-master's certificates, or doctorates. Despite calls for transition of APRN master's degree programs to the DNP, APRN education remains at the various graduate levels. Emergency specialty education for APRNs has yet to come to full fruition, but there are many other options available for competency of APRN practice in the emergency setting. For nurses who want a career in research, the PhD in nursing is the definitive route.

Last, but not least, continuing nursing education is a requirement for every emergency nurse. All direct-care emergency RNs and APRNs complete standardized courses, and many become instructors. Attending conferences, participating in specialty seminars, and reading peer-reviewed journals that relate to emergency care not only provide CE credit, but are also vital to nursing professionalism. And to validate the emergency nurse's knowledge, experience, and skills, specialty nursing certification is recommended for direct- and indirect-care roles for RNs and advanced certifications for APRNs, including the only advanced nursing emergency certification.

References

Accreditation Commission for Education in Nursing (ACEN). (2013a). *ACEN accreditation manual.* Retrieved from http://www.acenursing.net/manuals/GeneralInformation.pdf

Accreditation Commission for Education in Nursing (ACEN). (2013b). *Philosophy of accreditation.* Retrieved from http://www.acenursing.org/philosophy-of-accreditation/

Accreditation Commission for Education in Nursing (ACEN). (2013c). *Recognition.* Retrieved from http://www.acenursing.org/recognition/

American Academy of Emergency Nurse Practitioners (AAENP). (2015a). *ENP program info.* Retrieved from http://aaenp-natl.org/content.php?page=ENP_Program_Info

American Academy of Emergency Nurse Practitioners (AAENP). (2015b). *Fellowship programs.* Retrieved from http://aaenp-natl.org/content.php?page=Fellowship_Programs

American Academy of Emergency Nurse Practitioners (AAENP). (2015c). *Overview of emergency nurse practitioners (ENPs).* Retrieved from http://web1.amchouston.com/flexshare/002/AAENP/enpoverview.pdf

American Academy of Nurse Practitioners Certification Program (AANPCP). (2015). *AANPCP announces plan to offer emergency NP certification by exam.* Retrieved from http://www.aanpcert.org/ptistore/control/newsitem?id=68

American Association of Colleges of Nursing (AACN). (2001). *Indicators of quality in research-focused doctoral programs in nursing.* Retrieved from http://www.aacn.nche.edu/publications/position/quality-indicators

American Association of Colleges of Nursing (AACN). (2004, October). *AACN position statement on the practice doctorate in nursing* [position statement]. Retrieved from http://www.aacn.nche.edu/publications/position/DNPpositionstatement.pdf

American Association of Colleges of Nursing (AACN). (2006, October). *The essentials of doctoral education for advanced nursing practice.* Retrieved from http://www.aacn.nche.edu/publications/position/DNPEssentials.pdf

American Association of Colleges of Nursing (AACN). (2008). *The essentials of baccalaureate education for professional nursing practice.* Retrieved from http://www.aacn.nche.edu/education-resources/BaccEssentials08.pdf

American Association of Colleges of Nursing (AACN). (2010). *The research-focused doctoral program in nursing: Pathways to excellence.* Retrieved from http://www.aacn.nche.edu/education-resources/PhDPosition.pdf

American Association of Colleges of Nursing (AACN). (2011a). *Nursing fact sheet.* Retrieved from http://www.aacn.nche.edu/media-relations/fact-sheets/nursing-fact-sheet

American Association of Colleges of Nursing (AACN). (2011b). *The essentials of master's education in nursing.* Retrieved from http://www.aacn.nche.edu/education-resources/MastersEssentials11.pdf

American Association of Colleges of Nursing (AACN). (2012). *Clinical Nurse Leader frequently asked questions.* Retrieved from http://www.aacn.nche.edu/cnl/CNLFAQ.pdf

American Association of Colleges of Nursing (AACN). (2013). *Accelerated programs: The fast track to careers in nursing.* Retrieved from http://www.aacn.nche.edu/publications/issue-bulletin-accelerated-programs

American Association of Colleges of Nursing (AACN). (2014). *Fact sheet: The impact of education on nursing practice.* Retrieved from http://www.aacn.nche.edu/media-relations/EdImpact.pdf

American Association of Colleges of Nursing (AACN). (2015a). *Fact sheet: Accelerated baccalaureate and master's degrees in nursing.* Retrieved from http://www.aacn.nche.edu/media-relations/AccelProgsGlance.pdf

American Association of Colleges of Nursing (AACN). (2015b). *Fact sheet: Degree completion programs for registered nurses: RN to master's degree and RN to baccalaureate programs.* Retrieved from http://www.aacn.nche.edu/media-relations/DegreeComp.pdf

American Association of Colleges of Nursing (AACN). (2015c). *Fact sheet: The doctor of nursing practice (DNP).* Retrieved from http://www.aacn.nche.edu/media-relations/fact-sheets/DNPFactSheet.pdf

American Association of Colleges of Nursing (AACN). (2015c). *Fact sheet: The doctor of nursing practice (DNP)*. Retrieved from http://www.aacn.nche.edu/media-relations/fact-sheets/DNPFactSheet.pdf

American Association of Community Colleges, Association of Community Colleges Trustees, American Association of Colleges of Nursing, National League for Nursing, & National Organization for Associate Degree Nursing. (2012). *Joint statement on academic progression for nursing students and graduates*. Retrieved from http://www.oadn.org/files/resources-initiatives/140212_joint_statement_academic_progression_ana_endorsed.pdf

American Association of Community Colleges Health Professions Education Center [AACCHPEC]. (2011). *Community colleges: Keeping America healthy & safe*. Retrieved from http://www.aacc.nche.edu/Resources/aaccprograms/health/Documents/hpec_brochure2011.pdf

American Board of Nursing Specialties (ABNS). (2005). *A position statement on the value of specialty nursing certification* [position statement]. Retrieved from http://www.nursingcertification.org/pdf/value_certification.pdf

American Nurses Association (ANA). (2013). *Nursing education*. Retrieved from http://www.nursingworld.org/MainMenuCategories/Policy-Advocacy/State/Legislative-Agenda-Reports/NursingEducation

American Nurses Credentialing Center (ANCC). (2015). *Growth of the program*. Retrieved from http://www.nursecredentialing.org/Magnet/ProgramOverview/HistoryoftheMagnetProgram/GrowthoftheProgram

APRN Consensus Work Group & National Council of State Boards of Nursing APRN Advisory Committee. (2008). *The consensus model for APRN regulation: Licensure, accreditation, certification, education*. Retrieved from https://www.ncsbn.org/Consensus_Model_for_APRN_Regulation_July_2008.pdf

Association of Diploma Schools of Professional Nursing [ADSPN]. (2015). *About us*. Retrieved from http://adspn.org/about-US/

Augustana College Department of Nursing. (2012). *Bachelor of arts in nursing: Student handbook 2014–2015*. Retrieved from http://www.augie.edu/sites/default/files/u53/student%20handbook_2015_0.pdf

Catalano, J. T. (2015). *Nursing now! Today's issues, tomorrow's trends* (7th ed.). Philadelphia, PA: E. A. Davis Company.

Chism, L. A. (2010). *The doctor of nursing practice: A guidebook for role development and professional issues*. Sudbury, MA: Jones and Bartlett Publishers.

Commission on Collegiate Nursing Education (CCNE). (2013). *CCNE accreditation*. Retrieved from http://www.aacn.nche.edu/ccne-accreditation

Community College Baccalaureate Association. (2014). *Public community colleges conferring baccalaureate degrees*. Retrieved from http://www.accbd.org/wp-content/uploads/2013/10/Conferring-Institutions.pdf

Dreher, H. M., Donnelly, G., & Naremore, R. (2005). Reflections on the DNP and an alternate practice doctorate model: The Drexel DrNP. *Online Journal of Issues in Nursing, 11*(1). Retrieved from http://www.nursingworld.org/MainMenuCategories/ANAMarketplace/ANAPeriodicals/OJIN/TableofContents/Volume112006/No1Jan06/ArticlePreviousTopic/tpc28_716031.html

Emergency Nurses Association (ENA). (2008). *Competencies for nurse practitioners in emergency care*. Des Plaines, IL: Author. Retrieved from http://c.ymcdn.com/sites/www.nonpf.org/resource/resmgr/competencies/compsfornpsinemergencycarefinal.pdf

Emergency Nurses Association (ENA). (2011). *Competencies for clinical nurse specialists in emergency care*. Des Plaines, IL: Author. Retrieved from https://www.ena.org/practice-research/practice/quality/documents/cnscompetencies.pdf

Fitzpatrick. J. (2008). The DNP at the Bolton School: A historical perspective. *Case Western Reserve University: The Bolton School DNP program: Ahead of the curve*. Cleveland, OH: Case Western Reserve University. Retrieved from http://fpb.case.edu/DNP/documents/Magazine2008.pdf

Fulcher, R., & Mullin, C. M. (2011). *A data-driven examination of the impact of associate and bachelor's degree programs on the nation's nursing workforce* (Policy Brief 2011-02PBL). Washington, DC: American Association of Community Colleges. Retrieved from http://www.aacc.nche.edu/Publications/Briefs/Documents/2011-02PBL_DataDrivenNurses.pdf

Future of Nursing Campaign for Action. (2014). *Perspectives on education strategies to increase BSN-prepared workforce*. Retrieved from http://campaignforaction.org/sites/default/files/Campaign%20for%20Action%20BSN%20Report.pdf

Institute of Medicine (IOM). (2011). *The future of nursing: Leading change, advancing health*. Washington, DC: The National Academies Press. Retrieved from http://www.thefutureofnursing.org/sites/default/files/Future%20of%20Nursing%20Report_0.pdf

Keough, V. A., Cole, F. L., Jennrich, J. A., & Ramirez, E. (2003). Emergency nurse practitioners. In V. A. Keough (Ed.), *Advanced practice nursing: Current practice issues in emergency care* (pp. 57–62). Dubuque, IA: Kendall/Hunt Publishing Company.

Mason, D. J., Isaacs, S. L., & Colby, D. C. (Eds.). (2011). *The nursing profession: Development, challenges, and opportunities*. San Francisco, CA: Jossey-Bass.

McEwen, M., & Wills, E. M. (2014). *Theoretical basis for nursing* (4th ed.). Philadelphia, PA: Lippincott, Williams & Wilkins.

National Organization for Associate Degree Nursing [NOADN]. (2006). *Position statement of associate degree nursing* [position statement]. Retrieved from http://www.marylandnursing.net/PositionStatementADN.pdf

Northwest Nazarene University. (n.d.). *RN to BSN degree vs. RN to BS in nursing*. Retrieved from https://nursing.nnu.edu/rn-to-bs-in-nursing/rn-to-bsn-vs-rn-to-bs-in-nursing

St. Olaf College. (n.d.). Academic catalog (2014–15): Nursing. Retrieved from http://www.stolaf.edu/catalog/1415/academicprogram/nursing.html

Teachers College, Columbia University. (n.d.). *Nursing education*. Retrieved from http://www.tc.columbia.edu/hbs/NurseEd/index.asp?Id=Home&Info=Program+Home

University of Illinois at Chicago. (n.d.). *Graduate study at UIC*. Retrieved from http://catalog.uic.edu/gcat/graduate-study/graduate-study/

U.S. Department of Education, International Affairs Office. (2008). *Structure of the U.S. education system: Research doctorate degrees*. Retrieved from http://webcache.googleusercontent.com/search?q=cache:ox5EHkTuar4J:https://www2.ed.gov/about/offices/list/ous/international/usnei/us/doctorate.doc+&cd=1&hl=en&ct=clnk&gl=us

U.S. Department of Education, Office of Postsecondary Education. (n.d.). *FAQs about accreditation*. Retrieved from http://ope.ed.gov/accreditation/FAQAccr.aspx

CHAPTER 5

THE EMERGENCY NURSE AS A PROFESSIONAL

–Linda Laskowski-Jones, MS, APRN, ACNS-BC, CEN, FAWM, FAAN

In the general conversational sense, professionalism is often considered in the context of the behaviors and actions displayed by a nurse during an episode of care delivery or while working in a healthcare setting. However, the concept has significantly greater and far-reaching implications that extend well beyond the time a nurse is *on duty*. Professionalism involves a state of mind that manifests through intentions, words, actions, and deeds. It's intrinsically linked to an individual's core values as a human being and is connected to a moral code that is set within the context of societal expectations for ethical practice.

In this framework, you're a professional 24 hours a day, 7 days per week, whether you're working or not. A public expectation of professionalism is the basis for nursing licensure: a state or jurisdiction grants a license to practice nursing as long as the individual nurse demonstrates that he or she is worthy of the public trust. Any actions by the nurse while working or off duty that call that trust into question can be reported to the professional regulatory body and can result in discipline, including license revocation.

Categorizing professionalism only in the sense of licensure, however, is extremely narrow and limited. If there were to be a professionalism scale from basic to advanced, for example, those behaviors and actions that only meet the standards for licensure would be at the most basic level. Numerous other opportunities exist to advance along the scale to progressively higher levels of professionalism. These include making meaningful contributions to the profession through ongoing self-development, accountability, mentoring, advocacy, and involvement. Although professionalism is rooted in an individual's core values, it can be further developed through positive role modeling as well as through the learning and insights gained from lived experiences navigating complexity, conflict, adversity, challenge, and opportunity. The personal commitment to scholarship is a key component. According to Conard and Pape (2014), "Nurses demonstrate scholarly values as independent thinkers who engage in activities that advance teaching, research, and practice" (p. 88).

Professionalism is often considered in the context of goal achievement or reaching certain career milestones in nursing. Rather than simply identifying self-oriented career goals, however, Hinds et al. (2015) advocate that you develop a "legacy map" approach instead. A *legacy map* encompasses "the nurse's plan to contribute knowledge, practice changes, or other aspects of health care to benefit those who receive nursing care" (p. 212). These goals are considered to be of a higher order, more enduring, and intrinsically connected to a sense of professional wellbeing that stems from improving the experiences or outcomes of others (Hinds et al., 2015).

Use a legacy map as a personal guide to accomplish the legacy you want to leave on the profession of nursing and through your life overall. Hinds et al. (2015) suggest these key questions to explore when creating a personal legacy map (p. 213):

- What do you want to be better in nursing because of you and your efforts?

- What would you like best to be known for by others?

- What do you hope your legacy will be in life?

Given the myriad of professional opportunities available to emergency nurses today, the only real boundaries are the ones that you impose upon yourself. Howard and Papa (2012) maintain that "as emergency nurses of the future, it is essential to focus on the changing health care system, consider personal career paths, establish goals, and meet the challenge to accomplish these goals" (p. 551). This chapter seeks to explore activities that promote professionalism so that emergency nurses can map their own career path to fulfillment and success.

Fostering Evidence-Based Practice

There was a time not that long ago in nursing history when the accepted rationale behind nursing interventions was purely based upon concepts taught in nursing school or handed down as tradition by nursing "experts." According to Proehl and Hoyt (2012), "…nursing practice has always been based on some sort of *evidence*. It just was not necessarily good evidence" (p. 1). Similarly, nursing actions were often primarily guided by physician orders. For any given disease entity or injury, there were few if any research-driven, standardized approaches to the treatment plan among the various providers. The notion of employing outcome-based methods that were supported by scientific evidence in patient care was not part of the framework for typical day-to-day nursing practice.

The need for rigorous scientific inquiry to evaluate the validity and effectiveness of health-care interventions as the basis for modern-day practice has only gained widespread recognition in nursing within the last 30 years or so. Our professional culture is finally shifting to one that questions the efficacy and necessity of the strategies and methods of delivering care that frontline nurses employ. The value of research as an essential component in professional nursing practice is now well accepted and mainstream. Not only is scientific evidence required to serve as the rationale for nursing actions, but the strength of that evidence is also critiqued to give practitioners a sense of how well-supported any particular strategy is in the current literature (Rishel, 2013).

Times have indeed changed, but process and attitude changes have been slow to take root in day-to-day clinical practice. There are still substantial obstacles to applying research findings and incorporating evidence into practice at the point of care delivery. In a study that evaluated staff nurses' use of research to facilitate evidence-based practice (EBP), Yoder et al. (2014) found that although nurses' attitudes were positive about research, lack of time, resources, and knowledge were the most frequently identified barriers. They discussed a general theme in which staff nurses believed that unit educators or clinical nurse specialists—as opposed to themselves—were responsible for ensuring appropriate research utilization and incorporating EBP at the unit level.

Research and EBP are actually complementary but different entities. Research yields findings related to specific study questions and is a component of EBP. The concept of EBP involves reviewing research findings, evaluating the strength of the findings based on study design, and even taking into account expert opinion when research in a particular area is lacking or inconclusive. According to Yoder et al. (2014), "EBP models consider many types of evidence, including empirical research, clinical expertise, the expressed needs of patients, and the opinions of thought leaders" (p. 26). It's clear that EBP encompasses far richer sources of information than research results or scientific inquiry alone. Of significance is the integration of professional expertise, science, and patient-centeredness into the

EBP construct. In this regard, Salmond (2007) nicely summarizes EBP in the following manner:

> "Evidence-based practice (EBP) requires a shift from the traditional paradigm of clinical practice grounded in intuition, clinical experience, and pathophysiological rationale. In the EBP paradigm, clinical expertise is combined with integration of best scientific evidence, patient values and preferences, and the clinical circumstances." (p. 114)

Following Clinical Practice Guidelines

Ultimately, expert critical thinking is required to synthesize evidence into models or clinical practice guidelines (CPGs) that can be applied directly to patient care.

 Clinical practice guidelines—Documents that provide the framework to care for a particular clinical situation. Clinical practice guidelines provide an assessment of the benefits and harms of alternative care options and help to optimize patient care by standardizing care based on scientifically sound research.

Emergency nurses on the frontlines can support true EBP in a variety of ways. Using CPGs that contain the best available evidence to inform clinical decision-making is essential. CPGs serve to facilitate the translation of EBP into actual care delivery at the bedside (Clutter, 2009). Emergency nurses "...should have foundational knowledge of EBP CPGs and deliver care using EBP guidelines" (Clutter, 2009, p. 460). Because the quality and strength of the evidence are of paramount importance, pre-appraised evidence sources are available that have been rigorously evaluated to help busy frontline clinicians (Salmond, 2007). An excellent public resource that contains a very large collection of evidence-based CPGs is the National Guidelines Clearinghouse, sponsored by the Agency for Healthcare Research and Quality (AHRQ), available online at http://www.guideline.gov (AHRQ, n.d.). You can access this site, search, and download CPGs across a wide range of healthcare topics. The strength of the evidence to support interventions listed in the CPG is included. This site is an excellent repository of high-quality information that you can utilize instead of reinventing the proverbial wheel when the need arises for a new or updated CPG in your own practice setting.

Other valuable sites that offer access to a variety of evidence-based CPGs include:

- Centers for Disease Control and Prevention (CDC), which focuses on public health and disease prevention. This website can be accessed at http://www.cdc.gov/.

■ U.S. Preventive Services Task Force (USPSTF), which contains recommendations for preventive health services, can be accessed at http://www.uspreventiveservicestaskforce.org/.

■ The Emergency Nurses Association (ENA) has a dedicated "Practice Resources" section on its website that provides a host of excellent materials for EBP, including CPGs, position statements, standards of practice, and tool kits to help emergency nurses elevate their practice. These resources can be accessed at https://www.ena.org/practice-research/Practice/Pages/default.aspx.

Searching Evidence-Based Literature

Given the rapid pace of scientific advancement, you should strive to engage in practice with an open, inquiring mind that formulates questions and pursues answers to clinical and operational questions through searching evidence-based literature. Conard and Pape (2014) suggest that "nurse scholars immerse themselves in the literature and become experts in their topic" (p. 88). No longer should you simply accept at face value what is told to you as fact; nor should you depend upon long-held beliefs or view rituals in patient care as sacred truths. Salmond (2007) provides a different and much more robust EBP framework in which to consider all aspects of professional nursing care delivery:

> "The new values of EBP call for all practitioners to adopt a mindset of informed skepticism. The EBP clinician asks the wicked questions: Why are we doing it this way? Is there a better way to do it? What is the evidence for what we do? What practice guidelines are available to support my practice? Would doing this be as effective as doing that? and What constitutes best practice?" (p. 118)

To stimulate professional growth and foster a vibrant practice environment at work, you can pose such clinical questions or controversies and share results of the literature review with colleagues at staff meetings or through unit-based newsletters. Forming an ED journal club is an excellent strategy to communicate information from the literature, promote evidence-based practice, introduce the value and evaluation of research, and build interprofessional collaboration skills (Rishel, 2013). Questions can be developed which help to guide you in a critical review of the articles selected for discussion (Rishel, 2013). In this way, the staff-at-large can participate to the degree that they are comfortable, and new information can be appraised and carefully considered for possible integration into practice.

Applying Research to the Bedside

The critical competency for emergency nurses is the ability to effectively translate the results of evidence-based research from the literature to the bedside (Carman et al., 2013). Even though the study results might indicate that a particular intervention, process, or practice appears to be successful, Carman et al. (2013) caution that the quality of the study, the efficacy, and the applicability of the findings to a particular emergency department setting have to be carefully considered; the "fit" may or may not be appropriate, and adjustments may be necessary before implementation is attempted. Otherwise, unrecognized or under-appreciated differences in the ED environment from the study setting (such as the physical structure, culture, policies, resources, and politics) can affect the success of translating the research into practice. Similarly, Wolf et al. (2013) warn that practice changes are typically not made based upon a single study alone: "One should not take a single study and use the results to implement change, unless the study is so large and so well done that professional practice organizations are suggesting changes" (p. 199).

An excellent strategy to stimulate interest in evidence-based practice and apply the findings in the clinical setting is to have research experts involve emergency nursing staff directly in a research project. Based upon their interest and aptitude, staff can be invited to participate in any phase of the study process, from reviewing the literature to assisting research experts with study design considerations, implementing the intervention, collecting the data, or analyzing the results. Tanabe, Gisondi, Barnard, Lucenti, and Cameron (2009), for example, found that a staff-based participatory research methodology led to positive operational changes as a result of having charge nurses help to design, implement, and evaluate a process that involved closing the ED waiting room during certain hours of the day.

Academic teaching hospitals, particularly those that have achieved Magnet® designation, often employ PhD-prepared nurse scholars who can guide the design of a research project and help to obtain the necessary institutional review board (IRB) permissions to conduct the study. In Magnet® hospitals, these nurse scholars can advise and facilitate the work of frontline nurses who are members of evidence-based practice councils or research councils. Emergency nurses certainly have the option of joining these councils if they have a sincere interest in research, or they can participate in approved research by serving in a data-collection capacity. For the majority of hospitals that do not have research experts readily available, developing partnerships with nursing faculty in a university setting can be mutually beneficial for both the healthcare facility and the academic institution. When information on a particular subject is lacking in the literature, you can then pose a study question to experienced faculty as a means of stimulating a possible collaborative research effort. For more information on Magnet designation, see Chapter 7, "Types of Emergency Departments."

ENA also has an Institute for Emergency Nursing Research (IENR) that promotes EBP through advancing research efforts in emergency nursing. Its website (https://www.ena.org/practice-research/Pages/about.aspx) includes a listing of both current and completed research studies, CPGs, research priorities, requests for feedback via surveys, external research and funding opportunities, and white papers. In an article series written by members of IENR's Advisory Council to stimulate bedside nurses' interest in and understanding of research and EBP concepts, authors made a compelling argument as to why research is essential on the frontlines of care delivery: "As the most direct person providing care to persons in their most dire hour of need, it is imperative that we ask the questions, find the evidence, and translate it into the best of care" (Wolf et al., 2012, p. 591).

Seeking Lifelong Learning/Maintaining Competency

The pursuit of continuous learning is not only an obligation to maintain competency, but also the cornerstone of professionalism in emergency nursing. The Institute of Medicine's (2011) *Future of Nursing* report specifically cited lifelong learning as an essential component of nursing practice. Given the rapidly evolving healthcare system, professional and societal expectations also dictate the need for nurses to pursue lifelong learning (Rishel, 2013). It's important to recognize that lifelong learning and competency are fundamentally related. The Emergency Nurses Association's (ENA) *Code of Ethics* (2015a) explicitly identifies your obligations related to competency by stating, "the emergency nurse maintains competency within, and accountability for, emergency nursing practice" (p. 1). However, Harding, Walker-Ciollo, Duke, Campos, and Stapleton (2013) assert that "competence occurs not in isolation but needs to be tailored to the current best evidence, quality initiatives and indicators, and safety" (p. 255). Because maintaining competence is a duty for the duration of your career, and the science that underlies nursing theory and practice is being constantly updated, a commitment to lifelong learning is vital. As new knowledge is integrated into the literature and incorporated into standards of care, you must "remain abreast of new technology, treatments, and trends across health care" (Howard & Papa, 2012, p. 551).

In the fast-paced, highly acute, and complex world of emergency nursing, lifelong learning is especially relevant because the scope of practice encompasses the full range of illness, injury, and associated human responses from birth through death across the entire age spectrum. The knowledge necessary for expert emergency nursing practice is extremely broad. Because you deliver care to patients at some of their most vulnerable periods, time is often of the essence. You must possess a ready, actionable knowledge base that is up to date. Your initial actions can directly affect patient outcomes by what you do, or do not do. Harding et al. (2013) categorize emergency nursing competencies in the context of specific ED processes such as triage, the use of assessment tools like the Broselow Tape, and the ability to utilize commercial products such as a high-volume fluid infuser. Remaining current in regard to assessment techniques, priority setting, care delivery standards and tools, the patient's anticipated clinical course, diagnostic modalities, and outcome evaluation is critical to safe and effective nursing practice.

Equally important to safety and overall professionalism are the competencies related to maintaining collaborative inter- and intradisciplinary relationships, risk management, hand-off communication and care transitions, as well as efficient emergency department operations. All together, these aspects of the emergency nursing role clearly dictate the need for ongoing education to inform professional practice. You must make a conscious effort to assess your learning needs in an ongoing manner to have an accurate sense of the type of educational opportunities that you need to pursue. Scholarship and self-directed learning are hallmarks of professional practice.

Approach to Learning

Your core attitudes and beliefs about lifelong learning as a professional obligation are key determinants of professional success. From a worldview perspective, you may perceive learning as either a burden or a growth opportunity. This worldview influences whether you approach educational experience passively or actively:

■ **In the passive approach,** an educational activity is a job or licensure requirement that must be accepted, tolerated, or even endured. You only participate because you know the activity is required and not participating would likely result in a negative consequence. However, depending upon your overall interest in the topic and the effectiveness of the educator in stimulating new ways of thinking or practicing, your degree of engagement with the learning activity may be negligible.

 "Individual professional development starts when nurses acknowledge that they must be a life-long learner" (Rishel, 2013, p. 539).

■ **In the active approach,** you enter the learning event with an openness and intellectual curiosity that enables critical thinking and integration of new knowledge into practice. You also seek opportunities for ongoing learning. With an inquisitive mind, you pursue answers to the question *why* in clinical practice and research best practice approaches using high-quality, evidence-based resources and appropriate point-of-care references. An active pursuit of learning is both in the moment as well as deliberately planned to incorporate a variety of educational opportunities over the course of a career.

Learning Venues

There are multiple formal and informal learning venues for emergency nurses. These include hospital-based in-service education, both of the mandatory and elective varieties; conferences external to the healthcare institution; and academic programs that lead to a BSN, MSN, MBA, or doctoral degree (DNP or PhD). All certainly have significant value. Ideally, you should take advantage of the offerings as your professional needs, time, resources, and personal circumstances allow. Technology has added to the repertoire of available options. In the past, nursing education has been offered in lecture-based formats for learning. However, many nurses expressed a clear preference for hands-on or case-based learning opportunities. The growing popularity of simulation labs both in nursing schools and in hospitals speaks to the value of both learning and applying new knowledge in a realistic clinical scenario. High-fidelity manikins offer opportunities for full participant engagement in the scenario and hands-on competency development in relation to acquiring or honing practical skills. The use of healthcare actors who play a patient role provides nurses with challenging situations in which interpersonal communication skills may be challenged and ultimately improved. These types of learning experiences are frequently conducted using teams that include physicians, nurses, and allied health personnel to promote more effective teamwork, collaboration, and the development of interdisciplinary competence in patient care.

Stepping outside of your institution to attend local, regional, or national conferences, such as the Emergency Nurses Association Annual Conference, brings significant benefits. You have the chance to update your knowledge base regarding the latest developments and thinking about current topics in emergency nursing. You can also derive value by networking with colleagues from other facilities who may be dealing with similar issues or challenges. Professional relationships can form, which can evolve into long-lasting connections that are beneficial over the course of your career.

If the conference attracts international participants, you can come away with a very well-rounded view of current emergency nursing challenges and how they are addressed on a more global scale. Learning about the nursing or healthcare issues in another country helps place perspective on the significance of the issue and enables innovative approaches to problem solving. It's especially interesting and often eye opening to learn of the resource constraints that exist in other healthcare settings and how other emergency nurses deal with the situation. This cross-cultural exchange supports rich dialogue, deeper professional connections, and the ability to look outside of the usual ways of thinking about issues.

Funding Learning Opportunities

Unfortunately, institutional funds to support emergency nursing education may be limited in many settings. When they are available, the employer may only fund attendance at facility-based or local educational events. Participation in a regional or national conference often requires that you finance part or all of the expenses out-of-pocket. Typical costs include travel, meals, incidentals, as well as the fees associated with conference registration and any special pre-conference workshops. Although these costs may be prohibitive, several effective strategies can help to manage the financial impact:

- Set up a workable personal savings plan to fund attendance at a high-quality conference every 1 to 3 years. This strategy entails the ability to create a realistic budget for conference participation as well as the discipline to save the necessary amount of money, factoring in possible price increases.

- Itemize taxes to deduct costs as business or professional expenses. Personal recordkeeping is essential in this endeavor to show evidence of and validate legitimate tax-deductible expenses.

- Utilize frequent flier miles or hotel points that are part of brand loyalty plans to reduce conference travel costs. Check to see whether local hotels have arranged for reduced rates for those attending the conference. You could also consider sharing a hotel room with colleagues as a cost-saving measure.

- Join a professional organization that provides membership discounts for conference attendance. A benefit of active participation at the local chapter level is that it sometimes comes with opportunities to apply for conference scholarships. There might also be an option to serve as a chapter delegate at the conference itself with funding from the organization, particularly if you are a chapter officer.

The Internal Revenue Service (IRS) allows many legitimate educational expenses to be deducted from a nurse's income, reducing the amount of income subject to tax. To qualify, the education must be required either by law or the employer to keep present salary, status, or job and serve a bona fide business purpose to the employer or maintain/improve the skills needed to work as an emergency nurse (IRS, 2015). It's important to work closely with your tax professional to ensure that all deductions meet the requirements of the law.

- Apply to be a poster presenter or podium speaker. Such participation, particularly as a speaker, frequently leads to reduced or waived registration fees and perhaps even reimbursement for selected travel expenses within specified limits by the conference organizer.

The other benefit is the lifelong-learning opportunity to develop or refine skills in poster presentation, public speaking, and even publication that arise from this level of conference participation.

Completing an Academic Program

Academic programs are very much a part of a successful educational plan for lifelong learning. Pursuing baccalaureate education is a must if your entry-level nursing education was from a diploma or associate's degree program. The American Nurses Credentialing Center (ANCC, 2013) requires that all hospitals seeking Magnet® designation or re-designation must achieve an 80% rate of baccalaureate education in the nursing staff by the year 2020. Not having a baccalaureate degree in nursing will serve as a significant rate-limiting step for both jobs and career-enhancement potential. Nursing employers, particularly those with Magnet hospital designation, may offer some degree of tuition assistance to offset the costs of returning to school.

The baccalaureate degree is the springboard into master's, doctoral, and post-doctoral academic programs. Deciding how far to go in the academic realm is determined by your career aspirations and the corresponding formal educational preparation requirements. As you move through your career, scholarly aspirations may shift in different directions as new interests develop and personal or professional needs change. The key to success is to plan so that no barriers stand in the way of moving from one educational level to the next when the time is right. That means maintaining excellent grades, building lasting professional relationships with faculty, and selecting quality academic programs that support seamless transitions. For more information on various nursing degrees and how they apply to emergency nursing practice, see Chapter 4, "Education of the Emergency Nurse."

Gaining Certification

Certification in a nursing specialty area represents an objective mark of professional excellence and commitment for the emergency nurse. In the broad perspective, it validates that you've successfully acquired an up-to-date body of knowledge, skills, and experience that encompasses the scope and standards of practice for a particular nursing specialty (Rishel, 2013). Certification engenders a measure of professional recognition and achievement for the recipient. In that context, it may be a requirement for advancement or promotion if your healthcare facility has a nursing leadership structure that offers a formal clinical ladder. Attaining certification might also entitle you to receive a certification pay differential or a higher salary overall.

According to the Board of Certification for Emergency Nursing (2015), more than 30,000 emergency nurses are currently certified.

The healthcare institution also benefits from employing certified nurses. Certification serves as tangible evidence of your commitment to and individual responsibility for professional development (Kaplow, 2011). A high rate of professional certification is very favorably viewed and even expected by a number of hospital accrediting agencies such as The Joint Commission, the American College of Surgeons Consultation and Verification Program for trauma centers, and the American Nurses Credentialing Center's Magnet Recognition Program®. Patient outcomes are also positively affected: Kendall-Gallagher, Aiken, Sloane, and Cimiotti (2011) found that for every 10% increase in hospital nurses who had both their BSN and professional specialty certification, the risk of 30-day inpatient mortality and failure to rescue decreased. However, Altman (2011) found that some key barriers can negatively affect certification rates in the hospital: "Fear of test-taking or failure and lack of resources or organization recognition are reasons many nurses cite for not becoming certified" (p. 68).

Professional certification requirements vary depending on the type of specialty exam but typically include a practice requirement in the specialty, passing a standardized test, and either periodic re-testing or maintaining a specified composition of continuing education credits and professional activities, such as presentation or publication in every certification review cycle. Recertification intervals are dictated by the certifying body and generally fall in the 3 to 5 year range. Some certifications also mandate specific academic credentials like a bachelor's degree or master's degree in nursing as a qualifier to sit for the exam. For example, certification as a clinical nurse specialist or nurse practitioner requires a graduate degree in the appropriate nursing specialty area.

Each certification exam has its own unique application process and fee schedule. The application includes standard demographic and academic information. It may also contain questions about your practice setting and license or registration number. An unrestricted registered nurse (RN) license is an admission requirement. Depending on the exam, practice hours or years of service may be either recommended or required as a qualification to sit for the exam; a nursing supervisor signature may be needed to substantiate that the applicant has attained the specified work experience. Application fees vary by exam type and usually fall within a $200 to $400 range. If the certification exam is associated with a particular professional nursing organization, discounts on testing fees are usually available as a benefit for active membership. Some hospitals do offer reimbursement for exam fees and preparation expenses associated with the exam as both an incentive and a reward for successfully passing the test. In the same manner, institutions may also reimburse the expenses related to recertification.

Unrestricted license—A license to practice nursing without active disciplinary action by the professional licensing board.

Once the application is processed, you're sent a letter or electronic communication confirming that you can sit for the exam. Also included in the correspondence is pertinent information about how and where the test is offered and any special requirements such as having a valid driver's license with picture identification available for admittance to the testing site. Although some exams may still be offered in a paper and pencil format, the most common testing modality is via the computer in a designated, proctored testing center. Fear of test-taking is a common concern among nurses (Teal, 2011). The most important success strategy is devoting sufficient time and effort to test preparation. Exam preparation books, sample questions, review courses, and other educational resources should be obtained well in advance of the testing date to support test-taking readiness. Forming a study group is another excellent strategy to facilitate learning as well as build a peer support network for two or more emergency nurses studying for the same exam. For a listing of specific certification exams that may be appropriate for the emergency nurse, see Chapter 4.

Another common option if you have specialized training in forensic nursing is to obtain the Sexual Assault Nurse Examiner–Adult (SANE-A) and/or Sexual Assault Nurse Examiner–Pediatric (SANE-P) certification through the International Association of Forensic Nurses. There are also several certification exams available that cover a wide range of nursing specialties and have relevance to various aspects of emergency nursing practice, including adult or pediatric critical care nursing, gerontological nursing, nursing leadership, staff development, as well as a host of advanced practice certifications if you have a graduate degree. As long as the requirements are met for initial certification or recertification, you can achieve a number of certifications to represent your expertise. The challenge becomes the time, effort, and expense in maintaining all of them.

Adhering to Institutional Policies and Procedures

As an emergency nurse, you have a professional obligation to maintain knowledge of the institutional policies and procedures that govern practices and operations in your workplace. These policies and procedures are often established to meet regulatory requirements set forth by federal, state, and local government agencies as well as hospital accrediting bodies such as the Centers for Medicare & Medicaid Services (CMS), The Joint Commission, and the American College of Surgeons Committee on Trauma. Other policies and procedures may be connected to standards of care based on evidence-based practice sources as well as institutionally derived protocols and processes. At the most basic level, knowledge of the laws that govern nursing practice as well as institutional policies, procedures, and processes is an important defense against professional liability (Balestra, 2012).

In that regard, failure to follow institutional policies and procedures can lead to personal, professional, and institutional liability; regulatory consequences such as institutional citations or de-accreditation; and employer sanctions up to and including termination of employment. An important caveat, however, is that an institutional policy or procedure cannot override federal or state law or regulations if the documents are at odds. Laws and regulations supersede hospital policies.

 For example, if the Nurse Practice Act in a particular state does not allow nurses to delegate intravenous catheter insertion to unlicensed assistive personnel (UAP), but a hospital policy authorizes this practice, the nurse who follows the hospital policy could be found guilty of professional misconduct by the nurse licensure board.

Given the vast number of policies and procedures in most institutions, it's typically not possible to retain detailed information about all of them through memory alone. It's your professional responsibility to know how to locate the relevant policies and procedures and consult them as needed to inform practice and ensure that care delivery conforms to institutional expectations. The professional obligation does not stop there, however. In cases when the policy or procedure does not adequately address the issues at hand, use the ED's administrative chain of command to seek expert clarification of the appropriate course of action when needed. In this case, you're in an optimal position to raise awareness about gaps in policies and procedures that demonstrate the need for policy revision or development, and also participate in the effort to update or create the document based upon a review of current standards or best practices in the literature. This effort gives you an excellent opportunity to expand your knowledge base on the subject matter, take a leadership role in problem resolution, and become a resource for other staff on the topic. If the policy or procedure is not available at the point of care in a user-friendly format, you can also advocate for system changes that improve access to essential information when it is most needed in clinical practice.

Though the rationale underlying most institutional policies and procedures is rooted in good intentions, some may impose barriers to appropriate care delivery or add unnecessary burden. With that said, the policies or procedures cannot simply be ignored. Change is needed. When the policy or procedure is institutionally derived and not based on accreditation, regulatory requirements, or the latest best-practice evidence, the process simply requires that you make the effective argument for revision to the institutional leader(s) who maintain(s) the documents. Having data, current literature, or expert opinion to support your recommendations enhances the strength of your argument for change. This revision process may still take significant time, especially if new processes have to be developed, reviewed, tested, signed-off on by all key stakeholders, and then successfully disseminated to staff. If the policy or procedure that requires modification is linked to a regulation or statute promulgated outside of the healthcare facility, the change process is much more complex and time consuming. It may require statutory change that ultimately must undergo legislative action. The take-home point is that if you see a need for modifications in institutional policies and procedures, an important aspect of professionalism is advocacy for positive change.

Serving on Institutional Committees

Having the opportunity to serve on an institutional committee can significantly contribute to your professional growth. Emergency nursing leaders are often asked by organizational leaders if they can appoint one or more members of their staff to institutional committees or work groups. These committees are generally focused on system-level concerns that may also be relevant to various aspects of emergency care or operations. You can offer critical insights as an emergency nurse into issues as well as support the development of organizational strategies and goals. At the same time, "…soliciting staff input on goals, specific targets, and solutions may lead to an overall sense of ownership and investment," inspiring a culture of shared responsibility for achieving organizational goals in frontline nurses (Berkow et al., 2012, p. 167). Emergency nursing leaders may solicit participation from the nursing staff-at-large and then appoint a nurse in good standing who volunteers. The leader might also choose to select a nurse who has previously expressed a specific goal or interest area that fits well with the committee's mission or purpose, or one who has demonstrated a complementary skill or competency that will prove valuable to the committee.

Becoming a committee member enables you to step outside of the ED worldview, build new connections, and gain a broad-based perspective on issues pertinent to the healthcare facility, the community, the state, and perhaps the nation. This perspective can help you better understand key organizational initiatives and decisions as well as translate their relevance to ED co-workers. At the same time, your professional perspective contributes to a more robust approach to strategic analysis, planning, and problem resolution, especially when committee goals, objectives, or issues touch upon the ED in some way. Needleman and Hassmiller (2009) corroborate the value of frontline nurses' participation in decision-making:

"Nurses develop substantial knowledge of the strengths and weaknesses of hospital systems and how they fail … nurses' perspectives must be represented at the highest levels of hospital leadership and integrated into hospital decision making. In addition, consistent with process-improvement research that identifies the active involvement of front-line staff as a critical factor in making and sustaining change, processes for engaging nurses and other front-line staff also need to be expanded." (p. w627–w628)

When considering an appointment to an institutional committee, you should make a sincere effort to understand the goals and objectives of the group, as well as all of the expectations of the members, ahead of time. If the requirements do not appear feasible, it's best not to accept the appointment and allow another representative who can meet the expectations to serve.

 Common areas of focus for institutional committees that you may participate in as an emergency nurse include access to care, hospital operations, quality and safety, process improvement, infection prevention, human resources, patient flow, standardized care pathways, nurse staffing, employee engagement, electronic medical records, and accreditation.

To be successful as a member of an institutional committee, you should engage in professional meeting etiquette. It's extremely important to be present for the duration of each meeting. Depending on the committee, there may be a set standard for attendance. Failing to meet that standard can mean loss of membership. A proactive conversation with the ED manager or scheduler about the meeting requirements may help prevent scheduling issues. Like attendance, punctuality is expected. Although circumstances that cannot be predicted do occur, making a habit of arriving late is disruptive to the meeting proceedings and results in missing agenda content.

Expectations for behavior or ground rules are typically set by the meeting chair or through consensus with meeting members. Some meetings have a much more formalized structure based upon their purpose. For example, an institutional grievance committee or peer review forum may be run with a very rigid framework to ensure that all required administrative steps are taken in compliance with bylaws, hospital regulations, and any applicable employment laws. Similarly, institutional committees that include members of the board of directors or public officials may be run in a more conservative manner. On the other hand, there are also highly dynamic institutional committees where dialogue flows freely and the active exchange of thoughts and ideas is encouraged. Time is often allocated to discuss any issues that are not listed on the agenda in an open forum format.

The manner in which you conduct yourself at meetings can add value or detract from interactions at the table. During the meeting itself, you should be actively engaged in the proceedings. Set electronic devices to silent mode. Unless absolutely necessary, avoid checking email and text messages. If you anticipate multiple phone calls, arrange to have your phone calls covered while in the meeting. If you must answer a phone call, step away from the meeting so that the conversation cannot be heard. Direct your attention to those speaking. Body language should not convey disinterest, negativity, or hostility, no matter what the nature of the topic. If you have concerns about what is being said, ask clarifying questions and voice specific concerns in a professional manner when it is appropriate to do so.

Although you provide perspective on emergency department issues, it's important to take a balanced and wide-lens view to avoid being perceived as rigid or argumentative when challenging topics are raised. Focusing narrowly on how your ED has always done something as opposed to what might be a national best practice can inhibit effective dialogue and, ultimately, improvement efforts. At the same time, if the committee recommends actions that would pose significant concerns or will require changes in ED processes, you should enlist the active involvement of ED leaders as key stakeholders in the overall approval process. They can provide input and guidance, leverage resources, and plan strategies to facilitate the rollout of any mutually agreed upon process changes. If you're given an assignment with specific tasks to be completed (often referred to as *deliverables*) and an update or report is anticipated at the meeting, you are expected to either follow through or notify the chair in advance of any barriers or delays. The committee chair may be able to help you get the work done if aware in advance.

Overall, although taking on the responsibilities of committee membership will increase your workload, the professional benefits are significant. They include the satisfaction of having a designated place at the table in institutional decision-making, the opportunity to develop relationships and network with a wide variety of leaders and employees from other areas of the hospital, a chance to see healthcare from a wider perspective than may be experienced in a single department, and the chance to gain skills in problem solving and strategic planning. Serving on the committee builds personal leadership abilities and may qualify you for a higher performance rating or advancement on a clinical ladder. Participation can also help to position you for a new avenue in your career. For the healthcare facility engaged in quality initiatives, active nursing participation yields the best opportunity for successful outcomes. Needleman and Hassmiller (2009) assert that "improvement must be institutionalized in the day-to-day work of the front-line staff, with adequate time and resources provided and with front-line staff participating in decision making" (p. w631).

Joining Professional Organizations

Joining a professional organization is a voluntary activity that demonstrates your desire to connect with a nursing generalist or specialty group external to your workplace. In this regard, it can be viewed as evidence of commitment to the profession beyond that which is expected by the employer. According to Guerrieri (2010), "a professional organization often is the public image of the specialty or profession" (p. 47). Professional organizations perform several valuable functions for the members they serve. These functions vary somewhat with each individual group's mission and scope but generally have several roles in common:

- A forum for members to exchange ideas and collaborate through meetings, online forums, and blog posts

- Collective efforts to improve nursing practice

- Continuing educational opportunities

- Standards of care for generalist or specialty practice

- Areas for research as well as research funding opportunities available through grants

- Political advocacy and actions that support the mission of the organization

Many professional organizations also offer a complementary subscription to newsletters or a general or specialty journal. Other typical benefits include discounts on books and a variety of personal and professional resources (e.g., discounts on continuing education courses, certification fees, liability insurance, and home/auto/life insurance). The organization may also establish a clearinghouse or repository for institutional policies, procedures, protocols, and templates as resources for members trying to avoid "reinventing the wheel" when developing these documents for their own facilities.

Joining is generally very straightforward for most professional organizations—you usually only need to complete a membership application and pay the dues. For some professional organizations, however, membership is only granted after you meet specified criteria and are accepted through a specific review process, which may include having letters of endorsement or sponsorship from other active members. A good example of such an organization with restricted membership is Sigma Theta Tau International, the Honor Society of Nursing.

Membership in a professional organization demonstrates commitment and a willingness to be involved on a professional level beyond the typical workplace responsibilities. Joining is a voluntary act—you're choosing to support the mission of the organization through membership. By joining, you gain the membership benefits offered by the group and also support the mission of the organization through paying dues, making charitable contributions to fund special projects, and through active participation in the group's undertakings. Because strength lies in numbers, each individual member adds to the collective power of the organization. For those professional organizations that have local chapters, the opportunities for involvement increase and make active participation more feasible for some nurses.

The benefits you derive from a professional organization are very much dependent on your degree of involvement. You can choose to simply pay the dues each year and enjoy the publications, membership discounts, and continuing education offerings. This level of involvement is important and does support the organization through yearly dues but does not fully leverage all of the opportunities that a group offers. If you're a member of multiple professional organizations, choosing to only be a dues-paying member for some may be very reasonable, especially if you're highly involved in committees or projects of a particular organization at a local or national level.

Direct participation in the professional organization's meetings and events enables active networking, socialization, peer support, and leadership development (Guerrieri, 2010; Rishel, 2013). Socialization helps to instill professional values and perspective. You gain insights that extend beyond your workplace and find that many issues are actually quite common in the emergency environment or within the profession as a whole. In fact, there may be opportunities for collaboration to address shared concerns through local or national committee work. Collaboration confers a sense of professional satisfaction that stems from helping to shape the organization's direction or even by influencing health policy. In this regard, professional organizations serve to both inform members of current health policy or political issues and enhance their abilities to advocate (Wilmot, 2009). The Emergency Nurses Association (ENA), for example, nominates members to serve on federal advocacy groups and supports them through leadership education to enhance their confidence and competence in the political process (Howard & Papa, 2012).

Active involvement offers additional leadership development opportunities as well. Becoming an officer of the organization and engaging in governance activities at the local chapter, region, or national level builds leadership and administrative competencies. Achieving publication in the organization's journal confers professional recognition (Guerrieri, 2010). Likewise, annual conferences provide avenues for members to present posters or podium lectures and gain professional speaking experience. Exposure to professional achievement at these venues can inspire new goals for your own professional accomplishment (Guerrieri, 2010).

Professional organizations can be intradisciplinary or interdisciplinary:

- *Intradisciplinary* organizations include members from only one discipline, such as nursing. Some intradisciplinary organizations may extend associate memberships to individuals from other disciplines. Similarly, a nursing professional organization can have a generalist focus and address issues that span the universe of nursing practice and serve to elevate the profession as a whole, or it can have a specialty focus and concentrate on a particular area of nursing practice. An example of an intradisciplinary, generalist nursing organization is the American Nurses Association.

▪ *Interdisciplinary* organizations allow membership by a variety of disciplines (e.g., physicians, nurses, pharmacists, paramedics, etc.). An example of an interdisciplinary, specialty organization is the American Trauma Society.

Deciding what type of organization to join really boils down to your personal and professional goals. Ideally, the best option is to choose one or more professional organizations whose mission and member benefits align most closely with your interests and needs. There are several excellent and well-established professional organizations that are relevant to the specialty of emergency nursing.

The following list of professional organizations for emergency nurses is by no means all-inclusive or exhaustive but provides a flavor of the professional membership choices available for emergency nurses. Membership and active involvement at the local chapter level of a national professional organization may offer a more personal experience as well as the chance to directly influence chapter functions and strategic directions. This level of participation is exceptionally rewarding due to the peer interaction opportunities and the deep sense of accomplishment that stems from elevating emergency nursing practice.

Emergency Nurses Association (ENA)

The ENA is a widely recognized national intradisciplinary specialty organization for emergency nurses. This organization has a long and robust history of offering professional education to emergency nurses in support of lifelong learning (Howard & Papa, 2012). It also provides myriad opportunities for professional growth and development, as well as numerous resources and initiatives to elevate emergency nursing practice. ENA's official scientific publication is the *Journal of Emergency Nursing*. ENA is also the national provider of the Trauma Nursing Core Course (TNCC) and the Emergency Nursing Pediatric Course (ENPC).

 To learn more about the mission, resources, and activities of the Emergency Nurses Association, visit the website at www.ena.org.

Society of Trauma Nurses (STN)

The Society of Trauma Nurses (STN) is a national intradisciplinary specialty organization devoted to trauma nursing and improving trauma care delivery. This organization recognizes that "trauma nurses" work in a wide variety of settings across the trauma care continuum, from the pre-hospital realm through rehabilitation, injury prevention, and education. The emergency nurse who provides care to trauma patients in his or her ED would be viewed as a trauma nurse by this society. Like the ENA, STN offers its members substantial resources, education, and opportunities for involvement in a broad spectrum of activities related to trauma care. STN's official scientific publication is the *Journal of Trauma Nursing*. STN also provides the Advanced Trauma Care for Nurses (ATCN) course, which runs in conjunction with the Advanced Trauma Life Support Course for physicians.

To learn more about the Society of Trauma Nurses, visit the website at www.traumanurses.org.

International Association of Forensic Nurses (IAFN)

Some EDs have a forensic nurse examiner (FNE) team to both improve care delivery and evidence collection/preservation procedures for patients who are victims of sexual assault, domestic violence, child abuse, and elder abuse. Depending on the scope of the FNE program, these emergency nurses may also become involved in evidence collection/preservation during trauma resuscitation for patients who have sustained interpersonal violence, including gunshot wounds and stab wounds. The International Association of Forensic Nurses (IAFN) is a national nursing specialty organization that provides education, training, practice resources, and professional connections to forensic nurses. Their official scientific publication is the *Journal of Forensic Nursing*. They offer sexual assault nurse examiner (SANE) training and certification to nurses.

To learn more about the International Association of Forensics Nurses, visit the website at www.forensicnurses.org.

Influencing Legislation

Involvement in the political process as an advocate for legislative action or regulatory change is an important aspect of the emergency nurse's role. Understanding the political system and gaining skills in serving as a change agent in this arena enables you to expand your sphere of influence and make a positive impact on the profession as a whole or at a population level. Legislative action is a very effective strategy to hardwire change when other approaches fail. Whether you engage in advocacy activities to improve some aspect of health for individuals or direct efforts to better working conditions for nurses, the outcome can ultimately benefit patients (Oestberg, 2012). The key professional competency for effective advocacy is your ability to influence others. The American Nurses Association (ANA) *Code of Ethics for Nurses* defines advocacy as "the act or process of pleading for, supporting, or recommending a cause or course of action," and further states that "advocacy may be for persons (whether as an individual, group, population, or society) or for an issue, such as potable water or global health" (ANA, 2015, p. 41).

The ANA is also quite clear in defining your duty to engage in advocacy for political action:

> "Nurses must lead, serve, and mentor on institutional or agency policy committees within the practice setting. They must also participate as advocates or as elected or appointed representatives in civic activities related to healthcare." (ANA, 2015, p. 28)

The Emergency Nurses Association's (2015b) mission statement is consistent with this duty and reads: "The mission of the Emergency Nurses Association is to advocate for patient safety and excellence in emergency nursing practice." You can engage in advocacy activities in many different venues both inside the hospital and in the public domain. Hearrell (2011) asserts, "Emergency nurses have a diverse, professional background that provides the expertise and skills needed to take their profession out of the hospital and into the community, to the boardroom, and even the floor of the Senate" (p. 74).

Political action can advance the agenda of professional nursing organizations, improve access to care delivery, remove barriers that affect patient care, and enhance community health and wellness through illness and injury prevention. A legislative initiative that meets all three of these aims is the political effort to obtain full practice authority for advanced practice nurses (APNs) in states that do not currently recognize it, as well as enable all registered nurses to practice to the full extent of their education and training. This call to action charges nurses and other health policy makers to revise state statutes, regulations, and policies related to licensure and nursing scope of practice so that they are aligned with the Institute of Medicine's (IOM) recommendations contained in the *Future of Nursing* report (IOM, 2011). Howard and Papa (2012) contend that "the landmark IOM report provides the emergency nurse the opportunity to be the decision maker, the problem solver, the policy determiner, the legislative influencer, and the difference maker" (p. 551). As new treatment modalities develop and care models evolve, certain aspects of healthcare policy may no longer be relevant and will need to be updated or eliminated.

 Recently, emergency nurses have been actively lobbying state governments to make an assault against emergency nurses a crime. According to the Emergency Nurses Association (2013), as of February 2013, 37 states have enacted legislation making assaults against emergency nurses a misdemeanor or felony. This serves as proof of the power of emergency nurses to influence public policy.

Emergency nurses also have the ideal opportunity to back legislation targeted at specific illness- or injury-prevention strategies like supporting mandatory motorcycle helmet use or banning cigarette smoking in public areas. Statutory language typically sends a more powerful message and motivates the desired behavior change to a much greater extent in a population than traditional health teaching, because the law carries civil penalties for failing to meet the requirement. Addressing health inequalities is another ripe area for political action; in this scenario, you must be able to shift focus from the individual patient to the community (Carnegie & Kiger, 2009). This effort may also include influencing or guiding the development of health policy or regulations that serve to improve the health of specific populations.

The first step in any legislative involvement is recognizing that a compelling need for change exists and wanting to engage. How you proceed from that point depends upon the degree of personal commitment that you're willing and able to put forth in influencing health policy or the regulatory decision-making processes through advocacy activities (Hearrell, 2011). Fortunately, there is a wide range of options for involvement. One of the most fundamental forms of advocacy involves contact with a legislator through written communication via email, letter, or fax; and verbal communication through a phone call or a face-to-face meeting to discuss an issue and make recommendations. In this situation, you offer the legislator an expert perspective on issues pertinent to emergency nursing practice or healthcare in general.

If a change requires a more concerted group effort, you can connect with other emergency nurses on the issue, bring evidence to the table in the form of data and real stories that validate concerns and recommendations, and work to garner the support of key constituents in the healthcare facility, professional organization, or the community-at-large. Next steps might include proposing new regulatory language based upon the recommendations for change and then following them through the political process. You may be asked to attend a legislative meeting or hearing and provide expert testimony on the subject. The scale of this effort might involve advocacy on a regulatory board or coalition, local government, or state, regional, or national level (Hearrell, 2011). Being involved in these activities may sound daunting, but the professional growth experience is unparalleled, especially when your efforts serve to improve patient care.

Political involvement can represent new territory for some emergency nurses. Fortunately, there are many avenues to gain experience with the political process. As a good place to start, Oestberg (2012) recommends forming a mentor relationship with an experienced nurse advocate to learn the political process. There are also formal continuing education offerings as well as academic courses that teach concepts related to navigating the political system and gaining knowledge about how a bill becomes law. Master's or doctoral degrees in health policy or public health are available for those who want to develop significant expertise in this area. Many professional nursing organizations have a political action component or special interest group that provides templates to assist with letter writing campaigns (Montgomery, 2012). Some offer legislative internship opportunities that enable you to gain firsthand experience in the political arena.

You can also establish an ongoing connection with one or more political figures and serve as an expert in an advisory capacity on healthcare issues (Montgomery, 2012). Similarly, you might choose to build a more formalized relationship with a politician by supporting his or her campaign as a volunteer to learn about the political process from an insider's vantage point. This relationship can build effective political networks and lead to key connections when support for various types of legislative action is needed (Hearrell, 2011). After gaining experience in the legislative realm, you might even choose to run for political office. Oestberg (2012) places the need for nurses to become involved in the legislative process into perspective by asking a poignant question: "Do you really want someone that isn't a nurse (or who isn't getting input from a nurse) deciding how nurses do their jobs? Nurses need to have their voices heard!" (p. 49).

Volunteering

Volunteering is an element of professionalism that represents an orientation toward altruism and citizenship. It demonstrates a tangible commitment to service as an individual core value. For society, the knowledge base and abilities of emergency nurses make them a highly beneficial resource in a multitude of settings that range from clinical practice and public education to serving on boards of non-profit community organizations. Of course, there are those individuals who believe that financial compensation should be provided for all nursing-related activities or else the effort is not worthwhile. However, this mindset is extremely self-limiting. It fails to take into account how volunteer work can enhance your career as well as instill a deep sense of personal and professional satisfaction. Although you don't get paid in the monetary sense, the potential rewards are rich.

 According to the Bureau of Labor Statistics (2015), 62.8 million people volunteered between September 2013 and September 2014. The average number of hours spent volunteering per person was 50 hours per year. Volunteering is essential to the U.S. economy.

Volunteering offers opportunities for both life and work experience that may not be available in the typical employment setting. These can include gaining new competencies in varying aspects of teaching, leadership, clinical practice, finance, publication, and organizational skills. Volunteer work can also build networks and connections with individuals and organizations that can aid in career development. Service on community non-profit boards, for example, exposes you to health policy issues and offers opportunities for you to help shape future policy directions (Dawson & Freed, 2008). The travel involved in humanitarian or disaster-aid volunteer work affords contact with diverse cultures that can stimulate fresh thinking about innovative ways of delivering care. For those interested in research, the volunteer experience may yield questions and ideas for more in-depth study. Serving as a volunteer may qualify you for a higher rating on a performance evaluation or for promotion to the next level on a clinical ladder in the work place. Similarly, volunteer community service is often listed as part of the selection criteria for various honors and awards. It's an excellent avenue for professional recognition and may be a key differentiating factor when applying for highly competitive scholarship funding or a new professional role.

You have multiple options available to serve as a volunteer. Deciding which opportunities to pursue requires careful consideration. Dawson and Freed (2008) advise nurses to "match your passion and your available time, energy and money with an organization" in the context of pursuing an appointment to a community service board or agency (p. 268). This advice stands, however, as an ideal framework for assessing whether any particular type of volunteer work is feasible in relation to your current life circumstances. Understanding personal capacity is critical to avoid taking on unrealistic commitments that can overwhelm or lead to a failure to meet expectations. Fortunately, many volunteer choices are available that offer a wide range of commitment options for emergency nurses.

At a very basic but important level, there is often a great need for volunteer instructors to teach classes in cardiopulmonary resuscitation (CPR) or first aid to members of the general public. The commitment involves successfully completing the instructor classes through the sponsoring agency and meeting the ongoing teaching requirements to maintain instructor status. Similar short-duration and episodic opportunities can include participating in health screening and community education events, and manning first aid stations at fairs, summer camps, and athletic competitions, including adventure races and marathons. Longer-duration volunteer engagements that generally require more time and effort might involve supporting the activities of faith-based organizations by serving as a parish nurse, or staffing community clinics in resource-constrained areas. In remote locations, you may be called upon as a volunteer to aid the local emergency medical services workers during rescue operations or when prolonged patient transport is required.

If you want to travel, consider participating in national and international humanitarian aid as well as disaster response or relief efforts. These missions require a willingness to step out of a known comfort zone and work in extremely resource-limited environments with diverse cultures. Missions can last from 1 to 2 weeks or much longer, depending on the type of work to be done and the location. Spry (2009) advocates carefully researching the financial expectations, time commitment, working and living conditions, local practice standards and customs, safety considerations, and travel requirements before committing to go.

Many mission trips require the volunteer to use personal financial resources to fund a portion or all of the travel, including supply costs. It's also vital to make sure that your employer will support volunteer deployment if you're away from your regular job for an extended period. Employers have a duty to ensure that their own institutional staffing needs are met for patient safety. They are under no obligation to authorize participation in volunteer activities that may potentially jeopardize nursing services on the home front. You may be asked to find coverage for the shifts that you expect to miss. For more information on volunteering as an emergency nurse, see Chapter 3, "Unique Roles of the Emergency Nurse."

Working and living conditions may be very different from your usual experience in the United States, warranting careful consideration of personal factors such as stamina, health, flexibility, and adaptability to change. The volunteer hours may be long and the duty difficult; there may be no support services that you have come to expect, leaving you to perform tasks like housekeeping and instrument cleaning; single-use items may be in short supply and must be sterilized and reused (Spry, 2009). Personal safety is also a significant consideration. Food and water may be contaminated in areas that lack proper sanitation. Other threats to consider include crime and dangerous insects or animals.

A current passport or visa, a nursing license, and medical insurance may be required to gain entrance into the country. Customs regulations may also require proof of vaccination against endemic diseases. You must factor in the time necessary for immunity to develop before deployment. Prophylactic medications against malaria or other infectious diseases may be indicated. Travel and medical insurance is highly recommended in the event you require medical care or evacuation to home. You will also need to research language barriers, religious practices, and local customs, including the use of healers and folk remedies, to work effectively among people of a different culture. Spry (2009) places these issues into perspective by observing that "… most sites where volunteers are needed are not so fortunate. In these settings, basic skills, a commitment to making a difference, and a desire to help is what is needed most" (p. 195).

Having background education in wilderness medicine can be very helpful prior to embarking on a trip to an austere area, especially one in which the basic community infrastructure has been destroyed by a natural or man-made disaster. Wilderness medicine courses offer instruction to healthcare personnel on how to provide patient care in austere conditions, including strategies to improvise equipment and supplies while incorporating appropriate personal safety and survival skills (Wilderness Medical Society [WMS], n.d.).

Whatever venue is pursued, whether local or abroad, volunteer service promotes respect for nursing and widespread recognition of the positive contributions nurses make to society (Dawson & Freed, 2008). Perhaps most importantly, volunteering is exceptionally gratifying at the deeply human level; it can reinvigorate your passion for nursing and be a springboard for significant personal and professional growth.

Personal Professional Liability Insurance

The emergency department can be a high-risk and unpredictable work environment from a legal perspective. Although most nurses are not named in lawsuits, the question of whether or not to carry a personal professional liability insurance policy is one that is commonly considered by emergency nurses. Unlike physician policies that can be very expensive, the typical cost of a policy for a registered nurse is quite reasonable and is generally less than $200 per year. Advance practice nurses do pay higher premiums based upon their specialty and scope of practice.

 The cost of insurance and individual coverage is partially dependent on your state of residence and the malpractice burden the insurer must bear in that particular state.

When you're employed by a healthcare system, the facility's corporate liability insurance policy generally provides coverage for any malpractice claims that might be brought against you. Therefore, given the out-of-pocket costs, you might think that carrying personal professional liability insurance is an unnecessary expense. However, the decision to carry your own policy must be considered in the context of several very important factors:

- You're considered a professional 24 hours a day, 7 days per week. Any claims lodged against you for giving healthcare advice or rendering nursing assistance outside of the employer relationship would not be covered by the employer's liability policy and would be borne by you if a claim ensues.

- If a complaint is made to the professional licensing board about your professional conduct or failure to meet professional obligations in some way by the employer or by a member of the public, the employer's coverage generally does not cover defense costs for licensure protection.

- If you separate from an employer and a subsequent claim is made against you, the employer's policy may no longer cover your defense costs.

A personal liability insurance policy provides not only professional liability coverage but also licensure protection for professional regulatory claims. Depending on the insurer and the type of policy, it may also offer other valuable benefits such as legal representation during a deposition, defense expense reimbursement, and educational resources regarding risk-mitigation strategies. Of note, a professional liability policy does not typically cover expenses related to charges brought against you for criminal acts.

To protect themselves, RNs and NPs are encouraged to select an insurance company that (Balestra, 2012, p. 42–43):

- Supports RNs/NPs by providing an advisory board where they can present issues and seek solutions

- Includes license protection to help defend an RN/NP in an administrative or disciplinary situation

- Covers an RN/NP for incidents that occurred at a previous place of employment

- Provides adequate levels of coverage (i.e., malpractice coverage of $1 million/$3 million and disciplinary coverage of $25,000 per occurrence or aggregate). It's important to note that the state's attorney general's office will charge for its time representing the state's Board of Nursing (BON), and this is not covered by any insurance. Also, a complaint against an RN/NP in one state can have a domino effect in any other state in which he or she holds a license. This means the RN/NP will have to pay for defense costs in every state.

- Allows the RN/NP to select an attorney for representation in disciplinary actions

- Provides a website that addresses risk management issues and solutions

- Gives a discount if the RN/NP gets continuing education credits in a course related to risk management

Promoting Health/Injury Prevention/Community Education

One of the unique aspects of practicing as a frontline emergency nurse is the opportunity to care for patients experiencing the full spectrum of injuries and illnesses from birth through advanced age. So often the injury or illness may have been avoidable or of lower severity if the individual had made different conscious choices or engaged in behaviors that decreased health risks or promoted a healthy lifestyle. These encounters and insights make you exceptionally well-suited to play an active role in injury prevention, community education, and health-promotion efforts. A key aspect of professionalism in emergency nursing is the commitment to educating the public about strategies that decrease illness or injury risks and promote health. These efforts include education in both the clinical setting and in the community-at-large. The ENA *Code of Ethics* (2015) clearly articulates the emergency nurse's duty in this regard:

> "The emergency nurse is dedicated to providing care and knowledge to the public, which includes a healthy lifestyle, general well-being, and injury prevention. Through individual and institutional support, emergency nurses should become involved in strategies to educate the public, foster healthy lifestyles, and encourage legislative efforts that promote these ideas." (p. 3)

Although health promotion and injury prevention information is often incorporated into standardized or commercially available ED discharge instructions, the more comprehensive approach is to integrate it into the overall episode of care while the patient and family are in the ED whenever possible. In this way, you can leverage the teachable moment when there may be a higher level of motivation to make positive behavior changes because the patient or family member better connects the current health issue with the modifiable risks or problematic choices. In addition, you can spend more time assessing the patient's level of understanding and explaining concepts that are unclear, rather than rush through discharge instructions when the patient and family are impatient to leave the ED. Examples might include how dietary choices that are high in sodium can exacerbate heart failure, or how a high carbohydrate diet or failure to perform blood glucose monitoring can be a factor in poor glycemic control.

With a similar intent, the ENA has advocated implementing Screening Brief Intervention and Referral to Treatment (SBIRT) while the patient is in the ED to both identify problem drinkers who need substance abuse treatment and help patients to recognize at-risk drinking patterns (Désy, Howard, Perhats, & Li, 2010). In a quasi-experimental study evaluating the impact of ED nurse–delivered SBIRT, Désy et al. (2010) found that "... the SBIRT procedure conducted by existing staff nurses in the ED setting can also contribute to reducing alcohol consumption, drinking frequency, and repeat emergency care visits" (p. 543). Though not necessarily representative of all ED nurse–delivered SBIRT programs, their study results demonstrated the following positive outcomes:

> "Alcohol consumption decreased by 70% in the intervention group compared to 20% in the usual care group. Drinking frequency also decreased in both groups. Fewer patients from the intervention group (20%) had recurring ED visits compared to patients in the usual care group (31%)." (p. 538)

To learn more about SBIRT, visit http://www.integration.samhsa.gov/clinical-practice/SBIRT.

These researchers identified ED crowding from high patient boarding and lack of privacy as key factors that produced suboptimal conditions for implementing SBIRT. There are other factors to take into account that can also negatively impact effective implementation of SBIRT by frontline ED nurses. Ong-Flaherty (2012) identified "staff buy-in of the concepts" as one of the challenges to recognize when instituting an SBIRT program (p. 54). Quite frankly, staff buy-in is essential for the success of any initiative related to ED patient care. Overcoming staff resistance can be a significant hurdle for anyone attempting to elevate ED nursing practice. Here is where concepts of professionalism in emergency nursing must be leveraged to demonstrate that health promotion is indeed both a core competency and a role expectation of emergency nurses. With that said, it's incumbent on nursing and hospital leadership to support the staff by removing barriers to incorporating health promotion into ED care, such as provision of training programs, promoting ED throughput, and ensuring adequate staffing plans.

Pediatric emergency nurses have both the child and the family to consider in their health-education efforts. The habits and behaviors of the family can directly influence the health of the child. The parent's proper use of seat belts and child passenger safety seats, for example, is a good topic for discussion to promote injury prevention. Similarly, the smoking habits of people in the child's household represent another area of opportunity for both health promotion and disease prevention. Exposure to environmental tobacco smoke (ETS) poses significant health risks to children. According to Deckter, Mahabee-Gittens, and Gordon (2009), "when registered nurses (RNs) are caring for a child with an illness that may have been caused or exacerbated by ETS exposure, they are given the unique opportunity both to educate parents about the health effects of ETS on their child and provide parents who use tobacco with tobacco cessation advice" (p. 402).

Another area for health education of patients and families in the ED is related to the appropriate use of the healthcare system and resources for follow-up after discharge. Patients and families may need assistance to both understand and navigate the health system. In an effort to reduce the need for return visits to the ED, Gozdzialski, Schlutow, and Pittiglio (2012), emphasized the role of the ED nurse in discharge teaching:

> "Appropriate nurse-directed patient education after an ED visit may help both the patient and family better understand the challenges, needs, and expectations during the recovery process. In addition, this education can anticipate and assist in aiding patients and their families with physical limitations, role changes, and emotional struggles after injury or illness." (p. 293)

Although the ED does enable a point-of-care approach to health promotion, there may be very real barriers to effective screening and patient education that must be considered. There are challenges inherent in the ED setting as well as in the staff's willingness and ability to educate and the patient's personal capacity to engage in learning. The dynamic nature and demands of the ED environment, including high ED census and acuity, can pose challenges to an ED nurse's ability to educate effectively overall. Creativity and innovation are necessary to support health teaching, especially in challenging circumstances. Strategies might include selecting educational videos for the patient to view in the ED if available, providing quality printed educational materials written at the appropriate reading or health-literacy level, supplying contact information for health educators in the facility or community, offering information about community resources, and instituting a formal discharge phone call follow-up program for selected patients. For more information on discharge phone call follow-up programs, see Chapter 11, "Common Challenges Faced by Emergency Nurses."

When you choose to participate in community-based education programs, the opportunities to influence choices about health promotion and injury prevention expand dramatically from the single patient encounter in a challenging emergency environment to engaging a much broader audience. The community, in essence, becomes the patient. These programs are commonly offered through schools, faith-based groups, senior centers, police agencies, and non-profit community organizations such as local chapters of the American Heart Association, the American Cancer Society, or the American Trauma Society. Professional nursing organizations also typically sponsor programs that provide targeted health education to the general public as part of their mission. Offerings might include CPR classes, first aid courses, lectures or group discussions on healthy lifestyle choices or health risk mitigation strategies, disease management, substance abuse, fall prevention, and protective gear for sports.

Another possibility for community-based education is the creation of innovative programming by ED nurses in a specific hospital, community, or region that addresses health risks significant for that area. A great example of such an initiative came out of North Carolina. Nurses at an ED located close to the ocean noticed a very concerning number of drowning victims being brought into their hospital for resuscitation, as well as a rising incidence of marine-related injuries (Pelton, 2012). In response, several ED nurses and two of their support staff created the "ED Beach Reach" community outreach program. "Hydration, sun protection, child safety, marine life dangers, fishhooks, tetanus vaccinations, rip currents, and drowning prevention were identified as the highest priority for safety and injury prevention education" (Pelton, 2012, p. 79). They developed printed educational materials and give-away items as part of their strategy to educate the general public, and then went to the beaches to interact directly with beachgoers at various times over the course of the summer. Although they did recognize a slight decrease in the incidence of marine-related injuries that could have been the result of other factors, they did initiate a program with the potential to grow and make a more significant impact, especially since they took it to their ENA chapter for dissemination to a larger group (Pelton, 2012). Pelton (2012) makes a very compelling case for involvement in community outreach, which nicely sums up this aspect of professionalism in emergency nursing:

> "It takes time and energy to have an impact on a community. It takes passion and desire to effect change. All emergency departments are a reflection of the community they serve. It is our responsibility as emergency nurses to evaluate our communities to determine which risks are most prevalent."
> (p. 80)

In addition to the benefits for patients and communities, health promotion, injury prevention, and community outreach activities pose multiple opportunities for enhancing professional growth in emergency nurses. Presenting information to small or large groups builds public speaking skills. Interacting with event organizers and participants enables the development of new personal and professional connections and possible opportunities for a greater depth of involvement. Active community service may positively position you for a higher performance rating or for professional advancement. It may also help prepare you for a community education or outreach position within the healthcare facility. Community service is exceptionally rewarding because it offers the chance to help people avoid the situation that leads to an emergency department visit or a hospital admission. Ultimately, you can proactively prevent pain and suffering before it happens.

Summary

Nursing is a profession. That requires those in the practice of nursing to carry themselves as a professional. Yet asking individuals, even nurses, what the definition of *professionalism* is may conjure up responses as varied as the number of people asked. Understanding the concept of a profession and professionalism is challenging. This chapter provided a broad overview of the concept of professionalism. It's essential that emergency nurses, as members of the nursing profession, understand the professional responsibilities that go along with the title of "Registered Nurse."

References

Agency for Healthcare Research and Quality (AHRQ). (n.d.). *National guideline clearinghouse*. Retrieved from www.guideline.gov

Altman, M. (2011). Let's get certified: Best practices for nurse leaders to support a culture of certification. *AACN Advanced Critical Care, 22*(1), 68–75.

American Nurses Association. (2015). *Code of ethics for nurses with interpretive statements*. Retrieved from http://www.nursingworld.org/MainMenuCategories/EthicsStandards/CodeofEthicsforNurses/Code-of-Ethics-For-Nurses.html

American Nurses Credentialing Center (ANCC). (2013, June 7). *Magnet Recognition Program® FAQ: Data and expected outcomes*. Retrieved from http://nursecredentialing.org/Magnet/MagnetFAQs/MagnetFAQCategory/MagnetFAQs/MagnetFAQ-OrganizationalOverview#007

Balestra, M. (2012). The best defense for registered nurses and nurse practitioners: Understanding the disciplinary process. *Journal of Nursing Law, 15*(2), 39–44. Retrieved from http://dx.doi.org/10.1891/1073-7472.15.2.39

Berkow, S., Workman, J., Aronson, S., Stewart, J., Virkstis, K., & Kahn, M. (2012). Strengthening frontline nurse investment in organizational goals. *JONA, 42*(3), 165–169.

Board of Certification for Emergency Nursing. (2015). *BCEN spotlight*. Retrieved from https://www.bcencertifications.org/Home.aspx

Bureau of Labor Statistics. (2015, February 25). *Volunteering in the United States, 2014*. Retrieved from http://www.bls.gov/news.release/volun.nr0.htm

Carman, M. J., Wolf, L. A., Baker, K. M., Clark, P. R., Henderson, D., Manton, A., & Zavotsky, K. E. (2013). Translating research to practice: Bringing emergency nursing research full circle to the bedside. *Journal of Emergency Nursing, 39*(6), 657–659. doi: http://dx.doi.org/10.1016/j.jen.2013.09.004

Carnegie, E., & Kiger, A. (2009). Being and doing politics: An outdated model or 21st century reality? *Journal of Advanced Nursing, 65*(9), 1976–1984. doi: 10.1111/j.1365-2648.2009.05084.x

Clutter, P. C. (2009). Clinical practice guidelines: Key resources to guide clinical decision making and enhance quality health care. *Journal of Emergency Nursing, 35*, 460–461.

Conard, P. L., & Pape, T. (2014). Roles and responsibilities of the nursing scholar. *Pediatric Nursing, 40*(2), 87–90.

Dawson, S., & Freed, P. E. (2008). Nurse leadership: Making the most of community service. *The Journal of Continuing Education in Nursing, 39*(6), 268–273.

Deckter, L., Mahabee-Gittens, M., & Gordon, J. S. (2009). Are pediatric ED nurses delivering tobacco cessation advice to patients? *Journal of Emergency Nursing, 35*(5), 402–405.

Désy, P. M., Howard, P. K., Perhats, C., & Li, S. (2010). Alcohol screening, brief intervention, and referral to treatment conducted by emergency nurses: An impact evaluation. *Journal of Emergency Nursing, 36*(6), 538–545. doi: 10.1016/j.jen.2009.09.011

Emergency Nurses Association. (2013, February 25). *Workplace violence penalties and terminology database*. Retrieved from https://www.ena.org/government/State/Documents/WPVPenalties.pdf

Emergency Nurses Association (ENA). (2015a). *Code of ethics*. Retrieved from https://www.ena.org/about/Documents/CodeofEthics.pdf

Emergency Nurses Association (ENA). (2015b). *Mission statement*. Retrieved from https://www.ena.org/about/Pages/Default.aspx

Gozdzialski, A., Schlutow, M., & Pittiglio, L. (2012). Patient and family education in the emergency department: How nurses can help. *Journal of Emergency Nursing, 38*(3), 293–295. doi: http://dx.doi.org/10.1016/j.jen.2011.12.014

Guerrieri, R. (2010). Professional growth: Learn, grow and bloom by joining a professional association. *Nursing2010, 40*(5), 47–48.

Harding, A. D., Walker-Cillo, G. E., Duke, A., Campos, G. J., & Stapleton, S. J. (2013). A framework for creating and evaluating competencies for emergency nurses. *Journal of Emergency Nursing, 39*(3), 252–264. doi: http://dx.doi.org/10.1016/j.jen.2012.05.006

Hearrell, C. L. (2011). Advocacy: Nurses making a difference. *Journal of Emergency Nursing, 37*, 73–74.

Hinds, P. S., Britton, D. R., Coleman, L., Engh, E., Humbel, T. K., Keller, S., ... Walczak, D. (2015). Creating a career legacy map to assure meaningful work in nursing. *Nursing Outlook, 63*(2), 211–218.

Howard, P. K., & Papa, A. M. (2012). Future-of-nursing report: The impact on emergency nursing. *Journal of Emergency Nursing, 38*(6), 549–552. doi: 10.1016/j.jen.2012.08.001

Institute of Medicine (IOM). (2011). *The future of nursing: Leading change, advancing health.* Washington, DC: The National Academies Press.

Internal Revenue Service (IRS). (2015, January 15). *Tax benefits for education: Information center.* Retrieved from http://www.irs.gov/uac/Tax-Benefits-for-Education:-Information-Center

Kaplow, R. (2011). The value of certification. *AACN Advanced Critical Care, 22*(1), 25–32.

Kendall-Gallagher, D., Aiken, L. H., Sloane, D. M., & Cimiotti, J. P. (2011). Nurse specialty certification, inpatient mortality, and failure to rescue. *Journal of Nursing Scholarship, 43*(2), 188–194. doi: 10.1111/j.1547-5069.2011.01391.x

Montgomery, T. M. (2012). Health care and politics: Making your voice heard. *Nursing for Women's Health, 16*(3), 198–201. doi: 10.1111/j.1751-486X.2012.01730.x

Needleman, J., & Hassmiller, S. (2009). The role of nurses in improving hospital quality and efficiency: Real-world results. *Health Affairs, 28*(4), w625–w633. Retrieved from http://content.healthaffairs.org/content/28/4/w625.full.html

Oestberg, F. (2012). Policy and politics: Why nurses should get involved. *Nursing, 42*(12), 46–49. doi: 10.1097/01.NURSE.0000422645.29125.87

Ong-Flaherty, C. (2012). Screening, brief intervention, and referral to treatment: A nursing perspective. *Journal of Emergency Nursing, 38*(1), 54–56.

Pelton, M. M. (2012). Have fun, be safe: The start of an ED community outreach program. *Journal of Emergency Nursing, 38*(1), 79–80.

Proehl, J., & Hoyt, K. S. (2012). Evidence versus standard versus best practice: Show me the data! *Advanced Emergency Nursing Journal, 34*(1), 1–2.

Rishel, C. (2013). Professional development for oncology nurses: A commitment to lifelong learning. *Oncology Nursing Forum, 40*(6), 537–539.

Salmond, S. W. (2007). Advancing evidence-based practice: A primer. *Orthopedic Nursing, 26*(2), 114–123.

Spry, C. (2009). Volunteering speaks to the heart of nursing. *AORN Journal, 89*(1), 193–195.

Tanabe, P., Gisondi, M. A., Barnard, C., Lucenti, M. J., & Cameron, K. A. (2009). Can education and staff-based participatory research change nursing practice in an era of ED overcrowding? A focus group study. *Journal of Emergency Nursing, 35*(4), 290–298.

Teal, J. (2011). Certifiably excellent. *AACN Advanced Critical Care, 22*(1), 83–88.

Wilderness Medical Society (WMS). (n.d.). *Conferences/calendar.* Retrieved from http://www.wms.org/conferences/calendar.aspx

Wilmot, L. A. (2009). The power of nurses in the legislative process. *Journal of Emergency Nursing, 35*(2), 146–148.

Wolf, L. A., Carman, M. J., Henderson, D., Kamienski, M., Koziol-McLain, J., Manton, A., & Moon, M. D. (2012). Ten things we might not want to do anymore: How research changes nursing practice. *Journal of Emergency Nursing, 38*(6), 589–591. doi: 10.1016/j.jen.2012.09.003

Wolf, L. A., Carman, M. J., Henderson, D., Kamienski, M., Koziol-McLain, J., Manton, A., & Moon, M. D. (2013). Evaluating evidence for practice. *Journal of Emergency Nursing, 39*(2), 197–199.

Yoder, L. H., Kirkley, D., McFall, D. C., Kirksey, K. M., StalBaum, A. L., & Sellers, D. (2014). Staff nurses' use of research to facilitate evidence-based practice. *American Journal of Nursing, 114*(9), 26–37.

SELF-CARE AND THE EMERGENCY NURSE

–William Schueler, MSN, RN, CEN

What are you doing for yourself?

Emergency nursing can be a very rewarding career. The work can also be intense, laborious, and emotionally taxing. The very nature of the emergency working environment causes stress (de Souza Oliveira, Junior, de Miranda, Cavalcante, & das Gracas Almeida, 2014). When you understand the unique environment and culture of emergency nursing, you can employ strategies to deal with your emotional and physical wellbeing. The purpose of this chapter is to introduce you to some of these strategies. Many of the themes presented are interrelated, and you can discover how these themes influence each other and your role as an emergency nurse.

Each section starts with a question to help you reflect and analyze how you're currently taking care of yourself and your career. Come back to this chapter throughout your career to ask yourself these questions. The goal is to realize and fix ineffective self-care practices before they create a significant negative impact on your health and wellbeing. Anticipation, mitigation, and prevention of these work stressors can help you to have a prosperous career.

The Nurse-Focused Stressors Model, shown in Figure 6.1, visually represents the concepts discussed in this chapter and how they holistically relate to the nurse and his or her patients. Looking at this model, it's no wonder emergency nurses are under so much stress. This chapter also looks at various ways to reduce or handle the stress that is experienced in the emergency nursing profession.

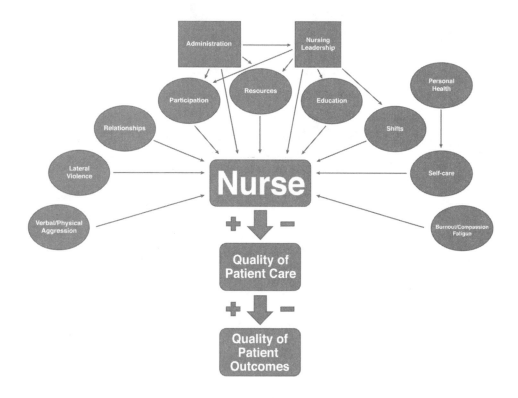

Figure 6.1   The Nurse-Focused Stressors Model
Developed and reproduced with the permission of William Schueler.

Emotional Health

Emergency nursing has the great potential to be emotionally and psychologically taxing. Time constraints, lack of emotional recovery time, staffing issues, peer and management support, verbal aggression, and physical aggression affect your emotional and physical ability to care for yourself and others. This section addresses the emotional health of the emergency nurse and how to overcome some of these challenges.

Maintaining a Healthy Work-Life Balance

Do you have a balance between work and home?

Work-life balance is the attempt to bring equilibrium between work activities and home life. For some nurses, it can be a constant struggle. Others might find that they might swing to either end of the spectrum within their career. Either way, time away from work is an important factor in preventing burnout and keeping a healthy relationship with the work environment.

Employers today are encouraging and promoting work-life balance. Some employers that promote a strong balance might be considered employee-friendly. Blazovich, Smith, and Smith (2014) found that employee-friendly companies had better financial performance and were at lower risk for bankruptcy. Healthier employees tend to equal healthier companies, and more prosperous companies could lead to prosperous employees. Employees have positive views of employers that offer compressed and flexible work weeks that are self-directed by the employee (Brough & O'Driscoll, 2010). The authors also mentioned the United Nations work-life balance initiatives, which include a compressed work week, job sharing, childcare facilities or allowances, overtime compensation, and specific work-life balance activities as the gold standard.

 Compressed work week—Instead of standard business hours, shifts are longer, allowing for more days off within the week or 2-week period.

Job sharing—Sharing the full-time work between two part-time workers.

Shift work has been found to help with the balance between work and home. According to Agosti, Andersson, Ejlertsson, and Janlöv (2015), flexible and part-time working hours encouraged employee wellbeing and work-life balance. The authors mentioned that part-time work allowed for adequate recovery between shifts. When looking at fixed versus rotating shift work, Shahriari, Shamali, and Yazdannik (2014) suggested that there might not be a perfect schedule. And curiously, nurses who work fixed shifts demonstrated more tendencies toward burnout than nurses working rotating shifts. We discuss the effects of shift work in "Physical Health," later in this chapter.

Fixed shift—Consistently working the same shift or work hours.

Shift work—A working schedule that is not 8am to 5pm or Monday through Friday.

Rotating shift—Hours of work change or cycle through day, evening, and night shifts.

It's important to look at nurses' engagement in their work as part of work-life balance. When assessing generational differences in nurses, Sullivan Havens, Warshawsky, and Vasey (2013) found that baby boomer nurses (born between 1946–1964) seemed to become bored in their work, while Generation X nurses (born between 1965–1980) were the least engaged. The authors also found that Generation Y (born between 1981–2000) nurses were the least dedicated and more prone to burnout and intention to leave, and yet the most highly educated, technologically proficient, and socially and culturally diverse. It's likely that the emergency department will have a mix of these generations, and it might be important to know the different motivations of each, especially in professional relationships and involvement. A mode of motivation for one generation might not appeal to another.

Other research shows that the working environment has an influence on nursing engagement. Adriaenssens, De Gucht, and Maes (2015) found that 53% of emergency nurses reported their work environment unfavorable, with contributions from problems such as understaffing, shift work, night shift work, lack of resources, poor organizational culture, and communication and collaboration problems. Low nursing engagement has been found to be a predictor of nurses intending to leave their current position (Sawatzky & Enns, 2012).

The Nursing Worklife Model (Roche, Spence Laschinger, & Duffield, 2015) is a great model to assess the multiple influencers of nurses and nursing quality. In this model, nursing leadership is the driver for the quality of nursing as well as the nurses' intent to leave their workplace. Other important interconnected components of this model include participation, collegial relationships, and resources that lay the groundwork for foundations for quality.

When taking the working environment and job demands out of the picture, Bargagliotti (2012) reported that trust and autonomy were paramount to the engagement of nurses. Because trust and autonomy are relational and not transactional, improving these two items between staff and nursing leadership carries no financial burden. The qualities of trust and autonomy were associated with increased personal initiative of the nurse, decreased patient mortality rates, and increased financial profitability of the employer.

Nursing engagement can be positively influenced by allowing nurses to help make policy and practice decisions, both at the unit and hospital level. The bottom-up approach to decision-making seems to be an attractive method. Allowing nurses to be more involved in their practice is a factor in preventing burnout. You can help yourself, your co-workers, unit, and hospital by participating in shared governance and committees both at the unit and hospital level. Yes, it might take some extra time beyond the regularly scheduled shifts, but the effort will be worth it.

 Shared governance—A staff-leader partnership that promotes collaboration, shared decision-making, and accountability.

Vicarious Traumatization, Nurse Burnout, and Compassion Fatigue

How does your work affect you?

Emergency nursing is unpredictable, hectic, and constantly changing, with a broad range of illnesses, injuries, and problems along with little time for recovery between urgencies/emergencies (Adriaenssens et al., 2015). From these qualities, burnout can manifest as a negative attitude toward patients and can be contagious among nurses (Hinderer et al., 2014). Burnout has been linked with obesity, depression, insomnia, alcohol intake, drug abuse, musculoskeletal disorders, intra-relational conflicts and aggression, as well as increased absenteeism, turnover, and healthcare costs (Adriaenssens et al., 2015). Those nurses with higher emotional exhaustion reported the greater intention to change their profession, and 56% of nurses surveyed had problems with negative interpersonal relationships (Beševi-omi, Bosanki, & Draganovi, 2014). The more activities a nurse is involved in, both in and out of work, increase the likelihood of burnout by not having an appropriate work-life balance (Ribeiro et al., 2014). Stretching yourself too thin by being involved in too many projects both inside and outside of work does not foster a healthy professional life. This then affects patients, because high levels of burnout correlate with decreased patient satisfaction (Hinderer et al., 2014; Hunsaker, Chen, Maughan, & Heaston, 2015).

 Burnout—Emotional exhaustion, cynicism, hopelessness, apathy, inability to be effective at work, and decreased personal accomplishment resulting from caring for people (Hunsaker et al., 2015; Sabo, 2011).

The major influencers of burnout are:

- Demographics
- Personality
- Coping strategies

- Exposure to traumatic events

- Job characteristics

- Organizational factors

Burnout and compassion fatigue are strongly correlated. A study by Hinderer et al. (2014) found that 35.9% of trauma nurses suffered some degree of burnout and 23.7% experienced compassion fatigue. It was also found that the increase in years in their position as trauma nurses correlated with an increase in professional burnout. Burnout can be associated with patient and family verbal abuse and complaints as well as unfavorable job outcomes (Van Bogaert et al., 2014). The authors suggest that if there seems to be an increase in family or patient complaints, the unit should be assessed for nurse burnout signs and symptoms. Decreased sleep has an influence on both personal and professional burnout (Chin, Guo, Hung, Yang, & Shiao, 2015). To make the point clear, burnout, compassion fatigue, and vicarious traumatization have negative effects on the nurse, which trickles down to the nursing care for patients and influences the outcomes of the patients as well.

Compassion fatigue—The negative consequences on the nurse due to witnessing suffering and working with traumatized people, along with the inability of the nurse to recover the energy expended (Hunsaker et al., 2015; Murphy, 2014).

Vicarious traumatization—The permanent alteration and lasting impression of the nurse's thoughts and behaviors from witnessing or participating in the trauma of others (Sabo, 2011; Short, 2012).

Interventions for the prevention and mitigation of burnout should be targeted to the nursing team (Van Bogaert et al., 2014). TeamSTEPPS (Agency for Healthcare Research and Quality [AHRQ], 2013) is one possible intervention for the prevention of burnout. The goals for TeamSTEPPS are: promoting a highly effective medical team with role clarifications, increasing team awareness, resolving conflict, and eliminating barriers to safety and quality. Nurses prefer innovative, supportive, dynamic, and entrepreneurial organizations. Changing the organizational culture and suggesting nurse-led initiatives could prevent burnout in nurses (Watts, Robertson, Winter, & Leeson, 2013). It might be safe to assume that if at least one nurse is suffering from burnout, other nurses on the same unit might feel the same.

Interventions for burnout include (Henry, 2014):

- Education on resilience

- Team-building

- Reflective practice

- Mindfulness stress reduction

- Employee assistance program

- Onsite or off-site retreats

- Expressive writing

- Onsite counseling

- Clinical ladder

- Rewards

- Walking

- Delegation

- Self-care outside of work

Because burnout is also related to personalities, Măirean and Turliuc (2013) suggest that interventions for vicarious traumatization be focused toward the nurses' personalities. The authors also report that focusing on the positive aspects of the profession and creating a positive reinterpretation of traumatic events might help with decreasing the negative side effects of repeated exposure to traumatic events. A professional might help with this interpretation, even better than co-workers. Seeking the help of a professional could be a great way to have customized therapy in order to help with the prevention and treatment of burnout.

Bringing it all into perspective, Maloney (2012) suggests that a good work-life balance and colleague support can decrease work stress. The take-away is that prevention of burnout in nurses needs to be action-oriented and purposeful. Stress will be present every day of work. Some days might be harder than others. Knowing this, there should be planned interventions for recognizing and mitigating the effects of nurse burnout in the emergency setting.

While employers have an effect on a nurse's work-life balance, the main responsibility for a healthy balance is on the emergency nurse. Juggling family, education, home life, health, and work responsibilities does require energy and careful planning. It is very easy to overextend yourself. Know your limitations. Learn to say "no" from time to time. It is OK to have some personal time and self-care, whatever that means to you.

Lateral Violence

How do colleagues interact with you? How do you interact with your fellow nurses?

Lateral violence is an unfortunately common occurrence in nursing. Multiple authors have presented that lateral violence will happen to nearly all nurses in their career. Ceravolo, Schwartz, Foltz-Ramos, and Castner (2012) found that 90% of nurses surveyed experienced verbal abuse from peers, which represents a significant risk to the emergency nurse.

 Lateral violence—Repeated, intentional confrontational behavior directed at an individual (Rainford, Wood, McMullen, & Philipsen, 2015).

Lateral violence is also known as *horizontal violence, vertical violence, workplace bullying, nurse-to-nurse violence, disruptive behavior, incivility,* and *nurses eating their young.* The symptoms of the aggressor can include impatience, anger, threatening behaviors, and even verbal and physical aggression. Nurses that experience lateral violence can have stress symptoms that present as decreased self-esteem with ineffective coping strategies, anxiety, sleep disturbances, and even physical health complaints (Christie & Jones, 2014). Elmblad, Kodjebacheva, and Lebeck (2014) found that incivility and burnout were related and that as the intensity of incivility increased, the likelihood of burnout increased as well. This is unfortunate because nursing leadership has the responsibility not to tolerate lateral violence, and leaders can be part of the problem instead of the solution.

Characteristics of lateral violence are:

- Loss of confidentiality

- Incorrect information

- Insults

- Eye-rolling

- Belittling

- Exclusion

- Jokes

- Excessive criticism

- Gossip

- Verbal aggression

- Sabotage

- Withholding information

- Gesturing when not looking

One theory as to why lateral violence occurs is the Oppressed Group Model, which poses that throughout history, nurses have been oppressed or dominated in relation to physicians and hospital administration. Through this model, lateral violence could be described as an expression of frustrations of lack of autonomy, worth, and power. Purpora, Blegen, and Stotts (2012) supported this model, finding that an increase in nurses with internalized beliefs of oppression also found an increase in horizontal violence.

Another theory that helps to explain lateral violence is the Nurse as Wounded Healer. Nurses receive wounds from both their personal and professional lives. After personal healing (transcendence), it is thought that nurses can use those experiences to help others. However, if the wounds are not realized or healed, self-destructive behaviors and emotional distress can result, influencing the nurse's response to bullying but also increasing the likelihood of the nurse becoming the aggressor (Christie & Jones, 2014; Mealer & Jones, 2013).

There are few well-studied interventions for reducing lateral violence. Coursey, Rodriguez, Dieckmann, and Austin (2013) highlight some interventions that might work better than others: management involvement and support, education, changing the culture, and involving individuals and teams in policy development. Some employees will try voicing their concerns and approaching management with them. When these measures fail, the employees may leave the workplace, viewing escape as the only alternative that would improve the situation (Sanner-Stiehr & Ward-Smith, 2014). Decreasing the intensity and size of the workload, improving the empowerment of nurses, and reforming nursing education were strategies offered by Rainford et al. (2015).

Crucial strategies such as enforcing the standards and code of conduct; empowering nurses within the organization; developing skills for conflict resolution, negotiation, and assertiveness; and addressing abusers' impairments (substance abuse, stress mismanagement, or mental illness) seem to be effective recommendations for nurses' accountability (Lachman, 2015). Dimarino (2011) also reports that strict enforcement of conduct behavior freed a work environment of lateral violence. The author promotes eliminating lateral violence with the responsibility starting with leaders and managers and ending with the staff members. Elmblad et al. (2014) also echo the enforcement of zero-tolerance policies, increased visibility of management, and in-services and workshops on communication skills.

Strategies to decrease lateral violence (Coursey et al., 2013):

- Executive leadership must be active participants

- Purposefully change the culture

- Feedback as a stimulus for improvement

- Involve individuals and teams in setting clinical policy

- Utilize best evidence

- Utilize education as a strategy along with audit and feedback

- Maintain a non-punitive process

After attending educational workshops to lessen lateral violence, nurses reported verbal aggression from peers decreased from 90% to 76% (Ceravolo et al., 2012). The authors also noted that nurses seemed to adopt a culture of empowerment and communicative problem-solving instead of lack of voice and conflict avoidance. Leinung and Egues (2012) also found similar positive anecdotal accounts after presenting workshops focusing on lateral violence recognition and mitigation along with self-care strategies.

Even in the face of limited research, there appear to be cost-effective strategies to mitigate lateral violence. Promoting self-care and including nurses in unit and hospital decision-making can decrease the perception of oppression and promote healing. Learning to exercise self-control, give and receive respect, and effectively communicate under stress and frustration can promote civility between emergency staff. The emergency department is already filled with stress and anxiety; there is no reason to make it worse with conflict between nurses.

Physical Violence and Aggression

Do you realize there is significant risk and your profession can be dangerous?

Both verbal and physical aggressions take a toll on the health of the emergency nurse. Many factors influence the risk of verbal and physical aggression in the ED. Emergency nurses do not know all the intricacies of the patients, the ED is open to any and all patients, there is frequent interaction with family members and visitors, the patient's treatment plan might not let him or her feel in control, and the environment is commonly stressful and highly emotional (Blando, O'Hagan, Casteel, Nocera, & Peek-Asa, 2013).

There might be physical environmental factors that can increase the likelihood of violence, such as lack of exits from rooms, insufficient surveillance of violent patients, and the inability to safely lock down an ED (Gillespie, Gates, & Berry, 2013). Nurses must also accept some responsibility in this problem of violence; they must speak up about previous or potentially violent episodes and people to the rest of the care team. If the problem is not verbalized, it can't be addressed or mitigated.

Factors influencing violence and aggression are (Pich, Hazelton, Sundin, & Kable, 2010):

- Prolonged waiting times

- Overcrowding

- Time pressure

- Distress

- Pain

- Mental disorders

- Drugs and intoxicants

- Lack of coping sills

- Unrealistic expectations

According to the Centers for Disease Control and Prevention (CDC) (2015), workplace violence almost doubled for nurses and nursing assistants from 2012 to 2014, and the assault rate is trending up for all healthcare professions. The Bureau of Labor Statistics (2013) reports that violence in healthcare is almost four times that of any other business in the private sector. Violence also accounts for 13% of injuries and illnesses requiring days away from work (Bureau of Labor Statistics, 2014). Another author poses that if you work in healthcare, you can expect to be assaulted at least once in your career (Henson, 2010). While nursing assistants and nurses are recipients of most healthcare violence, no occupation is immune to violence in the ED (Kowalenko, Gates, Gillespie, & Succop, 2013).

Nurses who have been exposed to violence suffer at least one symptom of stress (Gates, Gillespie, & Succop, 2011). Physical violence and the stress that follows negatively affect the working environment of the ED. It affects the nurses' abilities to care for patients and interrupts the flow of the department. It can even end an emergency nurse's career and, in rare occurrences, lead to death.

Emergency nurses experience verbal aggression more than physical violence. According to Stone, McMillan, Hazelton, and Clayton (2011), obscenities were directed at 29% of nurses one to five times per week, and 7% reported that they were continually the recipient of obscenities. This was described as "highly distressing," especially when coming from patients' families. The perpetrators of this verbal aggression tended to be mostly male and older than 18 years old. Those patients in acute psychosis tended to present with more verbal aggression than physical. With this in mind, violence-prevention training should focus on verbal de-escalation along with physical training for controlling, restraining, and self-defense. Although verbal aggression is more prevalent, physical violence presents a greater risk of harm and injury.

An international study by Spector, Zhou, and Che (2014) showed that violence against nurses is universal. The results showed that 36.4% experienced physical violence, 67.2% experienced verbal aggression, and 32.7% reported injury. This study captured rather small time frames; the rate of violence experienced by nurses is higher in the context of their entire career. Edward, Ousey, Warelow, and Lui (2014) found that up to 94% of nurses experience verbal aggression. Younger and less-experienced nurses as well as male nurses faced the most violence, and night shifts and weekend shifts tended to pose the greatest risk to the nurse.

Good practices to prevent violence include:

- Security presence

- Education for patients on the functions of the ED

- Signage of expected behaviors

- Identification and communication of violent/aggressive history

- A good work environment

- Adequate staffing

- Reporting all events

- Training in recognition and de-escalation

- Physical training including self-defense

- Post-incident debriefing and assistance

- Ongoing program evaluation

You should receive ongoing training on the early recognition and early intervention of anxiety and aggression with a focus on verbal de-escalation. One training session will not likely be enough, and therefore, education should be ongoing. De-escalation and management of verbal and physical confrontation are skills that need to be practiced to develop competency. Trainings have been found beneficial because nurses do report a heightened sense of awareness (Gerdtz et al., 2013) and significant retention of the training 6 months post education (Gillespie, Farra, & Gates, 2014).

On a higher level, it's imperative that hospitals and health systems support the prevention of violence. Nothing derails violence prevention programs quicker than lack of administrative and managerial support. Most states don't have mandatory education for violence prevention within healthcare, although a few do. Even in those few states, implementation is poor, and violence is still a problem (McPhaul, London, & Lipscomb, 2013). Violence prevention strategies given by professional and government organizations are just that—strategies and suggestions. However, it's the employer's responsibility to provide a safe work environment, which is supported by state and federal laws (Geiger-Brown & Lipscomb, 2011).

There might not be best practices for violence prevention, but there are guidelines for good practice from the international perspective. Blando et al. (2013) found that the same number of assaults happened even with the presence of metal detectors. Even interventions that seem to make the nurse feel safer did not actually decrease the number of assaults. Those facilities with security officers do experience less violence (Geiger-Brown & Lipscomb, 2011). However, education and training for recognizing and intervening in potentially physical situations are viewed as valuable and are a highly recommended strategy nationally and internationally. Although it's not at the root cause of violence in healthcare, the physical environment may need to be optimized for the safety and security of the emergency team. Posting signage of expected behaviors and informing patients and visitors of delays can be an effective strategy (Fulde & Preisz, 2011).

Nurses need to take ownership of the substantial lack of reporting of violence and aggression. Reporting violence in the workplace is essential for changing the environment. Not only does it gather data and present facts for legal aspects, it also stimulates further research, helps in education and training, and strengthens policies. Even with these benefits, nurses are reluctant to report violence (Gates et al., 2011; Kowalenko et al., 2013). One study showed that only 42% of healthcare workers reported violent acts at work and only 5% reported to law enforcement. If you want to receive better training and more resources to curb violence, you need to report. The excuses are numerous: no time, nothing will change, administration doesn't offer support. That does not excuse you from reporting acts that endanger the health and safety of you or others, or even criminal acts. Think of it like this: If you don't report, you're condoning and accepting the behavior.

You need to be involved in the assessment, development, implementation, and evaluation of violence prevention in your workplace. Reaction to a violent event is 100 times more costly than a proactive approach to violence in healthcare (Papa & Venella, 2013). There is a financial benefit to violence prevention as long as it involves careful assessment, planning, development, implementation, and evaluation. It's the right thing to do to protect nurses from this prominent work hazard.

Spiritual Care

How do you take care of yourself beyond the physical and emotional body?

You can't forget about your spiritual care. Good spiritual self-care is essential to providing spiritual care to people in times of distress. Helping patients with their spiritual and emotional needs can increase patient satisfaction. *Your* spiritual health also helps you cope with work stress and promotes resilience (Biro, 2012). The better you can take care of the spiritual self, the better you might be able to handle the stress that comes along with being an emergency nurse.

Short (2012) offered that spirituality can be nurses "getting out of touch with themselves, [getting in touch with] their god and their view of themselves in the world..." (p. 25). The author mentioned that lack of spirituality, as well as neglecting physical needs, could pose greater risk for vicarious traumatization of the nurse. Self-neglect could lead to a rather dangerous and permanent change in how you view patients that come to you for help, which is also known as *vicarious traumatization*. Ronaldson, Hayes, Aggar, Green, and Carey (2012) posed that spiritual needs can include giving and receiving love, discovering the meaning and purpose in your life, hope and creativity, help and support, respect and relationships. Self-neglect is very easy to fall into as an emergency nurse. There are many things to distract you from proper self-care and taking quiet time for your needs that are beyond emotion or physical health.

The ED operates at a fast pace. Biro (2012) found that there is lack of adequate training and time for acute care nurses to provide spiritual care. Biro also found the older nurses and those with a greater understanding of their own spirituality tend to provide more spiritual care. This is also supported by another study that compared the spiritual care of palliative care nurses and acute care nurses (Ronaldson et al., 2012). The authors found that the palliative care setting is more conducive to providing good spiritual care. Biro (2012) also posed that spiritual care is part of being a good nurse, and your actions, presence, and attitude influence the spiritual care that you give. Does this mean that you have to be in the palliative care setting and be an older nurse in order to give spiritual care to your patients?

Not at all. It might mean that you make your own spiritual care a priority while outside of the working environment. Practice and develop the healthy spirit so that you can bring it with you into your work.

Strategies to promote spiritual health are:

- Meditation

- Journaling

- Quietness

- Nature and creation

- Prayer

- Alone time

In terms of compassion fatigue, the spiritual symptoms can appear as lost sense of purpose, doubt, withdrawal, being non-reflective, and lack of joy (Murphy, 2014). The author offers that you should attend to your personal needs in order to be able to provide quality care to others. Mindfulness-based stress reduction has been shown to increase self-compassion and empathy, and decrease stress and anxiety. In other words, take care of yourself first, so that you can care for your patients with excellence.

Physical Health

Your mind and body are connected; if you do not have good physical health, it can affect your ability to care for your patients and yourself. The following sections talk about healthful eating, exercise, and trying to minimize the negative effects of shift work.

Body mass index (BMI) is often used to determine whether a person is underweight, normal, overweight, or obese. The measurement only takes into account weight and height. You should have a degree of skepticism with this measurement because it does not account for body fat percentage, lean body mass, or waist circumference, which are better indicators of excessive body fat. Think about it this way: A body builder would have increased weight due to increased lean body mass. However, by the BMI, the person might be considered overweight or obese, just by the measurement of height and weight. Or a person might have excessive body fat and be considered normal weight.

You should also be skeptical of the nutrition information you read or hear in the news. Many food studies are poorly designed and rely on people's recall of what they ate over a period of time, which is unreliable on its own. Associations between foods and diseases do not mean that foods cause certain diseases as some studies report. Hite et al. (2010) found contradictory evidence to the *Dietary Guidelines for Americans, 2010*; they found that the current science did not support (or directly contradict) the committee's recommendations, specifically on the topics of dietary fat, salt, fiber, carbohydrate, and protein.

Healthy Eating

How are you nourishing your body and mind?

People find benefits in many styles of eating. Some people do have naturally thin body types, no matter what they eat. Others can be extremely sensitive to food and how it relates to their weight. One style of eating might not be beneficial to another. Some science shows that restricting carbohydrates has a better influence on body weight than restricting calories or fat. Whatever the science, the data is inconclusive as to what is the best diet. And taking into account genetics, lifestyle, and metabolism, one diet does not fit all people. Hippocrates was known to say, "Let food be thy medicine and medicine be thy food." If you view your diet under this light, it could make sense that some ways of eating can harm you, while other ways can heal you.

Some general eating guidelines are (Lowden, Moreno, Holmbäck, Lennernäs, & Tucker, 2010):

■ No eating, or restricted intake, from midnight to 6am.

■ Eat at the beginning and end of your shift.

■ Avoid large meals 1 to 2 hours before sleep.

■ Eat complete meals without added sugars.

■ Allow meals to be eaten away from the work area.

■ Participate in regular exercise, regular meal times, and good sleep hygiene.

Nurses do not always practice what they preach or know about healthy lifestyles (Malik, Blake, & Batt, 2011; Nahm, Warren, Zhu, An, & Brown, 2012). In the few studies regarding nurses and eating, over 50% and up to 65.4% were considered overweight or obese. Long work hours, night shift work, work stress, and using eating to release stress were some of the barriers identified to healthful eating (Griep et al., 2014; Malik et al., 2011; Nahm et al., 2012). Increased weight has been linked to decreased productivity, increased risk of injury, problems with space and equipment, and decreased likelihood to seek a promotion or leadership role (Krussig, Willoughby, Parker, & Ross, 2012).

Unfortunately, eating was reported to be the top stress-relief activity (fortunately, it was closely followed by exercise). The limited studies also found that nurses working shifts, especially night shift, had eating styles that were higher in fat, sugar, and alcohol and lower in fiber, zinc, and vitamins A and D (Griep et al., 2014; Lowden et al., 2010). Irregular meal times and compressed time for eating don't help.

Following a specific diet program didn't seem to benefit nurses. There was weight loss initially, but it was not sustained after 6 months. Those that did successfully lose weight and keep it off followed a rather prudent approach. Making small lifestyle changes, adherence, persistence, and enthusiasm seemed to promote better weight maintenance than the diets themselves. It was also found that personality characteristics had no bearing on whether nurses lost weight or not (Zitkus, 2011).

There are some simple solutions to improve nurses' eating habits. Making a conscious effort to eat prepared meals, allowing adequate time for eating, and increasing the availability for healthy food at work can help to establish better eating patterns. It's bad enough that shift work and eating contribute to obesity, cardiovascular disease, ulcers, and metabolic syndrome. These risks are additive to the problems of decreased exercise, restless sleep, and disturbance of circadian rhythms.

If you're working shift, try these eating guidelines (Lowden et al., 2010):

- Eat breakfast before sleeping after working.

- Stay close to a normal day and/or night eating pattern.

- Balanced meals = three meals of 20% to 35% daily energy each.

- Don't rely on convenience foods.

- Schedule adequate time between shifts for sleep and meal prep.

- Decrease sugar intake, baked goods, and no-fiber carbohydrates.

The flip side of eating is fasting. Bodies are supposed to undergo periods of not eating. At night, muscle tissue is resistant to glucose, thereby increasing the risk of calorie intake being stored instead of used (Lowden et al., 2010). Fasting can help you utilize stored body fat for energy during exercise without significant changes to metabolism (Pilon, 2010). Contrary to popular belief, fasting doesn't change metabolism for up to 3 days.

Most of us could say that we need to eat better. It might take some experimentation to find which style of eating works best for you. In the ED, it's important to plan and have adequate time for meal consumption. Purposeful action by planning meals can win out over reactionary eating.

Exercise

How are you taking care of the only body you will ever have?

Along with not eating well, many nurses do not exercise. The few studies of nurses and exercise report 50% to 72.2% reporting lack of adequate exercise (Malik et al., 2011; Nahm et al., 2012). The common excuses are lack of time, being too tired, no easily accessible equipment, and no exercise partner (Yuan et al., 2009). Exercise has many benefits, from controlling stress, body weight, and stamina to improving performance and decreasing injury. And it has been known to make people feel good.

Many nurses think of exercise as running, jogging, or other cardiovascular exercises. But that may not be the best exercise for you. Try performing exercises that mimic or are closely related to your work. For example, weight lifting or resistance training may be more beneficial. You're generally not required to perform significant cardiac endurance while performing emergency nursing duties. You do, however, lift heavy objects and reposition, transfer, and assist people. Many musculoskeletal injuries can occur from these actions alone.

National Public Radio recently reported that even with proper body mechanics, the forces on a nurse's musculoskeletal system are enough to cause injury (Zwerdling, 2015). Healthcare in the U.S. is rated second-highest for the number of injuries, after the transportation and warehousing sector; Canada reported that healthcare workers account for the most workers' compensation claims (Bureau of Labor Statistics [BLS], 2014; Jordan, Nowrouzi-Kia, Gohar, & Nowrouzi, 2015). It was also found that for every 10% increase in physical workload, there was a 23% increase in reporting an injury. Working with adults, having lower co-worker support, and having a higher BMI also appeared to be risk factors for injuries.

 Resistance training—The use of resistance to muscular contraction to build the strength, anaerobic endurance, and size of skeletal muscles. (Also known as *strength training* or *weight training*.)

So maybe it would be more beneficial to utilize resistance training along with flexibility and cardiovascular training to produce a body more resistant to injury. The Occupational Safety & Health Administration (OSHA, 2015) has recommendations on safe patient handling, which includes the use of lifts. An active physical therapy program helped to decrease chronic back pain, improve body posture, and decrease disability (Jaromi, Nemeth, Kranicz, Laczko, & Betlehem, 2012). This intervention worked better than passive therapies such as massage, ultrasound therapy, and stretching. It was also shown to be a great therapy program for the prevention and rehabilitation of musculoskeletal injury.

It's no mystery that exercise is beneficial. Nurses that increased or started exercise reported better physical fitness, including lower BMI and improved grip strength, flexibility, cardiopulmonary durability, and abdominal and back muscle durability (Yuan et al., 2009). Nurses who live in denser communities that are friendly to walking seem to be more active and thus had a lower BMI (James et al., 2013).

Nurses who believe in healthy behaviors and practice them are more likely to coach others in those healthy behaviors (Esposito & Fitzpatrick, 2011; Zhu, Norman, & While, 2011). Some healthcare professionals who are not overweight practice prevention in order to remain at a healthy weight. Factors that seem to encourage and predict better exercise include positive social support from family, friends, and co-workers and the self-belief that they could actually exercise. The clinical area, age, nursing experience, or position did not have an influence on patterns of exercise for nurses (Kaewthummanukul, Brown, Weaver, & Thomas, 2006).

The official recommendations for exercise are about 30 minutes of moderate-intensity exercise most days of the week. Other recommendations for nurses from the scientific literature encourage three 10-minute periods of brisk walking during the working shift, increasing access to exercise equipment, allowing adequate time for exercise, and encouraging exercise while at the hospital (Esposito & Fitzpatrick, 2011; Lowden et al., 2010; Nahm et al., 2012; Yuan et al., 2009).

When comparing calorie restriction and exercise for weight loss, exercise produced better weight loss with greater reduction in visceral and intramuscular adipose (fat) tissue (Murphy et al., 2012). Female participants in a 12-week study found that those who combined cardiovascular and resistance training benefited from more weight loss, lower BMI, and lower body fat weight and percentage than either exercise alone (Ho, Dhaliwal, Hills, & Pal, 2012). A long-term regimen that combines cardiovascular and resistance training, versus either exercise alone, proved better at lowering blood pressure and improving blood lipid profiles (Sousa, Mendes, Abrantes, Sampaio, & Oliveira, 2013). Less physical activity combined with inadequate protein intake leads to decreased lean body (muscle) mass (Churchward-Venne, Breen, & Phillips, 2014).

Nurses who exercise have better morale and feel healthier (Yuan et al., 2009). Finding time for exercise can be difficult. If you work multiple shifts in a row, fitting exercise into that schedule can be an exercise in patience (pun intended). Find an exercise style that appeals to you and that you believe you can continue in the long term, along with some focus on resistance training. Some people prefer to exercise alone; some prefer group classes. Whatever you decide, it's important that you move. Remember the adage, "Move it or lose it." The same is true for exercise; if you don't use your muscles, they will atrophy.

Minimizing the Negative Effects of Shift Work

Are you working too much, too long, or too often?

Some studies regarding shift work found negative effects on nurses, and others reported the opposite. Some possible side effects to shift work include increased physical tension, work stress, sleepiness, weight gain, fatigue, sleep deprivation, and overtime. One nurse's husband brought legal action against her employer after she fell asleep at the wheel, crashed her vehicle, and died. The husband contended that the work demands of her employer caused her to fall asleep at the wheel (Debucquoy-Dodley, 2013). These side effects of shift work can reflect negatively on patient care, including increased errors, central line-associated blood stream infections (CLABSI), patient/family complaints, inconsistent policy judgments, pneumonia complications, and decreased quality of care (Harris, Sims, Parr, & Davis, 2015). Long work hours often interfere with healthy behaviors and increase obesity (Han, Trinkoff, Storr, & Geiger-Brown, 2011; Kim et al., 2013).

Good sleep hygiene habits:

- Use a regular bedtime for whatever shift you work.

- Eat regular/light healthy meals.

- Achieve regular exercise.

- Sleep 7 to 8 hours per 24-hour period.

- If you need sleep, sleep!

- Naps should be 20 to 40 minutes.

Although night shift is an essential component of healthcare, it has its own set of problems. Night shift tends to limit exercise; decrease sleep quality; increase accidents; increase risk for cardiovascular disease; increase BMI; increase gastrointestinal problems, diabetes, and cancer; decrease attention span and short-term memory; increase cortisol levels; promote hormonal and reproductive problems for women; and increase risk of breast cancer (Cassie, 2015; Griep et al., 2014; Lowson, Middleton, Arber, & Skene, 2013; Niu et al., 2015).

Nurses also lose the ability to quickly recover from night shift work as they age. Even though most nurses who work night shift tend to be younger, less experienced, and single, there is disruption to the nurse's social routine and an effect on the sleeping patterns of husbands and children for those who have families. One study showed that nurses sleep 2 hours and 20 minutes less during night shift work. This can also influence wakefulness and the ability to stay awake, with consecutive nights compounding the problem. Night shift also decreases cognitive function (Chang et al., 2014). If you also consider that staffing levels at night are decreased, the workload per nurse is increased. This increase in physical and psychosocial demands increases the risk for injury and is surmised to be the reason why night-shift nurses are more likely to visit a doctor and take painkiller medications (Buja et al., 2013).

Try these tips to get through a night shift schedule:

- Stay active during your shift.

- Keep lights bright while working.

- Consider short naps during breaks while working.

- Limit caffeine 5 to 8 hours before sleeping.

- Limit alcohol before sleeping.

- Wear sunglasses while driving home.

- Go to bed as soon as possible after a shift.

- Darken the room; use blackout curtains.

- Avoid blue light (TV, tablet, phone).

- Turn off the phone.

- Use the bedroom only for sleeping and sex.

Sleeping patterns of night-shift nurses were assessed in a recent study. The best adaptation by nurses was a pattern in which the nurse slept on a similar schedule regardless of work days. The second best adaptation was by nurses who switched their sleeping pattern for work days, but then switched back to their normal sleeping pattern on off days (Petrov et al., 2014). The results of this study support that consistent sleeping time seems to be the best for nurses. Sleep that is adequate both in quality and duration is essential for a healthy emergency nurse.

Not just night shift has a negative effect on the emergency nurse's health. Bae and Fabry's (2014) literature review found that 12-hour shifts have a negative effect on nurses' health, and working more than 40 hours within a week negatively affected patient outcome, but without a definite correlation. On the contrary, Clendon and Gibbons (2015) found that extended shifts do have a negative impact on patient outcomes, including medication errors, inappropriate judgment, and lack of attentiveness, intervention, and prevention.

Witkoski Stimpfel, Sloane, and Aiken (2012) found that extended shifts (those beyond 8–9 hours) had a higher relation to nurse burnout and patient dissatisfaction. Add onto this the fact that some nurses work more than one job or work excessive overtime, and it can be a recipe for poor nursing practice.

Even though most nurses work 12-hour shifts, is it best for nurses and their patients? Most nurses enjoy the opportunity to work and have more days off during the week. Maust Martin (2015) found that nurses who worked 8-hour shifts slept longer, experienced lower acute and chronic fatigue, and had better recovery between shifts in comparison to 12-hour shifts. Instead of working five 8-hour shifts in the week, nurses only worked four, which was considered full-time work by the employer. Some recommendations to minimize potential negative outcomes are encouragement of naps, extended rest periods, shorter working duration, and study of other professions and further research of the long-term effects of shift work.

Some consequences of working a night shift are:

- Chronic stress symptoms

- Fatigue

- Irritability

- Decreased work performance

- Presenteeism

- Absenteeism

- Decreased caregiver health

- Increased physical illness

- Post-traumatic stress, anxiety, depression

- Increased malpractice

Tips for surviving night shift are:

- At least 4 days off between consecutive night shifts for cortisol circadian rhythm normalization

- At least 2 days off between rotating shifts

- Consistent sleep pattern during day hours or adjust between shifts

Summary

Maintaining a healthy lifestyle as an emergency nurse will be a constant struggle, and some nurses may struggle more than others. There might be times when you might work extra, either requested or voluntarily. Long days of walking on your feet and increased physical and emotional demands do eventually take a toll. The constant influx of patients into the emergency department will never end. You only have one body and one mind, so make them a priority so that you can overcome the stress of being an emergency nurse. Learn early how to properly take care of yourself so that you can function at a high level for your family and career.

So: *How are you taking care of yourself?*

References

Adriaenssens, J., De Gucht, V., & Maes, S. (2015). Determinants and prevalence of burnout in emergency nurses: A systematic review of 25 years of research. *International Journal of Nursing Studies, 52*(2), 649–661. doi:10.1016/j.ijnurstu.2014.11.004

Agency for Healthcare Research and Quality (AHRQ). (2013). *TeamSTEPPS: National implementation.* Retrieved from http://teamstepps.ahrq.gov/

Agosti, M. T., Andersson, I., Ejlertsson, G., & Janlöv, A. (2015). Shift work to balance everyday life–A salutogenic nursing perspective in home help service in Sweden. *BMC Nursing, 14*(1), 55–77. doi: 10.1186/s12912-014-0054-6

Bae, S. H., & Fabry, D. (2014). Assessing the relationships between nurse work hours/overtime and nurse and patient outcomes: Systematic literature review. *Nursing Outlook, 6*(2), 138–156. doi:10.1016/j.out-look.2013.10.009

Bargagliotti, L. A. (2012). Work engagement in nursing: A concept analysis. *Journal of Advanced Nursing, 68*(6), 1414–1428. doi:10.1111/j.1365-2648.2011.05859.x

Beševi-omi, V., Bosanki, N., & Draganovi, S. (2014). Burnout syndrome and self-efficacy among nurses. *Scripta Medica, 45*(1), 26–29. doi: 10.7251/SMD1401025B

Biro, A. L. (2012). Creating conditions for good nursing by attending to the spiritual. *Journal of Nursing Management, 20*(8), 1002–1011. doi:10.1111/j.1365-2834.2012.01444.x

Blando, J. D., O'Hagan, E., Casteel, C., Nocera, M. A., & Peek-Asa, C. (2013). Impact of hospital security programmes and workplace aggression on nurse perceptions of safety. *Journal of Nursing Management, 21*(3), 491–498. doi:10.1111/j.1365-2834.2012.01416.x

Blazovich, J. L., Smith, K. T., & Smith, L. M. (2014). Employee-friendly companies and work-life balance: Is there an impact on financial performance and risk level? *Journal of Organizational Culture, Communications and Conflict, 18*(20), 1–13.

Brough, P., & O'Driscoll, M. P. (2010). Organizational interventions for balancing work and home demands: An overview. *Work & Stress, 24*(3), 280–297. doi:10.1080/02678373.2010.506808

Buja, A., Zampieron, A., Mastrangelo, G., Petean, M., Vinelli, A., Cerne, D., & Baldo, V. (2013). Strain and health implications of nurses' shift work. *International Journal of Occupational Medicine & Environmental Health, 26*(4), 511–521. doi: 10.2478/s13382-013-0122-2

Bureau of Labor Statistics (BLS). (2013). *Nonfatal occupational injuries and illnesses requiring days away from work, 2012 (USDL-13-2257).* Retrieved from www.bls.gov/news.release/archives/cfoi_08222013.pdf

Bureau of Labor Statistics (BLS). (2014). *Nonfatal occupational injuries and illnesses requiring days away from work, 2013 (USDL-14-2246).* Retrieved from www.bls.gov/news.release/pdf/osh2.pdf

Cassie, F. (2015, February). Coping with shiftwork: Is there a perfect roster? *Nursing Review, 15*(1), 4–7. Retrieved from http://www.nursingreview.co.nz/issue/february-2015-vol-15-1/coping-with-shiftwork-is-there-a-perfect-roster/#.VfQ8eBFVikp

Centers for Disease Control and Prevention (CDC). (2015, April 24). Occupational traumatic injuries among workers in healthcare facilities—United States, 2012–2014. *Morbidity and Mortality Weekly Report, 64*(15), 405–410.

Ceravolo, D. J., Schwartz, D. G., Foltz-Ramos, K. M., & Castner, J. (2012). Strengthening communication to overcome lateral violence. *Journal of Nursing Management, 20*(5), 599–606. doi:10.1111/j.1365-2834.2012.01402.x

Chang, Y. S., Chen, H. L., Wu, Y. H., Hsu, C. Y., Liu, C. K., & Chin, H. (2014). Rotating night shifts too quickly may cause anxiety and decreased attentional performance, and impact prolactin levels during the subsequent day: A case control study. *BMC Psychiatry, 14*(1), 126–146. doi: 10.1186/s12888-014-0218-7

Chin, W., Guo, Y. L., Hung, Y. J., Yang, C. Y., & Shiao, J. S. (2015). Short sleep duration is dose-dependently related to job strain and burnout in nurses: A cross sectional survey. *International Journal of Nursing Studies, 52*(1), 297–306. doi:10.1016/j.ijnurstu.2014.09.003

Christie, W., & Jones, S. (2014). Lateral violence in nursing and the theory of the nurse as wounded healer. *Online Journal of Issues in Nursing, 18*(4), 1. doi:10.3912/OJIN.Vol19No01PPT01

Churchward-Venne, T. A., Breen, L., & Phillips, S. M. (2014). Alterations in human muscle protein metabolism with aging: Protein and exercise as countermeasures to offset sarcopenia. *Biofactors, 40*(2), 199–205. doi:10.1002/biof.1138

Clendon, J., & Gibbons, V. (2015). 12h shifts and rates of error among nurses: A systematic review. *International Journal of Nursing Studies, 52*(7), 1231–1242. doi:10.1016/j.ijnurstu.2015.03.011

Coursey, J. H., Rodriguez, R. E., Dieckmann, L. S., & Austin, P. N. (2013). Successful implementation of policies addressing lateral violence. *AORN Journal, 97*(1), 101–109. doi:10.1016/j.aorn.2012.09.010

de Souza Oliveira, J. D., Júnior, J. P., de Miranda, F. N., Cavalcante, E. S., & das Graças Almeida, M. (2014). Stress of nurses in emergency care: A social representations study. *Online Brazilian Journal of Nursing, 13*(2), 146–153.

Debucquoy-Dodley, D. (2013, November 13). Lawsuit: Ohio nurse was "worked to death". CNN. Retrieved from http://www.cnn.com/2013/11/12/health/ohio-nurse-worked-to-death-lawsuit-says/

Dimarino, T. J. (2011). Eliminating lateral violence in the ambulatory setting: One center's strategies. *AORN Journal, 93*(5), 583–588. doi:10.1016/j.aorn.2010.10.019

Edward, K., Ousey, K., Warelow, P., & Lui, S. (2014). Nursing and aggression in the workplace: A systematic review. *British Journal of Nursing, 23*(12), 653–659. doi:10.12968/bjon.2014.23.12.653

Elmblad, R., Kodjebacheva, G., & Lebeck, L. (2014). Workplace incivility affecting CRNAs: A study of prevalence, severity, and consequences with proposed interventions. *AANA Journal, 82*(6), 437–445.

Esposito, E. M., & Fitzpatrick, J. J. (2011). Registered nurses' beliefs of the benefits of exercise, their exercise behaviour and their patient teaching regarding exercise. *International Journal of Nursing Practice, 17*(4), 351–356. doi:10.1111/j.1440-172X.2011.01951.x

Fulde, G., & Preisz, P. (2011). Managing aggressive and violent patients. *Australian Prescriber, 34*(4), 115–118.

Gates, D., Gillespie, G., & Succop, P. (2011). Violence against nurses and its impact on stress and productivity. *Nursing Economic$, 29*(2), 59–66.

Geiger-Brown, J., & Lipscomb, J. A. (2011). The health care work environment and adverse health and safety consequences for nursing. *Annual Review of Nursing Research, 28,* 191–231. doi:10.1891/0739-6686.28.191

Gerdtz, M. F., Daniel, C., Dearie, V., Prematunga, R., Bamert, M., & Duxbury, J. (2013). The outcome of a rapid training program on nurses' attitudes regarding the prevention of aggression in emergency departments: A multi-site evaluation. *International Journal of Nursing Studies, 50*(11), 1434–1445. doi:10.1016/j.ijnurstu.2013.01.007

Gillespie, G. L., Farra, S. L., & Gates, D. M. (2014). A workplace violence educational program: A repeated measures study. *Nurse Education in Practice, 14*(5), 468–472. doi:10.1016/j.nepr.2014.04.003

Gillespie, G. L., Gates, D. M., & Berry, P. (2013). Stressful incidents of physical violence against emergency nurses. *OJIN: The Online Journal of Issues in Nursing, 18*(1), Manuscript 2.

Griep, R. H., Bastos, L. S., de Jesus Mendes da Fonseca, M., Silva-Costa, A., Portela, L. F., Toivanen, S., & Rotenberg, L. (2014). Years worked at night and body mass index among registered nurses from eighteen public hospitals in Rio de Janeiro, Brazil. *BMC Health Services Research, 14*(1), 603–620. doi: 10.1186/s12913-014-0603-4

Han, K., Trinkoff, A. M., Storr, C. L, & Geiger-Brown, J. (2011). Job stress and work schedules in relation to nurse obesity. *Journal of Nursing Administration, 41,* 488–495.

Harris, R., Sims, S., Parr, J., & Davies, N. (2015). Impact of 12 h shift patterns in nursing: A scoping review. *International Journal of Nursing Studies, 52*(2), 605–634. doi:10.1016/j.ijnurstu.2014.10.014

Henry, B. J. (2014). Nursing burnout interventions: What is being done?. *Clinical Journal of Oncology Nursing, 18*(2), 211–214. doi:10.1188/14.CJON.211-214

Henson, B. (2010). Preventing interpersonal violence in emergency departments: Practical applications of criminology theory. *Violence and Victims, 25*(4), 553–565. doi:10.1891/0886-6708.25.4.553

Hinderer, K. A., VonRueden, K. T., Friedmann, E., McQuillan, K. A., Gilmore, R., Kramer, B., & Murray, M. (2014). Burnout, compassion fatigue, compassion satisfaction, and secondary traumatic stress in trauma nurses. *Journal of Trauma Nursing, 21*(4), 160–169. doi:10.1097/JTN.0000000000000055

Hite, A. H., Feinman, R. D., Guzman, G. E., Satin, M., Schoenfeld, P. A., & Wood, R. J. (2010). In the face of contradictory evidence: Report of the Dietary Guidelines for Americans Committee [Special article]. *Nutrition, 26*(10), 915–924. doi:10.1016/j.nut.2010.08.012

Ho, S. S., Dhaliwal, S. S., Hills, A. P., & Pal, S. (2012). The effect of 12 weeks of aerobic, resistance or combination exercise training on cardiovascular risk factors in the overweight and obese in a randomized trial. *BMC Public Health, 12,* 704. doi: 10.1186/1471-2458-12-704

Hunsaker, S., Chen, H. C., Maughan, D., & Heaston, S. (2015). Factors that influence the development of compassion fatigue, burnout, and compassion satisfaction in emergency department nurses. *Journal of Nursing Scholarship, 47*(2), 186–194. doi:10.1111/jnu.12122

James, P., Troped, P. J., Hart, J. E., Joshu, C. E., Colditz, G. A., Brownson, R. C., & ... Laden, F. (2013). Urban sprawl, physical activity, and body mass index: Nurses' Health Study and Nurses' Health Study II. *American Journal Of Public Health, 103*(2), 369–375. doi:10.2105/AJPH.2011.300449

Jaromi, M., Nemeth, A., Kranicz, J., Laczko, T., & Betlehem, J. (2012). Treatment and ergonomics training of work-related lower back pain and body posture problems for nurses. *Journal of Clinical Nursing, 21*(11/12), 1776–1784. doi:10.1111/j.1365-2702.2012.04089.x

Jordan, G., Nowrouzi-Kia, B., Gohar, B., & Nowrouzi, B. (2015). Obesity as a possible risk factor for lost-time injury in registered nurses: A literature review. *Safety and Health at Work, 6*(1), 1–8. doi:10.1016/j.shaw.2014.12.006

Kaewthummanukul, T., Brown, K. C., Weaver, M. T., & Thomas, R. R. (2006). Predictors of exercise participation in female hospital nurses. *Journal of Advanced Nursing, 54*(6), 663–675. doi:10.1111/j.1365-2648.2006.03854.x

Kim, M. J., Son, K. H., Park, H. Y., Choi, D. J., Yoon, C. H., Lee, H. Y., & ... Cho, M. C. (2013). Association between shift work and obesity among female nurses: Korean Nurses' Survey. *BMC Public Health, 13*(1), 1–15. doi: 10.1186/1471-2458-13-1204

Kowalenko, T., Gates, D., Gillespie, G. L., & Succop, P. (2013). Prospective study of violence against ED workers. *American Journal of Emergency Medicine, 31,* 197–205. doi:10.1016/j.ajem.2012.07.010

Krussig, K., Willoughby, D., Parker, V., & Ross, P. (2012). Obesity among nurses: Prevalence and impact on work. *American Journal for Nurse Practitioners, 16*(7/8), 14–21.

Lachman, V. D. (2015). Ethical issues in the disruptive behaviors of incivility, bullying, and horizontal/lateral violence. *Urologic Nursing, 35*(1), 39–42.

Leinung, E. Z., & Egues, A. L. (2012). Supporting the life balance, health and wellness of nurses through horizontal or lateral violence workshops. *International Journal of Health, Wellness & Society, 2*(3), 155–162.

Lowden, A., Moreno, C., Holmbäck, U., Lennernäs, M., & Tucker, P. (2010). Eating and shift work - effects on habits, metabolism and performance. *Scandinavian Journal of Work, Environment & Health, 36*(2), 150–162.

Lowson, E., Middleton, B., Arber, S., & Skene, D. J. (2013). Effects of night work on sleep, cortisol and mood of female nurses, their husbands and children. *Sleep and Biological Rhythms, 11*(1), 7–13. doi:10.1111/j.1479-8425.2012.00585.x

Măirean, C., & Turliuc, M. N. (2013). Predictors of vicarious trauma beliefs among medical staff. *Journal of Loss and Trauma, 18*(5), 414–428. doi:10.1080/15325024.2012.714200

Malik, S., Blake, H., & Batt, M. (2011). How healthy are our nurses? New and registered nurses compared. *British Journal of Nursing, 20*(8), 489–496.

Maloney, C. (2012). Critical incident stress debriefing and pediatric nurses: An approach to support the work environment and mitigate negative consequences. *Pediatric Nursing, 38*(2), 110–113.

Maust Martin, D. (2015). Nurse fatigue and shift length: A pilot study. *Nursing Economic$, 33*(2), 81–87.

McPhaul, K., London, M., & Lipscomb, J. (2013). A framework for translating workplace violence intervention research into evidence-based programs. *OJIN: The Online Journal of Issues in Nursing, 18*(1), Manuscript 4.

Mealer, M., & Jones, J. (2013). Posttraumatic stress disorder in the nursing population: A concept analysis. *Nursing Forum, 48*(4), 279–288. doi:10.1111/nuf.12045

Murphy, B. S. (2014). Exploring holistic foundations for alleviating and understanding compassion fatigue. *Beginnings, 34*(4), 6–9.

Murphy, J. C., McDaniel, J. L., Mora, K., Villareal, D. T., Fontana, L., & Weiss, E. P. (2012). Preferential reductions in intermuscular and visceral adipose tissue with exercise-induced weight loss compared with calorie restriction. *Journal of Applied Physiology, 112*, 79–85. doi: 10.1152/japplphysiol.00355.2011

Nahm, E., Warren, J., Zhu, S., An, M., & Brown, J. (2012). Nurses' self-care behaviors related to weight and stress. *Nursing Outlook, 60*(5), e23–e31. doi:10.1016/j.outlook.2012.04.005

Niu, S. F., Chung, M. H., Chu, H., Tsai, J. C., Lin, C. C., Liao, Y. M., & … Chou, K. R. (2015). Differences in cortisol profiles and circadian adjustment time between nurses working night shifts and regular day shifts: A prospective longitudinal study. *International Journal of Nursing Studies, 52*(7), 1193–1201. doi:10.1016/j.ijnurstu.2015.04.001

Occupational Safety & Health Administration (OSHA). (2015). *Worker safety in hospitals: Caring for our caregivers.* Retrieved from https://www.osha.gov/dsg/hospitals/

Papa, A., & Venella, J. (2013). Workplace violence in healthcare: Strategies for advocacy. *Online Journal of Issues in Nursing, 18*(1).

Petrov, M. E., Clark, C. B., Molzof, H. E., Johnson Jr., R. L., Cropsey, K. L., & Gamble, K. L. (2014). Sleep strategies of night-shift nurses on days off: Which ones are most adaptive? *Frontiers in Neurology, 51*(8). doi:10.3389/fneur.2014.00277

Pich, J., Hazelton, M., Sundin, D., & Kable, A. (2010). Patient-related violence against emergency department nurses. *Nursing and Health Sciences, 12*(2), 268–274. doi:10.1111/j.1442-2018.2010.00525.x

Pilon, B. (2010). *Eat stop eat: The radical new approach to nutrition that can burn fat, improve your health and might just save your life* [Electronic version]. Retrieved from www.eatstopeat.com

Purpora, C., Blegen, M. A., & Stotts, N. A. (2012). Horizontal violence among hospital staff nurses related to oppressed self or oppressed group. *Journal of Professional Nursing, 2*(8), 306–314. doi:10.1016/j.profnurs.2012.01.001

Rainford, W. C., Wood, S., McMullen, P. C., & Philipsen, N. D. (2015). The disruptive force of lateral violence in the health care setting. *Journal for Nurse Practitioners, 11*(2), 157–164. doi:10.1016/j.nurpra.2014.10.010

Ribeiro, V. F., Ferreira Filho, C., Valenti, V. E., Ferreira, M., de Abreu, L. C., Dias de Carvalho, T., & … Ferreira, C. (2014). Prevalence of burnout syndrome in clinical nurses at a hospital of excellence. *International Archives of Medicine, 7*(1), 1–14. doi: 10.1186/1755-7682-7-22

Roche, M. A., Spence Laschinger, H. K., & Duffield, C. (2015). Testing the Nursing Worklife Model in Canada and Australia: A multi-group comparison study. *International Journal of Nursing Studies, 52*(2), 525–534. doi:10.1016/j.ijnurstu.2014.10.016

Ronaldson, S., Hayes, L., Aggar, C., Green, J., & Carey, M. (2012). Spirituality and spiritual caring: Nurses' perspectives and practice in palliative and acute care environments. *Journal of Clinical Nursing, 21*(15/16), 2126–2135. doi:10.1111/j.1365-2702.2012.04180.x

Sabo, B. (2011). Reflecting on the concept of compassion fatigue. *Online Journal of Issues in Nursing, 16*(1), Manuscript 1.

Sanner-Stiehr, E., & Ward-Smith, P. (2014). Lateral violence and the exit strategy. *Journal of Nursing Management, 45*(3), 11–15. doi: 10.1097/01.NUMA.0000443947.29423.27

Sawatzky, J. V., & Enns, C. L. (2012). Exploring the key predictors of retention in emergency nurses. *Journal of Nursing Management, 20*(5), 696–707. doi:10.1111/j.1365-2834.2012.01355.x

Shahriari, M., Shamali, M., & Yazdannik, A. (2014). The relationship between fixed and rotating shifts with job burnout in nurses working in critical care areas. *Iranian Journal Of Nursing & Midwifery Research, 19*(4), 360–365.

Short, S. M. (2012). Vicarious traumatization and the call for universal precautions. *NENA Outlook, 35*(1), 25–29.

Sousa, N., Mendes, R., Abrantes, C., Sampaio, J., & Oliveira, J. (2013). Long-term effects of aerobic training versus combined aerobic and resistance training in modifying cardiovascular disease risk factors in healthy elderly men. *Geriatrics & Gerontology International, 13*(4), 928–935. doi:10.1111/ggi.12033

Spector, P. E., Zhou, Z. E., & Che, X. X. (2014). Nurse exposure to physical and nonphysical violence, bullying, and sexual harassment: A quantitative review. *International Journal of Nursing Studies, 51*(1), 72–84. doi:10.1016/j.ijnurstu.2013.01.010

Stone, T., McMillan, M., Hazelton, M., & Clayton, E. H. (2011). Wounding words: Swearing and verbal aggression in an inpatient setting. *Perspectives in Psychiatric Care, 47*(4), 194–203. doi:10.1111/j.1744-6163.2010.00295.x

Sullivan Havens, D., Warshawsky, N. E., & Vasey, J. (2013). RN work engagement in generational cohorts: The view from rural U.S. hospitals. *Journal of Nursing Management, 21*(7), 927–940. doi:10.1111/jonm.12171

Van Bogaert, P., Timmermans, O., Weeks, S. M., van Heusden, D., Wouters, K., & Franck, E. (2014). Nursing unit teams matter: Impact of unit-level nurse practice environment, nurse work characteristics, and burnout on nurse reported job outcomes, and quality of care, and patient adverse events—A cross-sectional survey. *International Journal of Nursing Studies, 51*(8), 1123–1134. doi:10.1016/j.ijnurstu.2013.12.009

Watts, J., Robertson, N., Winter, R., & Leeson, D. (2013). Evaluation of organisational culture and nurse burnout. *Nursing Management (Harrow), 20*(6), 24–29. doi: 10.7748/nm2013.10.20.6.24.e1113

Witkoski Stimpfel, A., Sloane, D. M., & Aiken, L. H. (2012). The longer the shifts for hospital nurses, the higher the levels of burnout and patient dissatisfaction. *Health Affairs, 31*(11), 2501–2509. doi: 10.1377/hlthaff.2011.1377

Yuan, S., Chou, M., Hwu, L., Chang, Y., Hsu, W. H., & Kuo, H. (2009). An intervention program to promote health-related physical fitness in nurses. *Journal of Clinical Nursing, 18*(10), 1404–1411. doi:10.1111/j.1365-2702.2008.02699.x

Zhu, D. Q., Norman, I. J., & While, A. E. (2011). The relationship between doctors' and nurses' own weight status and their weight management practices: A systematic review. *Obesity Reviews, 12*(6), 459–469. doi:10.1111/j.1467-789X.2010.00821.x

Zitkus, B. S. (2011). The relationship among registered nurses' weight status, weight loss regimens, and successful or unsuccessful weight loss. *Journal of The American Academy of Nurse Practitioners, 23*(2), 110–116. doi:10.1111/j.1745-7599.2010.00583.x

Zwerdling, D. (2015, February 11). Even "proper" technique exposes nurses' spines to dangerous forces [Special Series; Injured Nurses]. National Public Radio. Retrieved from www.npr.org/2015/02/11/383564180/even-proper-technique-exposes-nurses-spines-to-dangerous-forces

7

TYPES OF EMERGENCY DEPARTMENTS

–Aaron Wolff, BSN, RN, CEN

Different types of facilities deliver diverse practice and cultural environments. While the spectrums of human illness and injury are consistent across facilities, the resources used to treat them can vary tremendously based on facility size, organizational design, community need, and competitive focus. Selecting the right environment for your career interests contributes to the success of your professional expression. The different types of environments shape the career contexts in which you define your career.

Types of Hospitals

There are many organizational descriptions or combinations of descriptions used by hospitals to communicate how they serve patients and function within our financial systems. When understood, the terms provide insight as to how the hospital interfaces with the community as a business and as a healthcare-service provider. While clinical decisions are based in sciences, business decisions are made in a simpler model of ethics that is influenced by the organization's mission, vision, and values. By recognizing and considering the different types of hospitals, you can better identify which design fits the model of professional nursing that you want to pursue.

To be eligible to receive federal funds such as Medicare and Medicaid, hospitals with an emergency department (ED) must offer emergency and stabilizing treatment services to the public without bias or discrimination. The Emergency Medical Treatment and Active Labor Act (EMTALA) is a comprehensive federal law that obligates hospitals offering emergency services to do so without consideration of a patient's ability to pay. It's important to note that this obligation does not apply to inpatients or non-emergent conditions. The absence of bias in the delivery of care should not be misunderstood to suggest all hospitals must provide all medical services, but rather the services they choose to offer must be delivered without bias to the individual patient. For more information on EMTALA, see Chapter 12, "Risk Management and Quality Issues Affecting the Emergency Nurse."

EMTALA does not apply to inpatients or non-emergent conditions. Once a condition is stabilized to the extent of the capabilities of the facility, patients can be transferred elsewhere for more definitive care

The services provided at any facility are generally determined in consideration of community need, available financial and labor resources, and the mission of any sponsoring organizations.

Although the Affordable Care Act is improving the market presence of commercial insurance, locales with small employee populations may not have as many insured patients as suburban areas with large-volume employers. Higher percentages of commercially insured patients can represent better business opportunities for physicians and hospitals.

Although all EDs must respond to whatever emergent need may present to their doors, the expertise present can vary based on training available and frequency of skill exercise. For example, rural facilities may be better prepared to address crushing trauma/farm equipment injuries while inner city EDs frequently see more penetrating trauma. Both are likely similarly skilled in the emergency treatment of an acute myocardial infarction, but the rural facility is less likely to have the definitive interventional cardiac catheterization capability common in the Chest Pain Center ED. As you pursue your career passion, consider the varied resources and strategic positioning at the facilities you're considering. More importantly, contemplate the value you can bring to advance the capabilities of the facilities you join.

For-Profit

A *for-profit* hospital is, for tax purposes, no different from any typical commercial business. They sell products (healthcare services) with the intent of delivering the products for less than their cost to generate the service. The gap between the cost and the selling price is the profit, and taxes generally apply to the profit. This tax descriptor can apply to any size hospital or system of hospitals. The profitability of certain services, in combination with other organizational values, can be strong motivators for the development or closure of service lines offered by a hospital.

 Outlier payments are a federal subsidy that increases payment from federal payers when a facility can demonstrate a higher-than-typical cost to provide specific services (Centers for Medicare and Medicaid Services [CMS], 2013). This is intended to encourage the facility to continue to provide a service that may not otherwise be a sustainable business decision.

A for-profit hospital can be publicly or privately owned. This ownership can have significant implications for how the organization responds to market conditions and capital needs for equipment upgrades. Publicly owned for-profit hospital systems, such as Tenet, are owned through stock or shares of the company that are purchasable by the public via stock exchanges (e.g., New York Stock Exchange). Additional shares (ownership) or bonds (debt notes) can be released by the company for sale to the public to raise capital for purchases such as acquisitions and expansions. As with any publicly traded stock, investors buy it with the expectation that the value will grow. Increased value results from selling more services or delivering services at a lower production cost. For-profit hospitals must respond to revenue expectations of the investors as well as the expectations of patients; they are measured by their business outcomes as well as their patient outcomes.

Career context: For-profit facilities are typically quick to embrace new technologies and roll them out to the community with prominent marketing. Decisions about service expansion are usually done as a result of diligent exploration of the revenue growth that can be expected from the new or upgraded service. In other words, the new 64-slice CT prominently marketed on billboards and TV for coronary reconstruction images is expected to cause new patients to come to the facility.

? Regulations around primary marketing (marketing directly to the consumer) of prescription medical care began opening up in 1969. Before that, new medications were rolled out through medical journals and medical education, and the physician introduced the product to the patient. Now a TV ad tells the consumer to "ask your doctor if this medication may be right for you."

Non-Profit

Section 501 of the Internal Revenue Code allows organizations operating exclusively for charitable, scientific, religious, or public safety objectives to be exempt from paying property tax, sales tax, or income tax. The Affordable Care Act (ACA) has added new requirements for hospitals to sustain their 501 status (IRS, 2015). After paying expenses and direct employees, 100% of revenues must be kept within the organization for activity directly related to their mission. This is often demonstrated as service to their community and may be compared to the monetary value the community would have received from a for-profit business. Non-profits can and in fact must harvest a profit to survive, but they have greater control over how they make financial returns to the community. Non-profits can issue bonds (debt notes) to raise revenue, but they cannot issue stock (sell ownership). Their 501 non-profit tax status is increasingly challenged by politicians claiming not-for-profit hospitals behave no differently than for-profits in terms of meeting community need. As non-profit hospitals continue to group together, share resources, merge financial reserves, and leverage purchasing power (as is the standard in for-profit organizations), there will be continued political scrutiny.

Career context: Single facilities or small groups of hospitals may have a more local or community-based culture. They must rely on themselves in times of financial hardship. On the other hand, larger systems tend toward a more corporate culture, backed by more facilities and more diverse resources that can be very beneficial when weathering financial challenges.

Faith-Based

Faith-based is a common foundation of many non-profits. As an exercise of a faith belief, a vision is born to serve a community need. A prominent example in the United States are the Catholic faith-based facilities, which oversee one in nine inpatient beds and are involved with one in six patient contacts (Catholic Health Association of the United States, 2015). The original motive in faith-based hospitals was to meet a need through the exercise of faith, and that faith is typically reflected in how the organization makes decisions. All hospitals must harvest profit to sustain themselves, and in the faith-based facilities, profit yields opportunity to expand the mission of the faith.

Career context: Employees are not required to hold the faith of the sponsoring organization, but they are required to comply with its values when care is provided. When a faith opposes a procedure such as surgical sterilization, that service is typically not permitted to occur at that facility.

 Limitation of services in faith-based hospitals receiving government payment has drawn the opposition of the American Civil Liberties Union.

Teaching Facilities

Teaching facility resources and services are typically reflective of their more diverse mission. They seek to teach medical and/or nursing students in the professions of healing while also providing care to patients. This opens additional revenue sources to them for equipment upgrades because they have objectives broader than just direct patient care. These are the organizations that perform the majority of research and development of new treatments and testing of medical technology. They are known for offering leading-edge care, including research grant–funded trials before they are available outside of the research environment. Research trials are often funded from government or private grants. They are also supported by billing for services as well as from tax dollars flowing to them. An example of this reverse tax flow is a state university–based hospital: Tuition from students and tax support from the state flow into the organization to fund the innovation and research that is a leading objective of a teaching facility. Although not all innovation occurs in teaching facilities, a teaching facility that is not yielding new evidence would not be fulfilling its entire mission.

Career context: Teaching facilities have more professionals and typically more specialists on the care team overall. There are more people at the bedside as students seek opportunities to complete procedures. For example, morning rounds on the surgical floor may include the attending as well as multiple residents at varying stages of their education. These environments also receive referrals that concentrate the more rare conditions and treatments, making them seem more common in that facility than in the typical community. Staffing ratios and labor hours per patient visit may seem much higher because students are not counted in the labor model.

Critical Access Hospitals

Some rural facilities hold a "Critical Access" designation from the federal government that affords them a slightly higher reimbursement rate from federal payment programs. This is intended to facilitate their financial stability despite a size and location that may not otherwise be financially viable. Some of the requirements to be designated as a Critical Access hospital include the following (Department of Health and Human Services, Centers for Medicare and Medicaid Services, 2014):

- The hospital must be located in a rural area (some hospitals in urban areas are treated as rural under special provisions set out by the government).

- The hospital must be located more than a 35-miles drive from any other hospital (in mountainous terrain, the hospital must be more than a 15-mile drive to the next hospital).

- The hospital must either furnish onsite 24-hour emergency care services 7 days a week or have staff on call 24 hours a day to respond to emergencies in a timely manner.

- The hospital may have no more than 25 inpatient beds, and the average length of stay must be 96 hours or less per patient for acute care.

Veterans Affairs Facilities

Veterans Affairs facilities have been created to meet the needs of a specific population: those who have served their country though military service. They are by definition a government hospital, and therefore, their primary financial support results from revenue flowing to them from the government. These facilities can serve the comprehensive needs of their patients, and they often have exceptional skill in serving the unique needs of injured servicemen and women. These facilities can be research and teaching environments while they seek to accommodate the changing needs of wounded soldiers. A prominent example can be seen in the realm of prosthetic advancements and treatment of blast injuries resulting from the recent wars in the Middle East.

Career context: This is an ideal environment to serve the men and women who have served their country.

Active Military Facilities

Active military hospitals can be the leading edge of emergency-service innovation and research. As with other government hospitals, tax dollars flow *to* rather than *from* these facilities, and the populations and conditions served are more homogenous than the typical public hospital; this provides for more control in research. These facilities range from the forward battlefield units, through rotor and fixed-wing air transports, to the safe-zone hospitals. The science of trauma resuscitation and blood transfusion practices has been drastically rewritten by the experience and research of these hospitals. Their outcomes for major trauma have proven miraculous compared to civilian trauma centers. As a result of their research, we have seen the therapeutic deployment of tourniquets, advancements in damage control surgery, as well as changes in how we administer blood and fluids to maintain perfusion.

 Safe-zone hospital—Safe-zone hospitals were defined in the Geneva Convention as "hospital zones and localities so organized as to protect the wounded and sick from the effects of war, as well as the personnel entrusted with the organization and administration of these zones" (International Committee of the Red Cross, 2015).

Specialty Emergency Departments

There can be several different licensing levels of EDs that can vary by state and provide an escalating level of available services. These can include but may not be limited to:

- **Standby emergency department:** In a standby ED, nursing services are present onsite at all times, but the physician may have to be called in when a patient presents.

- **Basic emergency department:** The basic ED is the most common and must meet specific minimum requirements. Basic services in the United States typically include 24-hour onsite nursing, physician and diagnostic support services, and a varied complement of subspecialty physician services available upon call.

- **Comprehensive emergency department:** Comprehensive EDs are relatively rare but are typically supported by a comprehensive teaching facility with a volume of patients supported by onsite subspecialty physician services (Office of Statewide Health Planning and Development [OSHPD], 2012).

These license categories are issued by the state, and therefore, criteria can vary according to state law.

Trauma Designation: Level I, II, III, IV

Facility trauma designations are administered by states in accordance with published rules and requirements (similar to facility licensing's practices), but a successful trauma system functions independently of political or governmental boundaries (American Trauma Society [ATS], n.d.). Trauma systems are made up of collections of facilities offering varied levels of service. The goal of the system is to work collaboratively across facilities in a region to route patients to the resources necessary to achieve the best patient outcome. Systems are most effectively developed in response to geographic regions, population densities, injury patterns, facility resources, and especially transportation logistics rather than traditional jurisdictional boundaries. Most of the U.S. have a written trauma plan that defines how resources across jurisdictions or even state lines collaborate to deliver the best possible care for the injured patient.

In general, the state (and possibly adjacent geographic regions) is defined into smaller units with grouping of hospitals into trauma systems. Within those systems, different facilities hold varied levels of designations representing varied levels of available services. Trauma designations range from 1 through 4 and sometimes 5, with level 1s representing the highest level of resources. The designation comes from the state and should not be confused with a verification.

This pattern of level numbering is not universal across specialties and can easily create confusion. For example, the lowest level neonatal intensive care unit is described as a level 1, while in trauma, a level 1 describes the highest level of resources.

From a governance or regulatory view, the state administers or delegates authority to administer the trauma plan across regionally based systems. This authority can be delegated to the Local Emergency Medical Services Agency (LEMSA). This agency administers and regulates state requirements and can add additional regulations as it deems appropriate to best serve the patients within its regional responsibility. How it defines those regulations is up to the agency with the authority. Although the states (or their designated agency) have the authority to designate which facilities serve as different levels of trauma centers, other organizations are increasingly being contracted to verify the presence of services represented by the level of designation.

The state or an agency of the state appoints or designates which facilities will serve as a particular trauma level, but in pursuit of more standardized, evidence-based practices, there is an increasing trend toward using professional organizations to set the resource standards required for the designation. A common example is found in the standards set by the American College of Surgeons (ACS) for level 1, 2, 3, and 4 trauma centers. The ACS publishes and updates standards for trauma center resources approximately every 5 years. As a purchasable service, it also surveys hospitals to verify the presence of the resources it publishes as the standard for each particular level of trauma-center designation.

In an example of the hierarchy and checks and balances, the state delegates regulatory authority to an agency. The agency defines the regional requirements and regulates compliance to those standards. Its standards may be written only by the agency, or it may include an obligation for verification by an agency such as the ACS. The ACS (or other organizations), for a fee, would then come to the facility and verify the standard resources are present. If the standards are found to be present, the EMS agency would sustain the facilities designation. If the ACS finds the resources to be incomplete, it reports the finding to the EMS agency, which could then revoke the center's level designation. While a facility may be a designated trauma center, the gold standard is to have the resources represented by the designation to also be verified as compliant with the resources defined by an independent professional organization such as the ACS.

As the trauma level numeral decreases, the depth of services increases, and the level is not precisely comparable region to region unless it has been verified by an organization such as the ACS. Even without a trauma level verification, the facility is still required to treat trauma arrivals, but the facility is implying an absence of coordinated and consistently available trauma services. In the realm of ACS-verified centers, you can expect:

- Level IV represents the most basic level of coordinated trauma services and includes a typical ED and support services backed by an on-call trauma surgeon and an independent trauma-specific quality committee.

- Level III adds to the level IV resources continual call coverage of orthopedic surgical services but may not include comprehensive pelvic fracture surgical services.

- Level II represents a full complement of uninterrupted surgical services, including neurosurgery oral/maxillofacial/ENT, and many others. Level II trauma centers typically accommodate all but the most complex pelvic surgical services.

- At level I facilities, specialty services are often in-house as opposed to being on-call and are usually supported by a large university teaching facility. Specialty services like burn units, organ transplant, and limb implantation may be provided at level I or may be coordinated to other centers.

The ancillary services availability at all verified trauma centers also increases as the numeric level decreases, but the breadth of subspecialty surgical services offers the best overview of what is available at the different level trauma centers. See Table 7.1 for a review of requirements for various levels of trauma designations.

Table 7.1 Summary of Surgical Specialty Resources Represented by ACS Verified Trauma Designation Levels

Specialty Resource	Trauma Level I	Trauma Level II	Trauma Level III	Trauma Level IV
Internal medicine	X	X		
Pulmonology	X	X		
Cardiology	X	X		
Gastroenterology	X	X		
Infectious disease	X	X		
Nephrology	X	X		
Neurosurgery	X	X		
General trauma surgery	Within 15 minutes	Within 15 minutes	Within 30 minutes	
Vascular surgery	X	X		
Microvascular surgery	X	X		
Orthopedic surgery	Comprehensive pelvic surgery	Possibly limited pelvic surgery	Within 30 minutes	
Maxillofacial surgery	X	X		
Other resources	Cardiovascular surgery required	Bypass capability	ED MD onsite	Midlevel response or physician when available

Source: Adapted from American College of Surgeons, 2014.

 All verified trauma centers will have a state designation reflecting the level of service, but not all designated facilities have been verified by an independent agency such as the ACS. California, for example, is considering a statute that would require third-party verification before a designation can be issued by the state.

Pediatric Approved/Pediatric Specific

Pediatric emergency medical services readiness has been receiving increased attention since the Institute of Medicine released a report in 1993 (Millman, 1993). Similar studies have been completed by other organizations several times since, with the most recent including voluntary participation of 83% of EDs in 2013 (Pediatric Readiness Project, n.d.). In general, the reports illustrated that although they are improving, many EDs were not adequately prepared with staff training or equipment to deliver the standard of care recommended for pediatric populations. In response, the hospital industry, professional organizations, and regulatory agencies have developed courses and survey standards to bridge these gaps in resources. Terms and designations can vary by region and state, and many include designations such as Emergency Department Approved for Pediatrics (EDAP), verifications such as the ACS verification as a pediatric trauma center, or even a license as a pediatric-specific ED. The terms used can vary by state, but any verification by a professional organization such as the ACS represents achieving a standard typically in excess of the minimum state requirements. Thanks to national and international organizations such as the American Heart Association, the Emergency Nurses Association, the American College of Surgeons, and others, training and equipment resources are becoming more standardized and evidence-based. Courses like Pediatric Advanced Life Support (PALS), Emergency Nursing Pediatric Course (ENPC), and Pediatric Care After Resuscitation (PCAR) have been instrumental in setting the educational standards in evidence-based practice. If you're seeking a career focus in pediatric emergency care, begin by identifying the terms and titles that are specifically available or utilized in your prospective target region.

Career context: A typical pediatric patient volume in an average ED is around 25% to 35%, depending on community demographics (Schappert and Bhuiya, 2012). At a minimum, the professional nurse will facilitate the department commitment to maintaining the proper equipment and supplies. For increased pediatric exposure, seek a facility with a pediatric ICU, a pediatric trauma center, or a children's hospital.

Geriatric Emergency Department

Specialization in geriatrics is a need growing as rapidly as our geriatric generations. A written consensus guideline is published by emergency nurses, physicians, geriatric societies, and others detailing the characteristics of a "geriatric emergency department." Much of the content focuses on physical and environmental design features that better serve this population (American College of Emergency Physicians, American Geriatrics Society, Emergency Nurses Association, Society for Academic Emergency Medicine, 2013). There are also specialty clinical training and certifications that can be earned to bolster the clinician's knowledge about how to treat this unique population. Being first to deliver a geriatric focus in the proper demographic can yield a valuable advantage in a competitive environment.

Some of the recommendations laid out in the consensus guideline for a geriatric ED include (American College of Emergency Physicians, American Geriatrics Society, Emergency Nurses Association, Society for Academic Emergency Medicine, 2013):

- Staffing protocols that provide geriatric-trained providers (including physicians, nurse leadership, and ancillary services). The ED should have an identified geriatric emergency medicine medical director and a geriatric ED nurse manager.

- Discharge protocols that facilitate communication of clinically relevant information to patients, family, and other care providers to minimize admission rates as well as unnecessary returns to the hospital. All discharge instructions provided to the patient will be adapted to the needs of the elderly population, such as large-font discharge instructions.

- A Geriatric Program Quality Improvement Plan that encompasses all providers that care for patients and monitors factors such as geriatric volume, admission rate, readmission rate, deaths, abuse, neglect, transfers, and delivery of appropriate care. The hospital should not only track these factors but also put processes into place to ensure that there is intervention for parameters that do not meet minimum standards.

- Equipment and supplies designed for the geriatric population including (but not limited to) furniture from which the geriatric patient can exit easily, extra thick gurney mattresses, body warming devices, non-slip fall mats, bedside commodes, walking aids, appropriate lighting, and enhanced signage.

- Policies and procedures that address the specific needs of the geriatric population.

Career context: The percentage of patient volume fitting the "geriatric" definition is determined by the local demographics. You can anticipate this higher-than-average level of population commitment and likely an above-average patient percentage in facilities emphasizing a geriatric ED.

Disease Specific Centers, Certifications, and Designations

The favorable outcomes achieved by trauma-center designations has paved the way for a steady demand for other disease-specific designations, certifications, and verifications. Emergency Medical System design lends itself well to delivering patients to the facilities best prepared to deliver the best disease-specific care.

Disease specific certifications have proliferated for both the ED and across the hospital. Through EMS regulations, some destination decisions have protocols in place to bypass the closest facility in order to ensure the patient is received by the facility best prepared to deliver the optimal condition-specific outcome. Some dominant examples of this include Chest Pain Center or Stroke Center recognitions, but the list continues to grow, and resources behind those titles can vary based on which organization backs the designation.

Facility certifications and designations can give insight into the facility's focus or interest as well as what resources may be most abundant there. The Joint Commission offers a process for both basic and/or advanced certification specific to many different disease processes including chest pain, orthopedic and spinal surgery, sepsis, and literally dozens more. Cardiac- and stroke-specific certifications are also offered by the American Heart Association, and the Society of Chest Pain Centers is a prominent example of a reputable cardiac certification. The certification allows the facility access to benchmarking and best practices from other members as well as the right to advertise its resources and commitment to the specific patient population. The informed consumer can expect highly organized care delivery with an external oversight and validation that the facility is engaged in that specialty to a degree that exceeds the minimum requirements dictated by basic facility licensure.

Chest Pain Center and Other Disease-Specific Certification Details

All of the chest pain center designations (and any specific designation for that matter) serve the patient in a similar way: They ensure the center is well prepared to deliver optimal care for that condition. The consumer and the clinician can expect a designation to ensure technical and diagnostic capabilities on par with the industry best practice. These services are staffed at an acceptable standard and backed by protocols that facilitate timely care, which is monitored internally and externally to deliver benchmarked performance. In order to advertise as using any trademarked status such as Chest Pain Center, the facility must pay for and submit to regular survey by the external agency that issues the designation. Fees are paid prior to visit and are not refundable based on the outcome, so the surveying organization's decision is unlikely to be biased to overlook deficiencies. Most importantly, the certifying agency typically requires the organization's staff to have additional and recurrent disease-specific education to ensure their knowledge is kept up to date. Organizations that seek designations, certifications, and recognition above the minimum state law requirements can be fulfilling places to sustain professional motivation.

Although different organizations offer chest pain center designation, and each one may have its own specific requirements, the following list outlines the requirements necessary to be identified as a Chest Pain Center through the Society of Cardiovascular Patient Care (UNC Healthcare, 2012):

- The hospital must have a coordinated community education program that provides education about recognizing the signs of a heart attack and the importance of seeking immediate medical care.

- The hospital must demonstrate integration of ED services with pre-hospital services to ensure rapid transport and care of the patient with chest pain as well as the ability to share outcome data regarding patients with chest pain between the entities.

- The hospital must have written protocols and processes in place that allow for the timely recognition of patients experiencing acute coronary syndromes.

- The hospital must have processes in place to assess patients with chest pain, including biomarkers, 12 lead ECG interpretation, and stress-testing.

- The hospital must have a process improvement plan in place to evaluate the care provided to patients with chest pain.

- The hospital must have documented credentialing and training for all staff who are involved in care of the patient with chest pain.

- The administration of the hospital must be able to prove commitment to chest pain center accreditation.

- The hospital must have an appropriate design and signage for patients and pre-hospital providers to easily find access to services.

Career context: Facilities who hold specialty certifications have a data-driven focus on operations and outcomes for the specialties for which they hold a certification. These systems and outcomes are achieved as a result of increased education and meetings that evaluate and disseminate information regarding performance. A cardiac-designated ED in a facility with an interventional catheterization lab likely holds greater opportunity for the nurse who has a passion for treating patients experiencing acute myocardial infarctions.

Free-Standing Emergency Department

Free-standing EDs are delivering quality and competitive advantages in states that will license them. This is a great way to achieve a market presence in an area that cannot immediately accommodate or support a full-service hospital, as well as a way to get care to patients sooner for time-sensitive conditions. When an ED becomes impacted with large volumes of patients, opening a free-standing ED in another part of town can yield shorter door-to-doctor times. A free-standing ED, unlike an urgent care center, offers the same services as an ED, such as comprehensive radiology and laboratory services. But free-standing EDs are not physically attached to a hospital to provide care for the 12% of patients who will require admission; patients needing admission are transferred from the free-standing ED to a hospital with inpatient services (Centers for Disease Control and Prevention [CDC],

2015). Some non-emergent diagnostics and many invasive interventions, such as interventional cardiac catheterization lab services, commonly remain centralized in an associated comprehensive hospital. Advanced life support services are well-planned and organized to ensure optimal care during transfer, but in the case of time-sensitive interventions for critical conditions such as embolic stroke, the best clinical outcome can be achieved with CT and thrombolytic intervention, and an eventual transfer to the more distant intensive care unit can be clinically insignificant. Not all states currently license this model of service.

Career context: The free-standing ED would be an exciting place to work if you enjoy rapid intervention and transfer of the highest-acuity patients.

Urgent Care Center

Urgent care centers may be found as stand-alone entities in the community and do not undergo the rigorous licensing required by hospitals. They can also bypass architectural costs associated with overnight hospitals in many states. In other instances, they can be included as part of the main hospital, but in that case would incur more regulatory oversight. These facilities bridge the gap between primary care and the ED for non–life threatening needs such as lacerations and minor fractures while also accommodating no-appointment-needed, low-acuity medical needs such as minor illnesses. They are commonly staffed with family practice physicians and allied medical providers (nurse practitioners and physician assistants) as well as nurses. The equipment available is typically more like a doctor's office than an ED, but they will have the addition of basic radiologic imaging and possibly basic lab panels and urinalysis. Any inpatient need or specialty consultation requires transportation to a hospital. This can be an excellent milieu to gain exposure to episodic outpatient professional experience.

Career context: From this environment, you can expect a lower acuity and clinical intensity as well as shorter patient stays and fewer nursing interventions compared to an ED.

Lantern Award

Approximately 1% of the EDs in the United States have achieved prestigious recognition from the Emergency Nurses Association as Lantern Award facilities. This ED-specific award represents exceptional practice and innovative performance across multiple aspects of professional emergency nursing. These realms of excellence include leadership, clinical practice, education, advocacy, and research, all of which illustrate a commitment to an exceptional clinical practice environment (Emergency Nurses Association [ENA], 2015). As with the other certifications and recognition modalities, an organization must apply for survey once it is prepared to demonstrate the presence of the standards defined by the awarding organization. There is no higher honor or recognition for an ED than to achieve Lantern recognition, and reapplication is required annually to sustain the status.

Career context: An ED with Lantern Award designation is a demonstration to the public, as well as potential employees, that the ED provides an exemplary level of emergency care. If you're looking to work in a progressive environment in which you know you'll be part of a team that strives to provide emergency care that is truly exceptional, seek employment opportunities at a hospital with Lantern Award designation.

Magnet Designation

A Magnet® designation is achieved by the entire hospital, and therefore, it involves the ED. The award is administered by the American Nurses Credentialing Center (ANCC) as a result of application and survey proving excellent patient care across greater than 35 focus areas. These facilities are known for a highly empowered nursing culture steeped in evidence-based practice and registered nurse commitment to participation from the bedside, on quality and peer review committees, on through to the budgeting process. Professional nursing models and shared governance permeate all aspects of a Magnet hospital culture (ANCC, 2015). Achieving and sustaining Magnet status requires years of facility commitment and levels of professional commitment from the bedside nurses that are more likely to be described as ideal than common. A Magnet status for a facility could be roughly comparable to a Lantern designation for an ED.

Career context: Magnet facilities report some of the highest rates of professional nursing satisfaction. The name "magnet" refers to the fact that nurses are attracted to employment at the facility because of its dedication to quality and nursing-centered care.

Summary

The continuum of emergency nursing environments is as diverse as the spectrum of patients. Each department offers a customized response to community need, and no two EDs are identical. From the Critical Access–designated standby ED to the level I trauma center within the university teaching hospital, a professional emergency nurse can find the perfect fit to professionally serve the patient at every phase of his or her career. After you enter a phase of skill mastery in one environment, you can transfer some of that experience to a new environment and find there is more to learn. At each facility, you serve similar patients using a color palette of different resources. The professional, lifelong learner registered nurse will recognize opportunities to advance the care of patients regardless of the scope of capabilities present at his or her particular practice location.

References

American College of Emergency Physicians, American Geriatrics Society, Emergency Nurses Association, Society for Academic Emergency Medicine. (2013). *Geriatric emergency department guidelines.* Retrieved from http://www.acep.org/workarea/DownloadAsset.aspx?id=95365

American College of Surgeons. (2014). *Resources for optimal care of the injured patient* (6th ed.). (M. F. Rotondo, C. Cribari, & S. R. Smith, Eds.) Chicago, IL: American College of Surgeons.

American Nurses Credentialing Center (ANCC). (2015). *System eligibility requirements.* Retrieved from http://www.nursecredentialing.org/SysEligibilityRequirements

American Trauma Society (ATS). (n.d.). *Trauma center levels explained.* Retrieved from http://www.amtrauma.org/?page=traumalevels

Catholic Health Association of the United States. (2015, January). *Facts and statistics: Catholic health care in the United States.* Retrieved from https://www.chausa.org/about/about/facts-statistics

Centers for Disease Control and Prevention (CDC). (2015, April 29). *Emergency department visits.* Retrieved from http://www.cdc.gov/nchs/fastats/emergency-department.htm

Centers for Medicare and Medicaid Services (CMS). (2013, April 10). *Outlier payments.* Retrieved from https://www.cms.gov/Medicare/Medicare-Fee-for-Service-Payment/AcuteInpatientPPS/outlier.html

Department of Health and Human Services, Centers for Medicare and Medicaid Services. (2014, September). *Critical Access hospital.* Retrieved from http://www.cms.gov/Outreach-and-Education/Medicare-Learning-Network-MLN/MLNProducts/downloads/CritAccessHospfctsht.pdf

Emergency Nurses Association (ENA). (2015). *Lantern Award.* Retrieved from https://www.ena.org/practice-research/Practice/LanternAward/Pages/default.aspx

Internal Revenue Service (IRS). (2015). *New requirements for 501(c)(3) hospitals under the Affordable Care Act.* Retrieved from http://www.irs.gov/Charities-&-Non-Profits/Charitable-Organizations/New-Requirements-for-501(c)(3)-Hospitals-Under-the-Affordable-Care-Act

International Committee of the Red Cross (ICRC). (2015). *Practice relating to Rule 35. Hospital and safety zones and neutralized zones.* Retrieved from https://www.icrc.org/customary-ihl/eng/docs/v2_rul_rule35

Millman, M. (1993). *Access to health care in America.* Washington, DC: National Academies Press.

Office of Statewide Health Planning and Development (OSHPD). (2010). *Emergency room hospitals.* Retrieved from http://gis.oshpd.ca.gov/atlas/topics/er_dashboard

Pediatric Readiness Project. (n.d.). *Average pediatric readiness scores.* Retrieved from http://www.pediatricreadiness.org/State_Results/Average_Scores.aspx

Schappert, S. M., & Bhuiya, F. (2012, March 1). *Availability of pediatric services and equipment in emergency department: United States, 2006.* Retrieved from http://www.cdc.gov/nchs/data/nhsr/nhsr047.pdf

UNC Healthcare. (2012, November 8). *Working towards chest pain center accreditation.* Retrieved from http://news.unchealthcare.org/som-vital-signs/2012/nov8/working-towards-chest-pain-center-accreditation

CHAPTER 8

COMMON AREAS WITHIN THE EMERGENCY DEPARTMENT

–Debra Delaney, MS, RN, CEN; and
Jeff Solheim, MSN, RN-BC, CEN, CFRN, FAEN

Whether you call it the emergency department, the emergency care center, the emergency room, the ED, the ESD (emergency services department), or the ER, it's the place to go when you or a loved one is sick or hurt. It's also the place that the majority of emergency nurses call their "work home." Several different and unique areas that function together comprise what is commonly referred to as the emergency department.

Most emergency departments (ED) are on the ground level of the hospital to ensure ease of access for patients requiring emergent care. Clear red signs typically define the area of the hospital that is designated to provide immediate care for all emergencies. This chapter outlines what exactly you can expect to find within an ED.

Waiting Area (Lobby/Reception Area)

The waiting area is typically the first point of entry for patients and visitors arriving via private vehicle. Many EDs call this area the *lobby* or *arrival area* instead of the *waiting room* to avoid the stigma of asking patients to "wait" when they feel they're having an emergency.

Historical data suggest that waiting rooms have been designed as the gateway to the ED and should be able to accommodate the expected patients and their visitors. ED volume, although variable, does in fact follow a typical arrival curve, with the majority of the ED census arriving between the hours of 11am and 11pm (see Figure 8.1). Sometimes an "annex" location adjacent to the main waiting room is optimal for the peak hours, and it can be unofficially closed during the less crowded time periods. Because patient volume and waiting time vary by time of day, it's important to allow space for patients and families to sit during the ED visit.

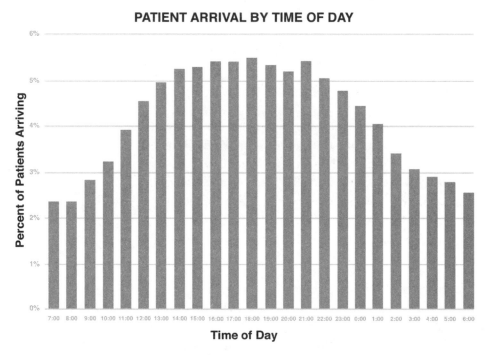

Figure 8.1   The peak times for an ED.

Some hospitals have divided the waiting area into smaller segments, which allows for private conversations among family members and can also be utilized for grouping similar patient populations (e.g., low acuity or vertical patients sit on one side of the partition while "sicker" patients stay closer to the nurses' view). Research has shown that seating that facilitates family and social support improves patient outcomes and satisfaction overall. Utilizing a sterile setting where chairs are aligned along the walls or in straight lines throughout the waiting area does not facilitate socialization and may serve to decrease satisfaction and increase anxiety regarding the ED visit (Malone & Dellinger, 2011). Rows of chairs also appear institutional and may force patients to focus on their health concerns.

 Vertical patients—Sometimes patients with lower acuities are referred to as vertical patients because they do not need to lie down on a stretcher (hence becoming horizontal) but instead are cared for in the upright (vertical) position.

Chairs should be durable and should have arms for those patients who may need assistance getting in and out (e.g., patients with weakness or limited mobility; the elderly). It's also optimal for the chair colors to contrast with the color of the rug or flooring for patients and visitors with vision and balance concerns. Chairs should lack sharp or hard edges that could injure individuals who fall. The furniture in the reception area must be durable, non-porous, and without surface joints or seams to facilitate cleaning to reduce the spread of infection (Malone & Dellinger, 2011). Ideally, furniture will have antimicrobial finishes to inhibit the growth of microbes as well. It's important for healthcare facilities to create and maintain a safe environment for patients and employees.

Bariatric Considerations

Recommendations from the Americans with Disabilities Act (ADA) suggest that at least 20% of seating be available for bariatric patients and visitors and that these chairs be integrated with the standard-sized chairs to prevent stigmatization. Bariatric seating includes love seats and oversized chairs with a reinforced structure to support up to 750 pounds (Kim, 2009).

 Bariatric— related to the individual with obesity.

Bariatric furniture is not simply bigger. There are many considerations including load limit, appropriate dimensions, and a design aesthetic that blends with the environment ensuring comfort and safety (InPro Corporation, 2012).

Standard chairs with arms are concerning for bariatric patients because they may not fit between the arms. They may be reluctant to sit for fear of not fitting into or breaking standard furniture. A larger seat width accommodates the greatest number of patients. Also, if the seat pitches forward slightly, it helps the patient exit safely from the chair. Elderly patients and others with limited mobility may benefit from the design as well (InPro Corporation, 2012).

Children's Waiting Area

Many ED reception areas have a separate area designed for children. This would include child-sized seating and play tables, video games, coloring books, and other age-appropriate modifications. Some facilities consider this a wonderful addition where children and their parents can be entertained while waiting; other departments find them underutilized and difficult to maintain, especially in terms of cleanliness. If the waiting room does not include a specific "play area" for children, it should still include smaller sections where parents can be with their children in a more comforting and private space.

Virtual Waiting Area

Some research suggests that traditional waiting rooms may be a thing of the past, recommending that traditional waiting rooms be replaced with simplified and space-efficient "pause" areas or "internal queues" strategically placed in different areas of the department (Dinardo, 2013).

There are also many models of a "virtual waiting room" and/or "call ahead" seating that include the use of technology to minimize the waiting experience. A relatively new concept to eliminate the wait, many hospitals are utilizing technology to improve the patient experience (Diane, 2014).

 Virtual waiting room—Involves adopting technology that allows patients to check in to the ED online. The system then notifies patients what their estimated time to be seen will be so they can go about other activities in the community, reporting to the ED at their estimated time to be seen. Not only is this potentially advantageous to the patient, but it may also give the ED a better indication of impending workload.

Signage in the Waiting Area

Requirements govern what signage must be located in the ED. Most of the mandatory information discusses patients' rights and the responsibility of the hospital in accordance with governing bodies such as CMS (Centers for Medicare and Medicaid Services). Some signs instruct patients and visitors of their rights to appropriate screening and/or care regardless of their ability to pay (EMTALA) and their right to privacy (HIPAA); see Figure 8.2. While some signage is mandated federally, state and local authorities may mandate other signage; therefore, it is incumbent on the hospital to know what signs are required in its locale.

```
+-----------------------------------------------------------+
|                       IT'S THE LAW                        |
|                                                           |
|  IF YOU HAVE A MEDICAL EMERGENCY OR ARE IN LABOR YOU       |
|  HAVE THE RIGHT TO RECEIVE, WITHIN THE CAPABILITIES OF     |
|  THIS HOSPITAL'S STAFF AND FACILITIES:                     |
|                                                           |
|      AN APPROPRIATE MEDICAL SCREENING EXAMINATION          |
|                                                           |
|   NECESSARY STABILIZING TREATMENT (INCLUDING FOR AN        |
|                      UNBORN CHILD)                         |
|                                                           |
|   AND, IF NECESSARY, AN APPROPRIATE TRANSFER TO ANOTHER    |
|                         FACILITY                          |
|                                                           |
|    EVEN IF YOU CANNOT PAY OR DO NOT HAVE MEDICAL INSURANCE |
|                                                           |
|     OR YOU ARE NOT ENTITLED TO MEDICARE OR MEDICAID        |
+-----------------------------------------------------------+
```

Source: EMTALA, 2012.

Figure 8.2 Sample signage for the waiting area.

Other Areas Associated with the Waiting Area

A number of different staff may be employed to help with the needs of patients and their visitors in the waiting room. Some EDs employ patient liaisons or customer service representatives to help meet the needs of those who are waiting and to provide some oversight while people wait. These individuals may have stations or offices in or near the waiting room. Other departments may include offices or podiums where case managers or social workers are stationed to provide assistance as needed.

Many EDs have a room designated as a "quiet room" or "grieving room" that allows families in need of support and/or consultation a place separate from the other visitors or patients. Sometimes an emotionally distraught individual may benefit from a quiet area away from others. If a public figure (VIP) were to present, he or she may prefer to have a private place to wait rather than be under the scrutiny of others in the waiting area. These rooms may be included within the main department. This also allows families of dying patients to be closer to their loved one.

Security/Safety Rooms

Because EDs are open around the clock, the waiting area is often the default entrance outside of standard business hours. Violence in the ED is surprisingly common, with one study indicating 1.8 physical assaults per nurse per year (Gillespie, Gates, & Berry, 2013). Staff in EDs can feel vulnerable in the triage area and may find this to be a security concern. To provide for the safety and security of staff and patients, many EDs have security presence in this area of the department.

Hospital security presence can vary greatly depending on the facility. Some hospitals include metal detectors, bulletproof glass, and surveillance monitors. Inner-city facilities may have visitors and patients scanned through metal detectors similar to an airport. Security officers might "wand" incoming patients. Some hospitals employ local police as uniformed officers in the department, and they might have an area designated for their officers to monitor security cameras and patient/visitor activity.

Patient Access/Registration Area

Often a space near the front entrance of the ED includes the registration or access services, an area usually operated by another department in the hospital. Optimally, registration or access services should not be a separate area of the ED; rather, it should be incorporated into the triage area. The registrar, working together with the triage nurse(s), is then able to quickly get the patient into the system and provide the wristband and patient labels that are required during the ED visit without requiring the patient to make multiple stops at different stations. Registration or access services is where patients are required to give pertinent demographic and insurance information. With electronic medical records in many places, the first step to the electronic record is obtaining the correct patient information in order to prepare the electronic record and patient tracking.

Some EDs are utilizing kiosks that allow incoming patients to register themselves, similar to many retail kiosks. Patients can enter demographic information that generates their electronic medical record. Some kiosks go a step further, asking patients a few additional questions utilizing a template asking triage questions. The kiosk can then place patients in an e-queue in accordance with their medical needs. In some places, if the patient's responses indicate a need for blood tests or X-rays, the kiosk can then alert phlebotomy or radiology (Agency for Healthcare Research and Quality [AHRQ], 2012).

Triage Area

The typical arrival process for ambulatory patients includes a visit through the *triage area*. The triage area is nearly always located within or adjacent to the waiting area. Although the word "triage" comes from a verb (trier) that literally means "to sort," most EDs utilize this area of the department to process the patient upon arrival and gather information, which is used to base the patient's care and priority in receiving further medical care. For more information on the process of triage, see Chapter 10, "The Emergency Nurse in the Role of Triage."

The triage area is often a booth or closed-off small room where the nurse can ask private questions and view the injured body part. Typically this area includes tools that help the nurse make the best decision on how to care for the arriving patients. Equipment maintained in this area to help make triage decisions includes vital sign monitors, ECG machines, computers, scales, etc. This area is also equipped with supplies used to provide emergency care such as gauze, gloves, eye wash stations, emesis bags, ice, etc.

The word *triage* is a verb, which means "to sort," yet virtually all EDs have a place (noun) called "triage."

The triage area is one of the areas of the ED that is being modified in nearly every ED throughout the nation. The process of triage has transformed over the years from a mechanism to sort arrivals into a cumbersome process that many departments consider an impediment to efficient patient care. Departments are trialing innovative solutions within the triage area to minimize waste, removing steps from this "linear process" to improve the arrival experience for the patient and the overall length of stay for each visit.

Many hospitals are responding to a patient-centered experience, which encourages the arrival process to be more welcoming for patients. The triage area in many EDs is modeled after a hotel experience, where the arrival seems friendlier and less intimidating. Often the nurse is stationed as close as possible to the entrance with a portable computer, tablet, or free-standing podium. This *nurse-first* process not only allows the patient to feel immediately attended to by a caring nurse, but the nurse can also start triaging incoming patients right away. This approach minimizes the risk for patients who would otherwise often be in a queue outside the vision of the triage nurses.

Some EDs utilize a *split flow* model of care in which a nurse greets patients upon arrival and "splits" the flow by sending patients with different acuity levels to different areas of the department to streamline and expedite care (see Figure 8.3). In these facilities, there may be additional rooms in which the patients are queued into segments of care. For example, they would be triaged and placed in a small "internal waiting room" that could be called the "awaiting evaluation" room. After being seen by a provider, they might be "awaiting tests" in another small area; after X-ray they may be seated in a "results pending" area. This process of moving patients through the system reduces the need for occupying treatment rooms in the department while waiting. This concept has been particularly successful for vertical patients (people who don't need to lie down in a room on a stretcher for a long duration).

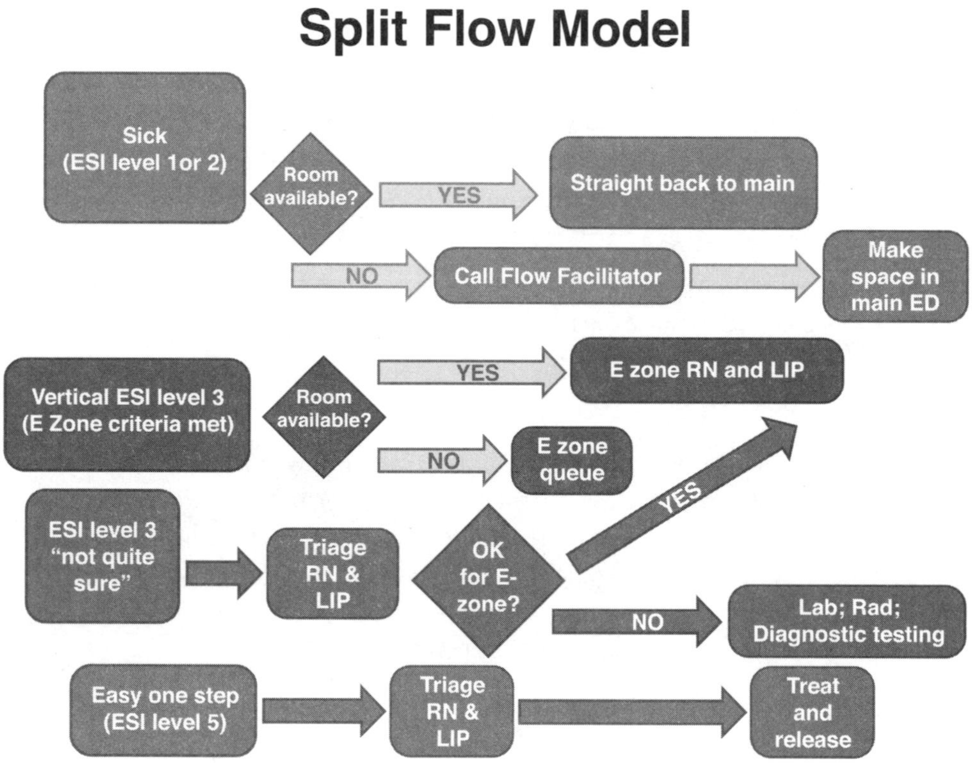

Split Flow Model

Figure 8.3   A split flow model where patients are sent to different places for different treatments.

Emergency Department Configuration

The number of beds required in the ED has historically been determined using a formula based on the assumption that one bed in the department could effectively accommodate approximately 2,000 annual visits (Zilm, 2004). This ratio continues to be re-evaluated as patient length of stay in the ED has increased, placing additional demands upon bed availability.

Additional demand on ED space is compounded as more and more admitted patients are "boarded" in the ED, awaiting transfer to their inpatient unit. Rather than building additional rooms to accommodate surges in patient volume, it's important for EDs to configure the department into pods or zones that can flex up and down to accommodate the ebb and flow of patient needs (Zilm, Crane, & Roche, 2010).

Of course, streamlining care is one way to improve patient flow, improve patient perception of care, and ultimately decrease demand on the beds needed. It's important to continue to trial ways to streamline care when planning the number of beds needed for care. By utilizing small internal waiting areas to cohort vertical patients, room utilization is greatly improved.

Throughput—The process by which patients are "put through" the ED. When one patient occupies an ED bed, another patient may wait for care.

Boarder—When a patient is admitted to the hospital, but a bed is not available on the inpatient unit, that patient is considered a "boarder" in the ED.

Length of stay—A measurement of time in minutes that it takes for each patient to arrive, be treated, and leave the ED.

Cohort—A group of people banded together or treated as a group.

Critical Care Area

A critically ill patient is a patient with a life-threatening illness. According to the Centers for Disease Control and Prevention (CDC, 2012), 2% of ED patients in the United States required care in less than 1 minute after arrival to the ED (defined as *immediate acuity*), and 10% needed care within 1 to 14 minutes after arrival to the ED (defined as *emergent acuity*). These are typically patients defined as critically ill, who would benefit from treatment in the critical care area of the ED.

This area may be a section of the ED that includes the trauma bay/code room and other similar rooms to care for the more critical patients. Smaller EDs may have one room that functions as trauma/resuscitation and critical care. Larger facilities can have more than one of each. These rooms are equipped with supplies needed to care for the sickest patients and staffed with emergency nurses who have the experience and training required to supply that care.

Trauma Bays

Many EDs (especially trauma centers) have a room or area specifically designated for the trauma patient(s). This area would have access to and be equipped with the supplies/equipment needed to care for the traumatically injured patient. Items found in this area vary but have the monitoring equipment needed for successful care of the trauma patient. In some hospitals, this room may also double as a resuscitation room.

The equipment normally kept in a trauma room depends on numerous factors. If the hospital is either verified or designated as a trauma center, then the regulating body providing that verification or designation mandates the specific equipment in the room. The trauma surgeons or the department of trauma in the hospital may request additional equipment be available in the trauma room above and beyond what is required for verification or designation as a trauma center. Here is a sample list of equipment that is required for designation as a trauma hospital in Arizona (Bureau of Emergency Medical Services and Trauma Systems, 2014):

- Airway control and ventilation equipment

- Pulse oximetry

- Suction devices

- Electrocardiograph-oscilloscope-defibrillator

- Standard intravenous fluids and administration sets

- Large-bore intravenous catheters

- Equipment to perform a cricothyrotomy

- Equipment to perform a thoracotomy

- Equipment to perform a venous cut-down

- Drugs necessary for emergency care of the traumatically injured patient

- A color-coded system for pediatric care such as a Broselow Tape

- Thermal control equipment to keep the patient warm as well as to warm fluids and blood

- A rapid infuser system to deliver large volumes of fluid rapidly

- Equipment to measure qualitative end-tidal carbon dioxide measurements

- A radio to communicate with local EMS

For more information on trauma designation and verification, see Chapter 7, "Types of Emergency Departments."

Caring for traumatically injured patients is challenging and requires skills and knowledge that may not be part of the routine experience that an emergency nurse gets working with other types of ED patients. Many institutions require specific training and experience to work in a trauma room. This training and experience may actually be mandated as part of the designation or verification process. At a minimum, you're usually required to successfully complete the Trauma Nursing Core Course (TNCC) (or a recognized equivalent) and may be required to participate in a minimum number of hours of continuing education annually in trauma-related education.

Resuscitation Room (Code Room)

A room set aside for the most critical of patients can be found in the ED. This room has the specific crash carts needed to perform life-saving measures on such patients as cardiac arrest, stroke, and other serious conditions requiring immediate intervention.

The American College of Emergency Physicians (2007) recommends the following equipment be made available in a resuscitation room (this is in addition to other equipment that should be available in all treatment rooms):

■ Adult and pediatric "code carts" with appropriate medication charts

■ Radiographic view boxes and a hot light

■ Bag-mask-valve ventilators for all sizes and ages of patients

■ Cricothyroidotomy instruments and supplies

■ Endotracheal tubes for all sizes and ages of patients

■ Fiber-optic laryngoscope

■ Laryngoscopes, straight and curved blades, and stylets

■ Alternate airways (laryngeal mask airways, oral and nasal airways)

■ Tracheostomy instrument and supplies

■ Equipment for a chest tube (closed-chest drainage system, chest tube instruments and supplies)

■ Emergency thoracotomy instruments and supplies

- End-tidal carbon dioxide monitor

- Nebulizer

- Peak flow meter

- Volume cycle ventilator and BiPAP ventilation system

- Cardiac monitors

- Blood/fluid infusion pumps and tubing

- Blood and fluid warmers

- Cardiac compression board

- Central venous catheter kits and monitoring equipment as well as cutdown instruments and supplies

- Intraosseous needles

- Defibrillator with paddles or pads for all sizes and ages, including internal paddles

- Pericardiocentesis instruments

- Temporary external pacemaker, and transvenous or transthoracic pacemaker

- 12-lead ECG machine

If the ED is recognized as a stroke center, a chest pain center, or a pediatric center, additional supplies may be required in the resuscitation room. The certifying body that designates the hospital in one of these specialties provides a list of the equipment required to safely and effectively care for these patients. For more information on specialty designations of emergency departments, see Chapter 7.

In the same way that special training is required in most institutions to work in the trauma room, specialized training and certification may be required to work in the resuscitation room. This training may include completion of the Advanced Cardiovascular Life Support (ACLS) course, the Pediatric Advanced Life Support (PALS) course, and other educational activities that prepare you for the advanced concepts required to care for critically ill patients. Working in the resuscitation room is often reserved for nurses who have experience caring for less acutely ill patients and have demonstrated exceptional critical thinking skills.

Acute Care Area

Most patients who present to the ED are not critically ill and do not require the resources and equipment needed in the critical care area. According to the CDC (2012), 41% of ED patients require care within 15 to 60 minutes of arrival (defined as *urgent acuity*) and would likely benefit from being placed in a room designed for an acute care patient. The majority of ED rooms are appropriate for caring for acute patients. Typical complaints cared for in this area include cardiac, abdominal, neurological, and other complaints and injuries.

EDs can be designed in a variety of ways. Some departments have pods or zones where several similar patient rooms surround a central station. At this station, care providers gather for recordkeeping and sharing information. This nurses' station area is generally off limits to patients and families, although conversations may be overheard by visitors and staff, which creates concerns about violations of privacy standards. When designing the ED, carpeting in the central area to absorb noise or glass partitions around the central area can help protect privacy. In the absence of these precautions, it's incumbent that you monitor what is said to reduce the flow of private health information to people who should not be hearing it. For more information on privacy and the emergency patient, see Chapter 12, "Risk Management and Quality Issues Affecting the Emergency Nurse."

Low Acuity Area

The CDC (2012) indicates that 35% of patients in the ED do not need to be treated for 1 to 2 hours (defined as *semi-urgent acuity*), and 7% do not need to be treated for as long as 2 to 24 hours after arrival (defined as *non-urgent acuity*). These patients often require minimal equipment to meet their health needs, may be cared for by staff who have less experience and training, and may not require the same number of resources as sicker patients. For that reason, it's often prudent to place them in their own area of the department—the lower acuity area.

Fast track, express care, acute assessment area, rapid treatment area, rapid clinical evaluation, and turbo triage are a few of the names given to this section of the department set aside from the main treatment area. This area is typically where the lower acuity patients are cohorted to receive prompt care, rather than continue to be skipped over as sicker patients continue to enter the department. Most prompt care areas are open during peak volume hours of the day (for example, 11am to 11pm).

Hallway Beds

Unlike an inpatient unit, which may refuse to accept additional patients when all the rooms are filled, patients continue to arrive in the ED long after every available bed is filled. Because of this, spaces not traditionally thought of as patient-care areas may be converted to patient-care areas to ensure everyone who presents to the ED receives the care needed. Although much less than ideal for many reasons, these spaces are usually not even within the confines of a room, but may be in hallways or other spaces without walls. A patient displeaser, hallway beds have become a necessity of many departments. As the name implies, these are locations strategically placed through the department in which stretchers or chairs line the hallway. They're used for patients waiting for transfer to their inpatient bed or discharge; sometimes care may actually be delivered while the patient is in a hallway bed.

Hallway beds create numerous challenges for the ED. The biggest challenge is providing the privacy that is required by law and owed to the patient. Another challenge is ensuring adequate staffing to care for additional patients. If patients are moved into hallway spots without expanding the staffing accordingly, the number of patients assigned to each emergency nurse will exponentially grow, exceeding a safe nurse-to-patient ratio. Hallway beds have to provide the same equipment needed in a traditional treatment room, such as ways for patients to summon help should they need it and patient-monitoring equipment. Numerous hallway beds can also clutter the area and create unsafe conditions for movement, especially in the case of an emergency such as a fire (Richards, van der Linden, & Derlet, 2014).

Rather than continuing to put more and more patients into the ED by expanding the number of beds to non-traditional areas such as the hallway, it's essential that efficiencies in patient throughput are continuously re-evaluated to minimize patient times in the department rather than just increasing patient numbers. Many creative strategies exist, including placing patients in the hallways of the inpatient unit rather than the ED. The advantage to this strategy is that patients are spread over numerous units rather than being consolidated in the ED, reducing overcrowding in one area and decreasing the demands on the staff in a single department (Viccellio et al., 2013).

Observation Area

Some EDs have another area that treats patients who might potentially be admitted. These areas have been described as an observation unit, overflow area, clinical decision unit, or acute admission area. In some EDs this area is staffed and run by the ED; in others, it's treated as a separate department. Regardless of who staffs the area, it's one way to decompress the ED by moving admitted patients out of the main emergency area. An example of a patient who might be appropriately relocated to an observation unit is a patient with intermittent chest pain who would benefit from repeated cardiac enzyme measurement over a period of 12 to 24 hours. It isn't appropriate use of ED staff and space to leave the patient in the ED for this extended period of time, but it would be expensive and provide minimal reimbursement to admit the patient for such a short period of time. An observation unit provides the bridge between these two options.

> The reimbursement rate to the hospital is different for patients classified as emergency department patients as opposed to those who are classified as observation patients. Therefore, if an ED has enough patients requiring lengthy stays for repeated diagnostic testing or further observation, it may be financially feasible to open an observation area so that the hospital can bill for the prolonged services provided to patients requiring prolonged lengths of stay for continued surveillance (American College of Emergency Physicians [ACEP], 2015).

Flex Rooms/Pods

Many EDs are moving away from the traditional "ballroom" design, which contains a main nurses' station in a central location and all the treatment rooms around this area. Research shows that one zone should be no more than 10 to 12 treatment rooms to maintain optimal efficiency (Zilm et al., 2010). As the volume of emergency patients continues to grow, the option to just continue building more rooms may not exist. Additionally, at lower volume times of day (i.e., 0300–0900), all the rooms may not be needed. The solution for many EDs is to move toward creating zones or pods. These treatment spaces of 10 to 12 rooms with smaller nurses' stations can open and close at appropriate times of the day to maximize patient care. This allows additional room space, and additional staffing can be flexed as needed to accommodate the ebb and flow of patient arrivals throughout the day. Some areas have seasonal fluctuations (beaches, college towns, etc.) that could utilize these areas seasonally and remain closed when not required.

Psychiatric Area

The ability to appropriately care for and find placement for the psychiatric population is a crisis in most EDs. Patients who are in danger because of violence place an added burden on the ED staff. Whether the patient is at risk because he/she has been a victim, or whether the patient is the perpetrator of violence, the ED staff must be available to care for the patient. It's important that the ED has a safe room or area. In some departments, this area may even be locked with security or police presence onsite. The psychiatric treatment room typically has no medical equipment within reach to minimize potential for self-harm. It's important to minimize supplies and equipment left in the area to prevent the patient from harming the staff as well.

Some safe rooms can also be used as standard patient care rooms if the typical equipment, monitors, blood pressure cuffs, and other equipment are enclosed behind a "garage door" type wall that can be pulled down and locked as needed for the safety of the psychiatric patient (Hernandez, 2014). The room has a window for observation that has blinds or curtains accessed from the outside for privacy as needed. The standard patient stretcher can be removed and a mattress can be placed on the floor. Some safe rooms have video surveillance as well. Often there are storage lockers outside the room in which to place patient clothing and belongings.

Psychiatric patients have unique needs that may be difficult to meet in the busy ED. Many emergency nurses do not feel they have the training to provide care to this unique patient population (Manton, 2013). While courses such as TNCC help prepare you to care for the trauma patient, and ACLS helps prepare you to care for the cardiac patient, similar courses that prepare you to care for the psychiatric patient are more difficult to access. Some departments employ psychiatric nurses and aides, social workers, and other allied health personnel to help the emergency nurse meet the demanding needs of this population.

Decontamination Area

When patients are exposed and potentially injured from toxic substances, the most likely place for them to report is the ED. Unfortunately, if they are brought into the ED with the toxic substance on them, everyone in the ED, including staff, other patients, and visitors, may be exposed to the toxic substance, quickly increasing the number of injured individuals. If the toxic substance is a gas or releases toxic fumes, those gases or fumes may be drawn into the ventilation system of the ED and disseminated to other areas of the hospital, creating a multi-casualty disaster.

The decontamination area is important to the ED to ensure that any patient arriving who is potentially contaminated can be decontaminated without exposing others to the toxic substance. It's ideally located outside but in close proximity to the ED, often near the ambulance entrance. Not all hospitals have permanent decontamination structures, and they may have to deploy temporary decontamination areas in the ambulance bay or ED parking lot. Some hospitals have a small room which is used for decontamination but may also double for other uses and can accommodate at least one or two casualties while the portable decontamination tent is being set up outside (California Hospital Association, 2011).

Decontamination areas have many specifications, including the ability for negative pressure, and are ventilated away from the hospital to reduce exposing others to the toxic fumes. The area should contain surface areas that can be easily cleaned (such as tile) after each use. If possible, there should be a movable shower/hose wand to wash down contaminated patients. A hose and wand attachment from a wall fixture at the head of the patient gurney is ideal so that the staff can wash down the patient, beginning at the patient's head, working down to the patient's feet. The wand provides a low pressure, small area spray. The water should be tepid, not too hot or cold (U.S. Department of Homeland Security, 2014).

A floor drain with chemical polyvinyl chloride (PVC) should be included to allow the drainage of the contaminated water to a hazmat-compatible holding tank. These are inspected and maintained by the hospital safety officer.

A hazardous waste drum should be in the room for contaminated patient clothing and belongings. Personal protective equipment, as well as medical and other decontamination supplies, should be stored in a cabinet in the vicinity of the decontamination area. These supplies should not be stored in the decontaminant area itself, because once a patient arrives it would be considered contaminated.

Decontaminated patients are not the only patients that could benefit from this space. It's optimal to utilize this area for activities such as burn debridement, rinsing dirt off of construction workers or farmers, patients needing hygiene such as homeless people, and even for cleaning trauma stretchers that are grossly contaminated with blood and bodily fluids. Because this area is often designed with negative pressure, it may also be ideal for the patients needing isolation.

Isolation Room(s)

EDs should have at least one room available to isolate infectious patients that may have contagious diseases. These rooms maintain negative pressure (or have the ability to become negatively pressurized). *Negative pressure* is created when the air from the room is exhausted directly outside or through HEPA filters to avoid recirculation. According to the American Institute of Architects, negative pressure rooms should be pressurized to –2.5 Pa relative to adjacent airways with 12 air changes per hour (Miller, 2014).

Satellite Laboratory and Radiology Services

Time is lost transporting patients to different departments for various diagnostic tests or to transport specimens to the laboratory for analysis. Transporting patients to ancillary departments also increases risks because fewer resources are available to deal with emergencies outside the ED. For this reason, some EDs have been designed with the inclusion of satellite laboratories and radiology services within the ED. Rooms within the ED may have a computerized tomography (CT) scanner or an X-ray machine. A small satellite laboratory may be found within the confines of the ED. Staff within this laboratory may actually collect samples from patients as needed and analyze those samples quickly within the ED, or ED staff may collect the samples and deliver them to the satellite laboratory for rapid analysis. The inclusion of these areas has improved access to care for emergency patients by reducing time away from the unit. This not only improves the patient's length of stay within the ED but also improves the safety of the patient by keeping the patient close to providers when needed.

In the same way that the standards in nursing units are regulated by bodies such as The Joint Commission, laboratories and radiology departments are overseen by regulations such as the Clinical Laboratory Improvement Amendments (CLIA). Because the experts in these regulations are people who work within these departments, it's essential that these areas are overseen and staffed by employees familiar with the regulating requirements.

Although a satellite laboratory is not found in many EDs, point-of-care testing may be available in most EDs. As the name implies, point-of-care testing occurs at or near the place where patient care takes place instead of in the laboratory. Examples of point-of-care testing include dipping a chemical strip into a sample of urine and analyzing the urine based on the changes of color on the chemical strip or testing a patient's serum glucose using a bedside glucometer. Although point-of-care testing is convenient and provides rapid results, if it's not done properly or the equipment is malfunctioning, aberrant results can cause an improper diagnosis and errant treatment. For that reason, point-of-care testing performed by nursing staff is overseen by the laboratory as well as CLIA standards. You must be properly trained in performing point-of-care testing and work with the laboratory to ensure all quality-improvement measures are maintained to ensure accuracy of the results.

Pediatric Area

Children get sick. Of the 128.9 million patients who visited EDs in 2010, 20% (25.5 million) were younger than 18 years of age (Wier, Yu, Owens, & Washington, 2013). It's almost impossible to work in the ED and not care for a pediatric patient. Pediatric patients have unique needs, including the environment in which they are cared for and equipment needed to take care of them.

Ideally, EDs will have unique areas to care for the pediatric patients. In a large facility, this may be a separate facility, a separate department (i.e., a pediatric emergency department), or a separate area of the existing ED. In smaller facilities, it may simply be a small part of the waiting room and a room that is deemed pediatric-ready.

If the ED has a separate area to treat children, it should be pediatric-friendly. A warm and welcoming environment must include not only the patient (child) but also the accompanying family members or caregivers. Care for the child in the ED must include care for the family unit as well, and the design must incorporate space for the visitors as well as the patient. The pediatric area design requires consideration for optimal staff visualization at all times, as well as a need for intimate spaces where families can wait in private.

This area should include child safety features as well as a design that is welcoming and soothing to children. Some departments have integrated technology into their pediatric areas; soft lighting, music, and movies or cartoons can help the children during this stressful period. Hospital-sponsored videos that provide information/education are often found in the pediatric areas and may provide diversion as well as information to the families. At least one treatment room should be readily available, or easily converted, to provide care for children with behavioral or mental health needs.

Pediatric play areas can include children's toys, play tables, and wireless Internet connectivity. Consideration for cleaning of these areas must be made because the area needs to remain free of contaminants and be strictly monitored to ensure the safety of all the children and families who utilize the play areas. Many pediatric areas utilize fish tanks to provide distraction and a source of relaxation; they also provide a visual divider between spaces and other anxious families.

Pediatric readiness goes far beyond a pleasant environment. It requires that staff who work this area are competent in care of the pediatric patient. At a minimum, staff in these areas should regularly take courses such as the Emergency Nursing Pediatric Course (ENPC) or the Pediatric Advanced Life Support (PALS). At least one individual should be identified within the department to coordinate care, training, and equipment needed to ensure pediatric patients receive the appropriate care. Equipment in sizes appropriate for all ages of children should be centrally located in the area where children are commonly cared for. For more information on caring for the pediatric patient, see Chapter 14, "Challenging Patient Populations Encountered by the Emergency Nurse."

The American Academy of Pediatrics, the American College of Emergency Physicians, and the Emergency Nurses Association have produced a checklist that should be utilized by all emergency departments to ensure they are properly prepared to care for pediatric patients. This checklist is available at www2.aaporg/visit/Checklist_ED_Prep-022210.pdf.

Geriatric Area

In 2009 and 2010, the number of patients 65 and older who visited EDs annually was 19.6 million, nearly as high as the number of pediatric patients (Albert, McCaig, & Ashman, 2013). Many EDs are converting areas of the department to be geriatric-friendly. Geriatric patients are a growing segment of the population with specific needs, making this area of the department one that is gaining popularity. Areas within the ED can be made geriatric-friendly with modifications to equipment and supplies typically found in the ED. Soft light is recommended, but exposure to natural light is also shown to be beneficial for recovery times and decreasing delirium (American College of Emergency Physicians, American Geriatrics Society, Emergency Nurses Association, Society for Academic Emergency Medicine, Geriatric Emergency Department Guidelines Task Force, 2014).

Stretchers should be left at levels low enough to allow for safe transfers. The mattress should be extra-thick or a pressure-redistributing foam mattress. Ideally, beds should have the ability to alarm should the patient be prone to wandering. Walkers and other mobility devices should be available. Monitors should be large enough for patients to view. Clocks and signage should be oversized. Rooms should be painted in contrasting colors so patients can differentiate where one wall ends and another begins. Floors should have a non-skid and non-glare finish and non-slip fall mats.

The ED designed for seniors should have warmer ambient temperature and include body-warming devices/warm blankets as well as additional space for family members to sit comfortably. The use of sound-absorbing materials such as carpet, curtains, and ceiling tiles may reduce background noise and can also increase patient privacy. The use of portable hearing assist devices for patients may also enhance communication. Sources of loud noise such as overhead paging and equipment should be reduced.

For less emergent presentations, large geriatric chairs may be more suitable for limited exams and easier for the elderly to transfer in and out of (American College of Emergency Physicians, American Geriatrics Society, Emergency Nurses Association, Society for Academic Emergency Medicine, Geriatric Emergency Department Guidelines Task Force, 2014).

Summary

Emergency nurses must care for patients with a wide variety of illnesses and injuries across the lifespan of the patient. This variation requires a workplace to be designed and supplied to facilitate a wide variety of conditions. You need to be familiar with all the areas in the

ED and ensure that each area is properly supplied and designed. A well-designed and supplied department not only ensures safer patient care but also creates a pleasant environment in which to work.

References

Agency for Healthcare Research and Quality (AHRQ). (2012). *Assessing utility of a "kiosk model" self-triage system in the pediatric emergency department of a tertiary care teaching hospital.* Retrieved from https://clinicaltrials.gov/ct2/show/NCT01515488

Albert, M., McCaig, L. F., & Ashman, J. J. (2013, October). *Emergency department visits by persons aged 65 and over: United States, 2009–2010.* Retrieved from http://www.cdc.gov/nchs/data/databriefs/db130.htm#how

American College of Emergency Physicians. (2007). *Emergency department planning and resource guidelines.* Dallas, TX: American College of Emergency Physicians.

American College of Emergency Physicians (ACEP). (2015, May 22). *Observation care payments to hospitals FAQ.* Retrieved from http://www.acep.org/Clinical---Practice-Management/Observation-Care-Payments-to-Hospitals-FAQ/

American College of Emergency Physicians, American Geriatrics Society, Emergency Nurses Association, Society for Academic Emergency Medicine, Geriatric Emergency Department Guidelines Task Force. (2014). Geriatric emergency department guidelines. *Annals of Emergency Medicine, 63*(5), e7–25. doi: 10.1016/j.annemergmed.2014.02.008. Retrieved from http://www.ncbi.nlm.nih.gov/pubmed/24746437

Bureau of Emergency Medical Services and Trauma Systems. (2014). *Trauma center designation scoring tool level IV.* Phoenix, AZ: State of Arizona. Retrieved from http://www.azdhs.gov/bems/documents/trauma/LevelIVScoringTool.pdf

California Hospital Association. (2011). *Decontamination.* Sacramento, CA: California Hospital Association. Retrieved from http://www.calhospitalprepare.org/decontamination

Centers for Disease Control and Prevention (CDC). (2012, August). *Wait time for treatment in hospital emergency departments: 2009.* Retrieved from http://www.cdc.gov/nchs/data/databriefs/db102.htm

Centers for Medicare & Medicaid Services. (2012). *Emergency Medical Treatment & Labor Act (EMTALA).* Retrieved from https://www.cms.gov/Regulations-and-Guidance/Legislation/EMTALA/index.html?redirect=/EMTALA/

Diane, A. (2014, October 1). Eliminate the waiting room. *InformationWeek.* Retrieved from http://www.informationweek.com/healthcare/patient-tools/eliminate-the-waiting-room/d/d-id/1316203

Dinardo, A. (2013, August 9). Waiting rooms: A thing of the past? *Healthcare Design.* Retrieved from http://www.healthcaredesignmagazine.com/blogs/anne-dinardo/waiting-rooms-thing-past

Gillespie, G. L., Gates, D. M., & Berry, P. (2013). Stressful incidents of physical violence against emergency nurses. *Onine Journal of Emergency Nursing, 18*(1). Retrieved from http://www.nursingworld.org/MainMenuCategories/ANAMarketplace/ANAPeriodicals/OJIN/TableofContents/Vol-18-2013/No1-Jan-2013/Stressful-Incidents-of-Physical-Violence-against-Emergency-Nurses.html

Hernandez, M. (2014, Spring). The new psych ED. *Emergency Physicians International.* Retrieved from http://www.cannondesign.com/assets/EPI-New-Psych-ED_Spring-2014.pd

InPro Corporation. (2012). *Bariatric design 101—An introduction to design considerations* [White paper]. Retrieved from http://www.healthcaredesignmagazine.com/sites/healthcaredesignmagazine.com/files/whitepapers/Bariatric-Design101.pdf

Kim, H. (2009). *Universal design: Meeting the needs of the bariatric population.* Retrieved from http://iwsp.human. cornell.edu/files/2013/09/Universal-Design-Meeting-the-Needs-of-the-Bariatric-Population-18360rc.pdf

Malone, E. B., & Dellinger, B. A. (2011, May). *Furniture design features and healthcare outcomes.* Retrieved from https://www.healthdesign.org/chd/research/furniture-design-features-and-healthcare-outcomes

Manton, A. (2013). *Care of the psychiatric patient in the emergency department.* Des Plaines, IL: Emergency Nurses Association.

Miller, S. (2014, October 4). *Temporary isolation rooms and their application to hospital surge capacity for infection control.* Retrieved from http://microbe.net/2014/10/04/temporary-isolation-rooms-and-their-application-to-hospital-surge-capacity-for-infection-control/

Richards, J. R., van der Linden, M. C., & Derlet, R. W. (2014). Providing care in emergency department hallways: Demands, dangers, and deaths. *Advances in Emergency Medicine.* Retrieved from http://www.hindawi.com/journals/aem/2014/495219/

U.S. Department of Homeland Security. (2014). *Patient decontamination in a mass chemical exposure incident: National planning guidance for communities.* Washington, DC: U.S. Department of Homeland Security.

Viccellio, P., Sayage, V., Chohan, J., Garra, G., Santora, C., & Singer, A. J. (2013). Patients overwhemingly prefer inpatient boarding to emergency department boarding. *Administration of Emergency Medicine, 45*(6), 942–946.

Wier, L. M., Yu, H., Owens, P. L., & Washington, R. (2013). *Overview of children in the emergency department.* Rockville, MD: Agency for Healthcare Research and Quality.

Zilm, F. (2004). Estimating emergency service treatment bed needs. *Journal of Ambulatory Care Management, 27*(3), 215–223.

Zilm, F., Crane, J., & Roche, K. T. (2010). New directions in emergency service operations and planning. *J Ambulatory Care Management, 33*(4), 296–306.

KEY PLAYERS IN THE EMERGENCY DEPARTMENT

–Pamela D. Bartley, BSN, RN, CEN, CPEN, CCRN;
Melanie Stoutenburg, BSN, RN, CEN; and
Jeff Solheim, MSN, RN-BC, CEN, CFRN, FAEN

The emergency department (ED) is often a chaotic environment requiring the collaboration of numerous healthcare professionals to care for the variety of patients who present for medical treatment. Gum, Prideaux, Sweet, and Greenhill (2012) noted that interprofessional collaboration often occurs between individuals from diverse professional qualifications who are actively attempting to provide services and resolve problems. Communication and teamwork are crucial for the delivery of safe, quality patient care (Gum et al., 2012). In order for communication and teamwork to be effective, nurses must maintain healthy work relationships between other nurses and healthcare providers in the ED.

This chapter gives you an overview of the various personnel you may work with in the ED and how they interact with each other.

Medical Care Providers

Medical care providers are important allies with emergency nurses in the ED. Medical care providers such as physicians, nurse practitioners, and physician assistants work alongside emergency nurses to ensure that the highest quality of care is provided to the acutely ill. Because there is an overlap between the role of medical care providers and nursing, the potential for friction between these two groups exists, but when medical care providers and nurses are able to work collaboratively, patient care excels. Because medical care providers are usually physically present in most EDs, there is frequently a stronger working relationship with nurses than what is found in other areas of healthcare.

Physicians

Physicians are healthcare professionals who complete an undergraduate degree, 4 years of medical school, internship, and residency. They graduate from an accredited medical school, complete national board examinations, and are licensed in the state in which they practice. Physicians practice the art and science of medicine.

Medical Doctor (MD)

Medical doctors attend traditional medical schools and deliver standard medical treatments, including medication and surgery. MDs practice allopathic medicine, a form of medicine focused on the diagnosis and treatment of human diseases. Physicians must complete undergraduate education, usually a bachelor's degree with a focus in the sciences, followed by 4 years of medical school. After medical school, they complete a residency program that can range from 3 to 7 years in length depending on the specialty they choose. Some go from residency to a fellowship to become proficient in certain specialized fields (Yang, 2014). The majority of physicians practicing in the United States are MDs.

 MDs focus on making a diagnosis and treating symptoms and diseases.

Doctorate of Osteopathy (DO)

A doctor of osteopathic medicine (DO) tends to focus on a holistic view of medicine, looking at the patient as a whole person rather than the symptoms apart from the patient. Osteopathic physicians are trained that stress or strain in the body's framework can directly influence diseases and conditions. They also prescribe medications but may also employ osteopathic manipulations for the whole body. Like an MD, a DO obtains an undergraduate degree before going to medical school for 4 years (American Osteopathic Association, 2015). DOs spend the same length of time in residency programs as MDs. Although a DO may approach a patient differently than an MD, both of these physicians receive very similar training and preparation to practice medicine and function in a similar manner in the ED.

DOs focus on the whole person and their lifestyle to prevent illness and treat diseases.

Both MDs and DOs complete medical school, internships, residencies, and fellowships. Both pass state licensing boards and are licensed to practice in all 50 states.

Attending Physicians/Consultants

Medical care providers employed in the ED only provide care for patients when they are in the ED and have generally not completed education or training to provide specialty care. When a patient requires specialty care or admission, an attending physician and consultant is called to assume the care of the patient. For example, although an emergency physician may reduce and immobilize a serious fracture during a visit to the ED, an orthopedic specialist provides the long-term complex care of that fracture. The patient may either be admitted to the hospital under the care of the orthopedic specialist as an attending physician or have a follow-up appointment established while in the ED for outpatient care with the orthopedic specialist as a consultant.

The ED requires an intimate working relationship with attending or admitting physicians (Beach et al., 2012). Attending physicians may be hospital-employed, such as hospitalists or internists, or they may be independent practitioners with privileges granted by the hospital to provide care in that institution. The physicians may see the patient in the ED to determine whether the patient should be admitted or discharged home. Some attending physicians may prefer to admit the patient without seeing the patient in the ED, utilizing basic inpatient orders, choosing to wait until they can arrive to the facility to examine the patient in the inpatient bed and formulate a more comprehensive treatment plan. Others may choose to visit the patient in the ED to determine whether admission is appropriate and provide thorough orders prior to the patient being transferred to the inpatient unit. Having multiple patients utilizing limited ED stretchers awaiting consultation and admitting orders by an attending physician has the potential to negatively affect efficient operations of the ED.

Hospitalist—A hospitalist is a physician, frequently employed by the hospital, to provide general medical care to hospitalized patients. Hospitalists frequently work shifts, like emergency nurses, and are generally available around-the-clock in the hospital to admit and care for patients on inpatient units.

Although referral of a patient to a consultant or attending physician usually occurs through the ED medical care provider, you'll frequently work with the consultant or attending physician to obtain orders for admission, establish an appointment for further patient follow-up, or provide necessary ongoing care in the ED collaboratively with the consultant or attending physician. Accurate and open communication between the nurse and the attending or consulting physician is required to avoid potential negative outcomes.

Medical Students

Medical school is generally 4 years in length. While an individual is in medical school, he or she will work in the clinical area, including the ED, to gain practical experience. Students who are still in medical school but working in the clinical area are *medical students*. Medical students have not yet completed their schooling and have limited ability to provide independent direct patient care. That care must always be supervised by a resident or physician. If you work in a teaching hospital, you'll frequently interact with medical students; you need to recognize the limitations of independent practice with medical students and work closely with the student's supervisor to ensure safe patient care.

Residents

When medical students successfully complete 4 years of medical school and graduate, they are *residents*. Traditionally, residents were referred to as interns during their first year out of medical school, but this term has been replaced with PGY-1 (post-graduate year one).

Because residents have graduated from medical school, they may assume the title of "doctor," but during their residency, they continue to practice under the direction of an experienced physician to ensure patient safety. Residents are referred to as "PGY-1" in their first year out of medical school; they will be referred to as "PGY-2" during their second year, and so on. It's common for residents with more experience to supervise the work of newer residents; a PGY-3 resident may supervise PGY-1 residents. It's also common for a senior resident to oversee all residents within the particular specialty in which they are working. All residents, including the senior resident, ultimately report to an attending physician who has successfully completed residency. If you work in a teaching hospital, you'll work directly with residents, both in the ED as emergency residents and residents who work for other specialties and come to the ED to consult or admit patients. Although residents generally have more experience than medical students, you need to recognize the hierarchical structure of residency and be prepared to take concerns about the practice of a resident to more senior residents or the attending physician when needed.

 Emergency medicine residency—A physician who plans to devote his or her life to being an emergency physician will usually choose an emergency medicine residency. Emergency medicine residencies take 3 or 4 years to complete, and the resident rotates through many different specialties in order to become the generalist that is required of an emergency physician, but much of the time will be spent working in the ED under the direction of the emergency physician.

Physician Assistants (PA)

Physician assistants are trained providers that complete a medical school–based curriculum and training but must work under the supervision of an attending physician (Kartha et al., 2014). Most PAs complete a bachelor's degree (often with a focus on the sciences) and have experience working in healthcare before attending PA school. PA school is 26 months in length and provides the graduate with a master's degree. PA school also involves more than 2,000 hours of clinical experience (American Academy of Physician Assistants, n.d.). EDs often utilize these practitioners to augment the rest of the medical team. PAs may be seen as a cost-effective strategy to manage patients with a lower acuity, thus expediting patient movement through an often overcrowded department. Kartha et al. (2014) confirm that care provided by a physician assistant is similar in quality to that of care by a physician. In addition to working in the ED, physician assistants may also be employed by primary care or specialty practitioners. Kartha et al. (2014) describe PAs in these instances as very task-oriented. They evaluate the patient, complete histories and physical examinations, and initiate orders for patients until the physician is able to make contact with the patient.

Nurse Practitioners (NPs)

A nurse practitioner (NP) functions similar to a PA and has overlying scopes of practice (Kartha et al., 2014). Whereas PAs complete a medical school–based curriculum, NPs are nurses who typically have completed a master's or doctoral degree. (For more information on educational requirements of the nurse practitioner, see Chapter 4, "Education of the Emergency Nurse.") The NP role may "cross the gap between nursing and medicine" (Li,

Westbrook, Callen, Georgiou, & Baraithwaite, 2013). These practitioners can often see patients who present to the ED with sub-acute conditions and can be employed by the hospital or attending providers to work in conjunction with them. NPs can also work more independently with less supervision than required for PAs in most states.

Major roles of physician assistants and nurse practitioners are to:

- Examine patients

- Order and interpret diagnostic tests

- Diagnose and treat medical disorders

- Educate patients

Scribes

Scribes work alongside staff, usually medical care providers, and function to facilitate the documentation of the patient record, including history and physicals, orders, and procedure notes. This allows the medical care provider more freedom to focus on patient care and needs without being burdened by tasks of documentation (Grimshaw, 2012). The medical care provider is still responsible for reviewing all documentation made by a scribe.

As the healthcare world has moved to electronic medical records, scribes have become less prevalent. Scribes are not taught to assess a patient and typically do not perform any hands-on medical training other than interviewing techniques and the use of basic personal protective equipment. Qualities of an efficient scribe include excellent listening skills, a good base knowledge of medical terminology, and the ability to type efficiently and spell correctly. Although some people choose to become a scribe as a career path, many scribes are students who plan on becoming PAs or physicians, using this job to earn money while developing skills they can use in their future career. Many universities give higher consideration to applicants applying for nursing or medical school who have experience working as a scribe (Scribe America, n.d.).

Overall, you'll have little professional interaction with scribes in the ED. Because the role of the scribe is to assist the medical practitioner with documentation as opposed to providing direct patient care, it is generally best for you to work directly with the medical practitioner as opposed to communicating through the scribe to ensure safe and efficient care.

Communication Between the Emergency Nurse and Medical Staff

The Joint Commission reports that communication failures are a leading cause of sentinel events in healthcare institutions (The Joint Commission, 2015). One foundation of safe care is clear oral and written communication. Many factors lead to breakdowns in communication in the ED. The chaotic and busy nature of the ED is an obvious cause. In some EDs, an outmoded model of care in which the physician is the "captain of the ship" may also contribute to communication breakdowns. RNs may be wary of approaching physicians or residents about concerns or assessment findings, and they may not question treatments when this environment exists. Similarly, if the medical staff does not pay close attention to written communication entered into the patient's record by the emergency nurse, this communication breakdown may be detrimental to the patient. It is incumbent on all members of the emergency care team to communicate frequently and clearly as well as welcome communication from other team members to ensure patient safety. For more information on the effects of communication failures on patient care, as well as strategies to improve these, see Chapter 12, "Risk Management and Quality Issues Affecting the Emergency Nurse."

Positions Frequently Supervised by the Emergency Nurse

The emergency nurse is responsible for providing care to assigned patients. That includes collecting patient data and developing, implementing, and evaluating a plan of care. Some EDs have sought to maximize the efficiency of their healthcare teams. Evans (2014) discussed how this effort to increase productivity and efficiency has led to the expansion of the roles of many healthcare workers with varied educational backgrounds, including those without higher educational degrees or certifications. "Supervision of unlicensed personnel is a growing responsibility of the licensed practitioner" (Hammond & Zimmermann, 2013, p. 3). The registered nurse (RN) must often delegate appropriate tasks to other healthcare workers. It is important to remember that as an RN, there are some nursing functions, such as assessment, planning, and evaluation, that cannot be delegated to unlicensed personnel (Hammond & Zimmermann, 2013).

Unlicensed Assistive Personnel (UAPs)

Unlicensed assistive personnel (UAPs) can come from varied educational backgrounds. They may be given a variety of titles in the ED including technician (ED tech), monitor technician (monitor tech), and nursing assistant. Some may only receive on-the-job training; others receive formal training as a certified nursing assistant (CNA) or a medical assistant (MA);

yet others receive training from nursing or medical school programs. Some healthcare facilities and organizations have developed their own specific requirements, role definition, and education for these personnel (Jenkins & Joyner, 2013). With appropriate teamwork and supervision, UAPs can be valuable team members. UAPs can alleviate the nursing workload, freeing up the RN to perform more complex patient care (Hammond & Zimmermann, 2013). Be familiar with your own state's Nurse Practice Acts and laws to verify what may and may not be delegated to a UAP. Some things commonly delegated include obtaining vital signs, splinting or casting with training and competency, minor wound care, monitoring intake and output, and activities of daily living such as eating, bathing, and positioning. Some organizations allow UAPs to perform phlebotomy and monitoring of cardiac rhythm strips, with specialized training and education (Jenkins & Joyner, 2013). Even though care is delegated to another healthcare worker, the nurse is still responsible for ensuring that the quality of care is maintained and the tasks are appropriate for delegation.

Unit Secretaries

Unit secretaries are often another type of unlicensed assistive personnel that are utilized in the ED. These individuals are the hub of communication for the department. The unit secretary is often the person who answers the patient call bell system and relays information to the nurses (Digby, Bloomer, & Howard, 2011). Other duties might include facilitating communication between departments for patient studies and results, paging and contacting various consulting physicians and other healthcare providers, assembling patient charts, and entering patient orders. Just as with other UAPs, the supervising RN is responsible for ensuring the quality of the unit secretary's work.

Licensed Practical Nurses (LPNs) and Licensed Vocational Nurses (LVNs)

Licensed practical nurses (LPNs) and licensed vocational nurses (LVNs) may also work in the ED. Although they are licensed personnel, they may not perform all the functions of a registered nurse. LPN's typically work under the direct supervision of an RN. LPNs usually complete a 2-year diploma level program (Whittingham, 2012). Scope of practice for the LPN may vary by state, and both the RN and LPN should become familiar with their state's regulations.

Paramedics/Emergency Medical Technicians (EMTs)

Paramedics and emergency medical technicians (EMTs) may work as care providers in the ED, even though they traditionally work as pre-hospital providers. (More information on the role of paramedic and emergency medical technicians in the pre-hospital setting is provided later in this chapter.) With the push to increase efficiency and productivity, some organizations have included them as part of the ED team. Although they can be invaluable members of the emergency care team, their role can also create challenges within the department.

While working with an ambulance service provider, these personnel can perform advance procedures, monitoring, and medication administration that they may not be able to perform when working in an institution. Laws vary by state as to what they are able to perform in the hospital or ED setting. It's important that you know the laws of your state to know how much patient care a paramedic or EMT can perform. Some states allow these healthcare workers to initiate IV therapy and administer certain medications when working in the ED setting; others classify them as UAPs with a very limited scope of practice.

Educational preparation of an EMT is variable depending on the state and the level at which the EMT is practicing. An EMT-Basic, for example, requires 120 to 150 hours of training. An EMT-Intermediate has additional training, often 300 to 350 hours of classroom and clinical instruction. An EMT-Paramedic is a 2-year program (EMS1.com, 2011; Study.com, n.d.).

 Even when care is delegated to another healthcare worker, you're still responsible for ensuring the quality of care is maintained and the tasks are appropriate for delegation.

Allied Personnel an Emergency Nurse Frequently Encounters

In addition to personnel that frequently work in the ED, there are numerous departments that play a major role in patient care in the ED setting. Again, laws vary by state, so be sure to investigate the scope of practice for staff of ancillary departments working with the ED.

Respiratory Therapists (RTs)

Respiratory therapists (RTs) are healthcare professionals specially trained in evaluating and providing respiratory-related patient care. Commonly you see RTs obtaining arterial or venous blood gases, administering nebulized medication treatments, assessing breath sounds and pulmonary function, and managing oxygen administration. Barnes, Gale, Kacmarek, and Kageler (2010) discussed that the role of the RT will continue to expand as organizations look for cost-effective ways to deliver care. Some states and facilities also allow RTs to perform advance procedures such as endotracheal intubation, monitoring of moderate sedation, and administration of emergency cardiac medications. RTs should be able to "administer and interpret the results of basic respiratory care techniques, pulmonary function, radiographic and laboratory studies" (Barnes et al., 2010, p. 601).

Pharmacists

Pharmacists are relatively new team members in many EDs. In fact, many EDs do not have a pharmacist in the department and rely on assistance and advice from pharmacists working in a pharmacy department that is in a different physical location than the ED.

Although physicians, advanced practice nurses, and registered nurses all receive training in pharmacology, the amount of time spent learning about medication pales in comparison to the 6 to 8 years required to become a pharmacist (Different Medical Careers, 2014). For that reason, having a pharmacist with such an in-depth knowledge of drugs physically present in the ED can significantly enhance medication safety and patient outcomes. In one study, medication errors dropped from 16.09 per 100 medication orders (before a pharmacist was present in the ED) to 5.38 medication errors per 100 medication orders after a pharmacist was introduced to the ED (Brown et al., 2008). Some of the roles that pharmacists play in the ED include (American Society of Health-System Pharmacists, Inc. [ASHP], 2011):

- **Direct patient care:** When pharmacists don't work in the ED, they rarely see the patients for whom they prepare medication; therefore, they're unable to determine the appropriateness of the medication order and the effectiveness of the medication regimen. When pharmacists can visit the bedside of patients, they may be able to make recommendations for improved therapeutic pharmacological regimens based on their assessment and can better assess the effectiveness of the medication administered.

- **Medication order review:** Medication orders must be reviewed to meet federal, state, and local regulations and accreditation guidelines. It's always safer to perform this review before the drug is administered rather than afterward. Pharmacists in the ED can review medication orders before administration and add an extra layer of security into the process to reduce the likelihood of an error.

- **Patient care involving high-risk medications and procedures:** The very nature of the ED makes it more vulnerable to medication errors. Life-saving drugs that have the potential to be fatal if given incorrectly must be administered rapidly in high-stress situations. Dosages, especially when caring for pediatric patients, must be calculated in real time. Utilizing the expertise and knowledge of the pharmacist to help oversee, prepare, and sometimes even administer these drugs decreases the risk for medication errors. The addition of the pharmacist to a resuscitation or other life-saving event provides an extra set of hands (along with exceptional knowledge) to handle medications, freeing up other health team members to perform other necessary tasks.

- **Toxicology emergencies:** The expertise pharmacists bring to the ED when caring for emergencies involving drugs—such as overdoses—is invaluable. The ability of the pharmacist to recognize toxidromes and recommend treatment may be indispensable to both the ED team and the patient.

- **Medication procurement and preparation:** When a pharmacist is in the department, he or she may be able to mix or prepare medications immediately. This reduces the time it would normally take to transport those medications from the pharmacy department.

- **Education:** The knowledge of a pharmacist can be invaluable to the entire ED. Pharmacists can serve as resources to prescribers, nurses, patients, and families. The education can be formal, such as providing discharge instructions to patients and their loved ones regarding medications or pharmaceutical in-services to the healthcare team. The education may be much less formal, including introducing a prescriber to a new medication alternative or offering advice to the emergency nurse on safer or alternate ways to administer medication.

Social Workers/Case Managers

Social workers and case managers represent another type of healthcare worker you interact with in the ED. The population visiting the ED, often laden with health disparities, has increased the need for intervention in the social circumstances of patients (Craig & Muskat, 2013). The social worker has historically performed this vital role in the care and disposition of ED patients. Social workers are prepared minimally with a bachelor's degree, and many have master's degrees. Case managers may come with a variety of educational backgrounds but are often nurses who have received additional training and experience in case management. With increasing disparities in healthcare, these personnel are often looked to for creative and alternative solutions for patients. Nursing-home placement, follow-up care, arranging home-health services, coordination of primary care services, facilitation in obtaining medication and other medical supplies, and discharge planning are just a few of the roles social workers and case managers fulfill.

Hospital Chaplains

True emergencies can precipitate crisis and emotional distress. Chaplains can be an integral member of the emergency team and can assist with providing comprehensive crisis care. Chaplains can sit with patients' family members and provide emotional and spiritual support while allowing nurses and physicians to focus on the medical aspects of treatment for the patient.

The Joint Commission requires healthcare facilities to provide a spiritual assessment and to help the patient to meet her or his spiritual needs (Saguil & Phelps, 2012). Chaplains nearly always have education and experience in this area, making them the ideal individuals to meet the intent of these Joint Commission standards. Chaplains not only focus on the needs of patients and their families but may also be called upon to assist staff in times of crisis. Hospital chaplains may be trained in critical incident stress management and be called to the ED to work with staff after a particularly difficult event. You should consider seeking the services of a chaplain when the stress of this demanding career takes its toll. For more information on spiritual care of the emergency nurse, see Chapter 6, "Self-Care and the Emergency Nurse."

Phlebotomists

Phlebotomists are often trained in formal programs and receive a certificate of completion for their program, but requirements vary by state. These healthcare workers usually have received numerous hours of training and are extremely proficient in obtaining venous or capillary blood from patients for various laboratory tests, blood typing, and blood cultures. Some organizations employ full-time phlebotomists in their EDs, while others only use phlebotomists from the laboratory department in certain situations.

Radiology Technicians

Radiology technicians are healthcare workers whose duties range from basic radiology technicians that perform standard X-rays to specially trained technicians who perform advanced or complicated radiology exams such as computerized tomography (CT), magnetic resonance imaging (MRI), ultrasounds, and/or nuclear medication studies. Some radiology technicians have also been trained to initiate IV access to administer contrast dye for studies and/or to place urinary catheters required for specific tests. Educational requirements for a radiology technician are greatly varied and can range from 1 year to an associate or even bachelor's degree, which may take 2 to 4 years of schooling.

Admission Clerks

Admission clerks have a variety of titles depending on the institution. Aside from an admission clerk, they may be known as registrars or access services personnel. They play an integral role in helping the institution to meet a variety of regulatory requirements, such as determining advance directives, as well as ensuring the hospital will be reimbursed for care by obtaining the patient's identifying and insurance information. This job class starts the medical record process. Clerks must have a solid medical terminology base and adhere to patient confidentiality. This job also requires strong computer and interpersonal skills. Admission clerks in the ED must also have a solid understanding of the Emergency Medical Treatment and Active Labor Act (EMTALA) to ensure that they do not inadvertently violate this law, prompting a potential investigation of the hospital. For more information on EMTALA, see Chapter 12.

Support Services

Other personnel, often known as support services, are vital to the ED. Support services can include housekeeping and dietary personnel. Although not medically trained, these team members can be invaluable to the overall functioning of the department.

Housekeeping

Housekeepers provide routine and extensive cleaning, which may be challenging in the ED due to its inherent busy atmosphere. Housekeepers clean surfaces and empty trash and linen hampers, keeping the department clean and tidy. Housekeepers may also be utilized to thoroughly decontaminate an area after use by a patient with a highly contagious or infectious diagnosis. Housekeepers can be trained to use advanced technology such as ultraviolet light disinfection systems (Schwartz-Cassell, 2015). The relationship you have with the housekeeping department may be integral to ensure a rapid throughput of patients as well as a reduction in transmission of infectious diseases.

Dietary Services

Dietary services may vary based on the size or location of the ED. They deliver various staples such as crackers, peanut butter, and ginger ale, and they may be responsible for delivering meal trays for ED patients for an extended period of time. Depending on facility policies, dietary staff may be limited in their patient interaction and may rely on the nursing staff to interact with the patients to meet their dietary needs. Although dietary services personnel and especially hospital dieticians rarely interact with the ED, you should always consider the contribution they can have in the ED. The dietician, for example, can provide consultation and education to the patient whose illness may be directly or indirectly related to diet, such as diabetes or obesity.

Pre-hospital Personnel

Pre-hospital personnel are key stakeholders in emergency care (Dawson, King, & Grantham, 2013). These include paramedics, emergency medical technicians (EMTs), first responders, firefighters, and police officers. Paramedics complete rigorous programs that prepare them to monitor, stabilize, and provide life-saving measures while transporting patients to medical facilities. First responders and firefighters receive some degree of training and basic resuscitation and first aid and are often the first people on the scene of a medical emergency. Laws, policies, and scopes of practice vary by state and organization. Most have standing orders and protocols that they can initiate to provide care during a transport to a facility. All of these personnel are vital to patient outcomes.

Maintaining healthy working relationships with allied health personnel is a necessity in the ED. Staff in the ED rely on the network of health personnel to effectively collaborate to provide quality patient care. This requires clear communication and trust, feedback, and ongoing learning. The care team must rely on pre-hospital personnel to accurately assess and relay pertinent information as well as provide stabilizing care (Dawson et al., 2013). The care team must also be able to effectively work together to provide the highest level of care to ensure positive patient outcomes. Although everyone has different roles and responsibilities in the ED, they must function together as a team.

Summary

Providing care to patients with emergency medical conditions is a complex task that requires multiple people with unique skills and training working collaboratively together to be successful. The emergency nurse is often the central hub coordinating the various individuals needed to provide thorough care to patients. Therefore, emergency nurses should have an in-depth knowledge of the key players that work in the ED and how they contribute to patient care.

References

American Academy of Physician Assistants. (n.d.). *Becoming a PA*. Retrieved from https://www.aapa.org/what-is-a-pa/

American Osteopathic Association. (2015). *Frequently asked questions*. Retrieved from http://www.osteopathic.org/osteopathic-health/about-dos/about-osteopathic-medicine/Pages/frequently-asked-questions.aspx

American Society of Health-System Pharmacists, Inc. (ASHP). (2011). ASHP guidelines on emergency medicine pharmacy services. *American Journal of Health-System Pharmacy, 68,* e81–95.

Barnes, T., Gale, D., Kacmarek, R., & Kageler, W. (2010). Competencies needed by graduate respiratory therapists in 2015 and beyond. *Respiratory Care, 55*(5), 601–616.

Beach, C., Cheung, D. S., Apker, J., Horwitz, L. I., Howell, E. E., O'Leary, K. J. … Williams, M. (2012). Improving interunit transitions of care between emergency physicians and hospital medicine physicians: A conceptual approach. *Academic Emergency Medicine: Official Journal of the Society for Academic Emergency Medicine, 19*(10), 1188–1195. doi:10.1111/j.1553-2712.2012.01448.x

Brown, J. N., Barnes, C. L., Beasley, B., Cisneros, R., Pound, M., & Herring, C. (2008). Effect of pharmacists on medication errors in the emergency department. *American Journal of Health System Pharmacy, 65*(4), 330–333.

Craig, S. L., & Muskat, B. (2013). Bouncers, brokers, and glue: The self-described roles of social workers in urban hospitals. *Health & Social Work, 38*(1), 7–16.

Dawson, S., King, L., & Grantham, H. (2013). Review article: Improving the hospital clinical handover between paramedics and emergency department staff in the deteriorating patient. *Emergency Medicine Australasia, 25*(5), 393–405. doi: 10.1111/1742-6723.12120

Different Medical Careers. (2014, January 22). *How long does it take to become a pharmacist?* Retrieved from http://differentmedicalcareers.com/how-long-does-it-take-to-become-a-pharmacist/

Digby, R., Bloomer, M., & Howard, T. (2011). Improving call bell response times. *Nursing Older People, 23*(6), 22–27.

EMS1.com. (2011, February 6). *What are the requirements to become a paramedic?* Retrieved from http://www.ems1.com/careers/articles/1058465-What-are-the-requirements-to-be-a-paramedic/

Evans, M. (2014). Expanding the team. Care delivery reforms create new roles for less-credentialed staff in patient care. *Modern Healthcare, 44*(38), 16, 18, 20.

Grimshaw, H. (2012). Physician scribes improve productivity. Oak Street Medical allows doctors to spend more face time with patients, improve job satisfaction. *MGMA Connexion / Medical Group Management Association, 12*(2), 27–28.

Gum, L. F., Prideaux, D., Sweet, L., & Greenhill, J. (2012) From the nurses' station to the health team hub: How can design promote interprofessional collaboration? *Journal of Interprofessional Care, 26*(1), 21–27. doi:10.3109/13561820.2011.636157

Hammond, B. B., & Zimmermann, P. G. (Eds.). (2013). *Sheehy's manual of emergency care, 7th ed.* St. Louis, MO: Elsevier Mosby.

Jenkins, B., & Joyner, J. (2013). Preparation, roles, and perceived effectiveness of unlicensed assistive personnel. *Journal of Nursing Regulation, 4*(3), 33–44. doi: http://dx.doi.org/10.1016/S2155-8256(15)30128-9

The Joint Commission. (2015, April 24). *Sentinel event data: Root causes by event type: 2004–2014.* Retrieved from http://www.jointcommission.org/assets/1/18/Root_Causes_by_Event_Type_2004-2014.pdf

Kartha, A., Restuccia, J. D., Burgess Jr., J. F., Benzer, J. K., Glasgow, J. M., Hockenberry, J. M., … Kaboli, P. J. (2014). Nurse practitioner and physician assistant scope of practice in 118 acute care hospitals. *Journal of Hospital Medicine, 9*(10), 615–620. doi: 10.1002/jhm.2231

Li, J., Westbrook, J., Callen, J., Georgiou, A., & Braithwaite, J. (2013). The impact of nurse practitioners on care delivery in the emergency department: A multiple perspectives qualitative study. *BMC Health Services Research, 13*, 356. doi: 10.1186/1472-6963-13-356

Saguil, A., & Phelps, K. (2012, September 15). The spiritual assessment. *American Family Physician, 86*(6), 546–550.

Schwartz-Cassell, T. (2015). Technology can improve housekeeping practices. *Long-Term Living, 64*(1), 22–23.

Scribe America. (n.d.). *What we expect.* Retrieved from https://www.scribeamerica.com/what_we_expect.html

Study.com. (n.d.). *EMT requirements and qualifications overview.* Retrieved from http://study.com/emt_requirements.html

Whittingham, K. (2012). Assistant practitioners: Lessons learned from licensed practical nurses. *British Journal of Nursing, 21*(19), 1160–1167.

Yang, K. (2014, October 24). *How long does it take to become a doctor?* Retrieved from http://www.medschoolpulse.com/2014/09/09/long-take-become-doctor/

THE EMERGENCY NURSE IN THE ROLE OF TRIAGE

–*Rebecca S. McNair, RN, CEN; and
Jeff Solheim, MSN, RN-BC, CEN, CFRN, FAEN*

The function of triage is unique to the practice of emergency nursing. Although nurses practicing in all clinical areas will have to perform assessments and are frequently forced to prioritize care based on those assessments, the additional challenges faced by the triage nurse in making complex assessments, taking independent actions based on those assessments, and making decisions that can have profound effects on the individual patient and the functioning of a department as a whole are unique to the emergency nurse. This chapter provides a brief overview of the role of the triage nurse and the process of triage.

The demanding role of triage requires an understanding of not only the functions of the triage nurse but also the underlying concepts involved. The complexity of a triage system implies that education and standardization are the best path to providing quality care in this arena. The Emergency Nurses Association's (ENA) *Standards of Practice* states clearly:

"The emergency nurse triages each patient and determines priority of care based on physical, psychological and social needs, as well as factors influencing flow through the emergency care system" (ENA, 2011a, p. 21).

Understanding What Triage Is

The word "triage" originates from the French verb "trier," which means "to sort" or "to choose." In the United States, it was first used as a medical term in the military in the 1930s. In the decades that followed, more physicians moved away from individual practice, house calls, and perpetual availability, causing patients to seek care in emergency departments (EDs). As hospital-based care grew, so did the number of patients waiting for that care. A new system for determining who needed immediate care in EDs became necessary, and the civilian world began adopting the triage system from military models to ensure that the sickest patients received the timeliest care. In the 1950s and '60s, triage principles were developed and adopted to address many of the same challenges facing EDs today. Currently, triage is performed in nearly every ED in the United States. This is a skill that is predominately specific to the profession of emergency nursing and not a skill required in most other nursing specialties. Triage is difficult, and if it is not carried out competently, it can result in dire consequences for the patients under your care.

 Triage—Noun: The assignment of degrees of urgency to wounds or illnesses to decide the order of treatment of a large number of patients or casualties. Verb: To assign degrees of urgency to wounded or ill patients (Triage, n.d.).

Triage should be a flexible and dynamic process because a patient's status can change dramatically and rapidly. It's a process by which patients are classified as to the type and urgency of their presentation to get the right patient to the right place at the right time with the right care provider, all the while allocating limited resources.

In the 1980s, due to evidence of "patient dumping," the U.S. Congress passed the Emergency Medical Treatment and Active Labor Act (EMTALA), which has had a profound regulatory impact on all aspects of emergency care, including triage. With the adoption of EMTALA regulatory standards, the U.S. Health Care Financing Administration (HCFA) made it clear that the triage examination in the ED was distinct and different from the mandated medical screening examination as defined by the statutes and accompanying regulations. For detailed information on EMTALA, see Chapter 12, "Risk Management and Quality Issues Affecting the Emergency Nurse."

Triage Nurse Qualifications

Staff in the triage role are usually geographically isolated and make critical decisions that affect not only the health of the patients, but also the health of the working environment of the treatment team as a whole. The triage team provides care for all patients and their significant others in the waiting area until additional ED resources are available. This makes the role of the triage nurse inherently autonomous and critical to the functioning of the ED as a whole. Therefore, it's essential to ensure the correct people are appointed to work in this area.

This is not to say that certain nurses only perform triage and take no other assignments while working in the ED, but rather that only a certain group of nurses, meeting specific requirements, are able to perform triage. This group may be small initially but should (with time, education, and mentoring) grow to include a larger number of the emergency nurses.

The general qualifications you need to be a triage nurse are (ENA, 2011b):

- Registered nurse who has completed a standardized triage education course that includes a didactic component and a clinical orientation with a preceptor prior to being assigned triage duties

- Current certification in CPR and ALS

- Completion of Emergency Nursing Pediatric Course (ENPC)

- Completion of Trauma Nursing Core Course (TNCC)

- Completion of Geriatric Emergency Nursing Education (GENE)

- Credentialed as a Certified Emergency Nurse (CEN) or Certified Pediatric Emergency Nurse (CPEN) (preferred)

- Diverse knowledge base

The personal qualifications you need to be a triage nurse are (ENA, 2011b):

- Strong interpersonal skills

- Excellent communication skills

- Strong critical thinking skills

- Ability to conduct a brief, focused interview

- Strong physical assessment skills

- Ability to make rapid, accurate decisions

- Ability to multitask yet focus

- Ability to provide patient education throughout the triage process

- Ability to work collaboratively with interdisciplinary team members

The Emergency Nurses Association position statement on qualifications of a triage nurse does not delineate a specific length of time (experience) as an emergency nurse prior to assuming the role of triage but states, "A specific amount of time and experience in emergency care alone may not ensure that a registered nurse is adequately prepared to function as a triage nurse" (ENA, 2011b, p. 1).

The triage nurse should embody "clinical expertise accompanied by an empathetic approach to patient care in the emergency department" (McNair, 2012, p. 7). Here are some critical-thinking qualities that will enhance the triage interview (Facione, 2011):

- **Inquisitive:** Ask appropriate questions. During the triage interview, seek further information from the patient or accompanying person(s) as appropriate to the patient's presentation and history.

- **Systematic:** Use a systematic approach to gather and consider information provided by the patient or the person(s) accompanying the patient. This decreases the likelihood of not obtaining information necessary to make the best decision possible.

- **Analytical:** Anticipate what happens next. For example, you should recognize the need to prepare for intubation in a patient in respiratory distress who has a sudden decrease in respiratory rate.

- **Truth-seeking:** When triaging patients, the truth must be sought with objectivity. For example, it's not difficult to lose objectivity in seeking the truth when interviewing a caregiver who presents with a child who has injuries that are consistent with non-accidental trauma.

- **Open-minded:** Eliminate bias, prejudice, and stereotyping when triaging patients.

- **Self-confident in the ability to reason:** Self-confidence enables you to make autonomous decisions.

- **Maturity:** Be willing to reconsider and revise views based upon new or more complete information.

Triage Systems

Triage nurses work within the triage system adopted by the institution in which they are working. There is a difference between a triage acuity scale and a triage system. A *triage acuity scale* is a sorting and prioritizing tool. A *triage system* may include a triage acuity scale, but it is much more than this. A system of triage not only *begins* the process of patient throughput, but it also, in many ways, *defines* the goals and outcomes of ED operations. A triage system is the basic framework in which patients are sorted, using one of the triage acuity rating scales, to determine priority of treatment. As early as 1982, Thompson and Daines described the three most common types of triage systems in use (Thompson & Daines, 1982), which are discussed in the upcoming sections.

Traffic Director

The *traffic director system* is the most basic form of triage in which little information is gathered except for the patient's presenting complaint. Assessment of the patient is minimal. Non-licensed staff without formal medical training or training in triage carry out this form of triage. Documentation is minimal. This system of triage is not recommended by the ENA. In fact, this system would be frowned upon by the federal government, because EMTALA makes it illegal for a clerk to obtain demographic or financial information if it delays the medical screening exam (MSE).

 EMTALA (Emergency Medical Treatment and Active Labor Act) —Part of COBRA (Consolidated Omnibus Budget Reconciliation Act of 1985), the EMTALA says that every person who comes to the ED shall receive a medical screening exam. EMTALA was passed by Congress in 1986 due to a growing concern regarding the availability of emergency healthcare services to the poor and uninsured.

MSE (medical screening exam)—An MSE is the process required to reach, with reasonable clinical confidence, the point at which it can be determined whether an emergency medical condition exists or a woman is in labor.

Spot Check

Spot check triage is carried out by a registered nurse who collects the patient's history as it relates to the chief complaint as well as limited subjective and objective assessments. At the completion of the process, the most seriously ill patients are given the highest priority for further care. Although established standards and protocols are utilized, variations in staff experience and ability may result in inconsistent triage decisions. This form of triage does not incorporate formal reassessment criteria for patients who may experience waits in the waiting area after triage. Documentation requirements vary.

Spot check triage is the most commonly used type of triage. Its priority is to identify the sickest persons and get them to the treatment area. However, the reality is that in many facilities using this approach, there remains a first-come, first-served mentality, with the use of sign-in sheets and other queuing devices.

The fact that there is little standardization with regard to triage reinforces the idea that ED triage nurses are an unprofessional "rag-tag bunch in the basement." This should serve as a strong incentive to continue to professionalize this approach in a scientific manner, committing to best-practice, evidence-based standards.

Comprehensive Triage

The most advanced form of triage is *comprehensive triage,* which is performed by registered nurses with appropriate education and experience. For this reason, ENA supports comprehensive triage. In order to make an informed triage decision, the triage nurse utilizes subjective and objective data including a medical history, health status, psychosocial components, and health behaviors to determine holistic healthcare needs. Discriminating categories for patient prioritization and acuity as well as written standards for assessment, planning, and intervention help ensure accurate triage decision. Protocols are in place to allow the initiation of diagnostic tests, selected treatments, and reevaluation of patients. Requirements for documentation help ensure this is properly carried out.

Implementing a Triage System

Regardless of the triage system utilized, certain industry standards can be used to evaluate the effectiveness of that system. A rapid triage assessment should be accomplished within 60 to 90 seconds; when necessary, a comprehensive assessment should be consistently performed within 2 to 5 minutes. Many studies have shown that a comprehensive triage assessment takes longer than these recommendations. The problem may be that too many triage nurses are attempting a comprehensive triage assessment without the necessary support systems in place, such as proper documentation tools, a controlled interview, discriminating categories for patient priorities, and appropriate use of treatment protocols and guidelines, as well as criteria for determining whether to use immediate bedding or perform a comprehensive triage assessment.

Immediate bedding—Placing the patient in a treatment bed prior to a comprehensive triage assessment. This can only occur when there are treatment beds available in the ED and a triage assessment would simply delay movement to the treatment area.

The following list summarizes the components that need to be in place to maximize the success of a triage system:

- **Physical plant:** An efficient triage area must be appropriately placed and have the tools necessary to perform the triage assessment.

- **Documentation tools:** Documentation is an important step in the triage process, and having the appropriate documentation tools that enhance rather than slow down triage is essential.

- **Acuity category scale:** A standardized acuity scale must be utilized to ensure consistency between providers.

- **Clinical expertise and systematic decision-making skills:** Triage nurses must have the skills and competencies to carry out the process.

- **Hospital and federal mandates:** Requirements by outside agencies and the institution for collecting information must not be onerous or it may slow down the triage process.

- **Appropriate use of protocols, clinical algorithms, and standing orders:** Triage nurses must have the tools to implement interventions in a timely manner to ensure rapid patient movement through the system.

- **Violence prevention and de-escalation training:** Because of the vulnerability of the triage nurse in an isolated area of the department, he or she must be given the training to feel safe enough to be effective in the role.

- **Customer service:** The role of customer service affects the patient's perception of the entire ED visit and even the entire hospital experience, so customer service cannot be stressed enough.

- **Pain management:** The triage nurse must be provided with the tools and knowledge to provide pain relief in a timely fashion.

- **ED triage concepts and process education:** Success in triage requires education to ensure success.

- **Effective patient throughput:** Effective triage requires not only the ability to manage the triage area but also the ability to understand and manage flow into the department; this includes patient chart management, appropriate disposition, patient tracking, outcomes measurement, bed management, and communication technology.

- **A thorough review of the literature:** Research reveals certain key strategies necessary for efficient clinical triage and point-of-entry processes.

- **A systematic, progressive, and reasonable approach.**

- **A controlled interview.**

- **Rapid and comprehensive assessments based on strict criteria for immediate bedding.**

- **A five-level acuity category scale:** Including discriminating categories for patient priorities.

- **Protocols, standing orders, clinical algorithms, and reassessment standards:** These must be developed and implemented appropriately.

- **Evaluation and support of triage competency.**

The Triage Process

A triage system determines the broad framework in which triage is carried out, but the way that you perform within that triage system is the *triage process*. The key to an efficient triage process is systematic data collection and the recording of that data. Triage education should focus on the nurse-driven interview, the systematic physical assessment of the patient, and the documentation of both the interview and the objective findings.

"Triage is not a PLACE...it is a PROCESS" (McNair, 2006, p. 11). Triage is one of several "point-of-entry processes" in an ED. And whether patients walk in to the ED, arrive by ambulance, or by privately owned vehicle, they still need to be prioritized, sorted, assigned appropriate acuity and disposition, and cared for utilizing the nursing process. Whether a rapid (focused) or comprehensive triage assessment is employed, a systematic decision-making process should be utilized as an overarching framework: across-the-room assessment (critical look), triage history (patient interview or subjective assessment), physical (objective assessment), triage decision (acuity and disposition). (See Figure 10.1.) The process of triage continues until the patient is placed in the treatment area and care is assumed by an appropriate care provider (an RN or an advanced practitioner) (McNair, 2012).

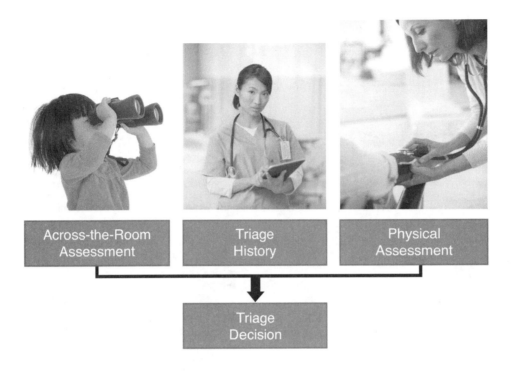

Source: McNair, 2012.

Figure 10.1 The triage process.

Here are the steps of the triage assessment process (see Figures 10.2 and 10.3):

1. **Take a critical look** (assess patient from across the room).

2. **Obtain the chief complaint from the patient.**

3. **Perform and document rapid triage assessment on all arriving patients** (identifying and facilitating placement of patients who meet immediate bedding criteria).

4. **Perform and document comprehensive triage assessment** (if patient does not meet immediate bedding criteria).

5. **Determine and document acuity level and disposition,** using a specific triage acuity scale.

6. **Initiate appropriate nursing interventions and/or diagnostics** (by common nurse practice or advanced triage protocols, or under the direction of a licensed independent practitioner [LIP]).

7. **Reassess patient according to specific triage acuity scale objectives and/or reassessment policy.**

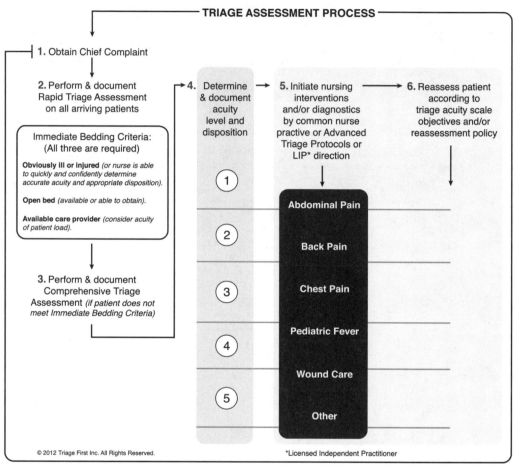

Source: McNair, 2012.

Figure 10.2 The triage assessment process.

Immediate bedding criteria (all three are required):

- Obviously ill or injured (or nurse is able to quickly and confidently determine accurate acuity and appropriate disposition)

- Open bed (currently available or able to obtain rapidly)

- Available (nursing or physician) care providers (consider acuity of current patient load)

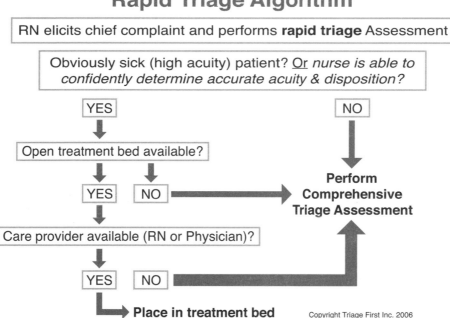

Source: McNair, 2012.

Figure 10.3 The rapid triage algorithm.

The Critical Look (Across the Room Assessment)

An astute triage nurse can make many observations before the patient even arrives in the triage area or the initial assessment has begun. The part of the triage assessment that is accomplished without obtaining subjective data from the patient is sometimes referred to as an *across the room assessment*. Some of these initial observations may be utilized to make a rapid triage decision. The triage nurse should utilize nearly all of the senses as part of this decision:

- **Sight:** Everything from skin color (pink versus pale versus cyanosis) to facial expression (relaxed versus stressed versus pain) can help the triage nurse begin the process of sorting the sick from the less-sick. The patient's method of arrival (ambulatory versus wheelchair versus stretcher) and the way the patient interacts with those that accompany him or her will also give some clues before any words are exchanged.

- **Hearing:** Certain sounds heard during the "critical look phase" may give the triage nurse hints as to the acuity and final destination of the patient. Sounds such as stridor, wheezing, muffled voice, halting speech patterns, quality of the cough, and auditory indications of pain may give clues to the need for a higher acuity.

- **Smell:** A fruity odor on the breath indicates potential ketoacidosis, whereas the smell of coal gas on the breath can be indicative of carbon monoxide poisoning. The smell of poor hygiene may indicate a lack of resources to maintain hygiene, but it can also indicate an individual who is too ill to be able to provide for basic hygiene needs. Your nose can be a strong tool during the across the room assessment.

- **Touch:** A good rule of thumb is to touch every patient. Is the skin warm? Dry? Cool? Clammy? What is the patient's reaction to being touched? Many findings that may influence the triage decision can be partially formed through the sense of touch.

- **Intuition:** Your sixth sense should never be overlooked as an important tool in the arsenal needed during the triage assessment. Always pay attention to that "unsettled" feeling of intuition and consider a higher triage priority when you feel it.

The Chief Complaint

While an across the room assessment is being performed, you must find out why the patient is in the ED. There are times that this step alone may bring an end to the triage process and require immediate movement of the patient to the treatment area. Even if this is not the case, eliciting the chief complaint helps guide the assessments to follow.

A patient walks into triage, and when the triage nurse asks what brings the patient to the department, he relates that he has this "excruciating ripping and tearing pain" in his chest that radiates through to his back. Would this change the urgency of the triage process to follow?

Rapid and Comprehensive Triage Assessment

How we look at the world determines what kind of world we find. As Werner Heisenberg (1962), a theoretical physicist and one of the key pioneers of quantum mechanics, cautions us: "We have to remember that what we observe is not nature itself but nature exposed to our method of questioning" (p. 56). As you engage with patients when performing triage, you must recognize that what you discover in your questioning is not the patient's situation itself but the patient exposed to your method, or line of questioning.

Excellent triage nurses learn how to elicit information by asking the right questions in the right way. The use of open-ended questions reduces error and improves accuracy during patient interviews. This is not necessarily a skill that most triage nurses bring to the role with them. It must be learned and honed, but once mastered, it can yield some of the most accurate triage decisions.

Open-ended question—A question that cannot be answered with a "yes" or a "no." Consider the following two questions: "Can you describe your pain to me?" versus "Would you describe your pain as crushing?" The first question is open-ended; the second question is not.

There are times when you should gather not only information about the current illness but also data about the patient's past medical history, especially if it is likely to pertain to the patient's presenting complaint. Remember, however, that triage should ideally occur in a short period of time, and the history you gather should be limited to things that are pertinent to the triage decision. Here's a mnemonic device that can be used as a reminder of the components of a patient's history that may be useful in the triage process (Gurney & Westergard, 2014, p. 48):

S: Symptoms associated with the injury

A: Allergies and tetanus status

M: Medication history

P: Past medical history

L: Last ... oral intake, menstrual period

E: Events leading to the illness or injury

The triage assessment should also include a limited physical exam as necessary. Whenever possible, visualize the area of the complaint, comparing assessment findings bilaterally for symmetry or lack thereof.

An important component of the assessment process is documentation of findings. Efficient documentation and process flow largely determine in what manner and how rapidly the data is recorded. The hallmarks of good triage documentation are both brevity and clarity.

Determine and Document Triage Acuity

Because triage is ultimately about sorting out patients, assigning a triage acuity is an important component of the triage process. Currently, there is not one specific triage rating scale identified as a national triage scale for the United States.

An acuity categorization scale is never absolute; it must be flexible to take into account your own judgment. And although the balance of subjective and objective information will often lead triage nurses to agree on the acuity of certain presentations, due to all the variables of the human condition, acuity categorization should not (at this time at least) be considered an exact science.

If the goal of triage is to just grab the "sickest" persons and take them to the treatment area, you'll succeed in a prioritization of the obvious, but assigning accurate acuity and appropriate disposition is a much more complex task for the majority of patients presenting to EDs, and this task must be accomplished in a rapid, efficient, and expert manner.

Clinical prioritization strategies in triage include:

- Systemic over local
- Life before limb
- Acute over chronic pain

Since 2005, the Emergency Nurses Association (ENA) and the American College of Emergency Physicians (ACEP) have continued to support the migration to a uniform national five-level triage system (Fernandes, 2005). The ENA and ACEP currently do not endorse a specific five-level system but simply recommend a statistically valid and reliable five-level system.

Because the United States has not adopted a standardized triage acuity system, individual institutions may choose which acuity system they want to adopt. There are many acuity systems currently available, and while an institution may choose to adopt any of these systems, it's imperative that the institution provide training to all staff who use the system to ensure it is used uniformly. The following sections discuss a few current triage acuity systems.

Canadian Triage and Acuity Scale

The Canadian Triage and Acuity Scale (CTAS) is a robustly developed tool as a triage system and acuity scale and conceptually supports nurse-led triage, provides the ability to assign acuity based on symptomatic presentations, and does not take into consideration the patient's likely diagnosis or expected diagnostic/treatment resources.

CTAS guidelines allow users to reference each "usual" presentation of the patient in connection with a specific list of chief complaints. For example, people who are diagnosed with acute myocardial infarction (AMI) or acute coronary syndrome (ACS) usually present with chest pain along with visceral symptoms; therefore, these presentations fit into the emergent category. The same presentation of chest pain without associated visceral symptoms, risk factors, or severe pain might receive a lower acuity categorization.

The CTAS provides operational objectives (the recommended time that a patient is triaged and receives appropriate care) and fractile responses, both of which are valuable for benchmarking. (See Table 10.1.) When any facility is unable to meet these objectives, root cause analysis can be employed effectively, resulting in either individual practitioner education, process redesign, or proper allocation of resources.

 Fractile responses—The fractile response is a way of describing how often a system operates within its stated objectives. CTAS also provides reassessment guidelines per acuity level.

 CTAS implementation guidelines and revisions are available at www.caep.ca/resources/ctas.

Table 10.1 Canadian Triage and Acuity Scale

Level	Description
I – Resuscitation	Should receive medical care immediately 98% of the time (fractile response), and 70%–90% of these patients are likely to be admitted.
II – Emergent	Should receive medical care within 15 minutes 95% of the time (fractile response), and 40%–70% are likely to be admitted.
III – Urgent	Should receive medical care within 30 minutes 90% of the time (fractile response), and 20%–40% are likely to be admitted.
IV – Less Urgent	Should receive medical care within 60 minutes 85% of the time (fractile response), and 10%–20% are likely to be admitted.
V – Non-urgent	Should receive medical care within 120 minutes 80% of the time (fractile response), and 0%–10% are likely to be admitted.

Source: Canadian Association of Emergency Physicians [CAEP], 2008, 2013.

Emergency Severity Index

Emergency Severity Index (ESI) is also a research-based, descending, algorithmic, five-level acuity scale, based on evaluating both patient acuity (for the top two levels) and then expected resource needs (for the bottom three levels). The original concept of ESI was developed by Drs. Richard Wuerz and David Eitel and brought to its present state (Version 4) by the ESI Triage Group, which consists of "emergency nursing and medical clinicians, managers, educators, and researchers" (Gilboy, 2012, p. v).

 For more information, see the *Emergency Severity Index (ESI): A Triage Tool for Emergency Department Care Version 4.* Implementation Handbook 2012 Edition. For access, email AHRQPubs@ahrq.hhs.gov or download at www.ahrq.gov/research/esi.

The Australasian Triage Scale and Manchester Triage System

The Australasian Triage Scale (ATS) and the Manchester Triage System (MTS) are also fully developed, valid, and reliable five-level, symptom-driven, nurse-led triage systems and acuity scales. The ATS uses a conceptual line of questioning, and the MTS uses a symptom-specific algorithmic approach with over 50 flow charts.

Initiate Appropriate Nursing Interventions and Diagnostics

The role of the triage nurse extends beyond assessment and assigning a triage priority. Frequently, you must provide care to patients who present to the triage area. Nurse-initiated interventions may be employed, of course, at any step in the triage process. It's appropriate to consider this step whether the patient is taken immediately to a treatment bed, remains in the triage arena, or is placed in a formal Rapid Medical Evaluation zone.

 Rapid Medical Evaluation—A licensed independent practitioner (LIP) performs an evaluation and orders diagnostic procedures while keeping the patient from entering the main ED treatment area. Usually situated near the point of entry, kept vertical, and sometimes returned to the waiting area while awaiting return of diagnostics.

If beds and/or resources are not available, many effective patient throughput strategies have been employed such as Team Triage, Rapid Medical Evaluation (RME), and Advanced Triage/Advanced Initiatives (AT/AI) utilizing protocols, clinical pathways and guidelines, and standing orders.

 Team Triage—A physician-and-nurse team assess the patient together and determine if lab work is needed. The patient goes directly to a phlebotomy chair where laboratory studies are drawn, and he can have his lab work processed while he waits for a treatment bed to become available.

Advanced Triage/Advanced Initiatives—The combined application of first aid, common nurse practice acts, and treatment protocols or standing orders.

First Aid and Comfort Measures

Interventions must begin with the basics, the non-negotiable provisions of supportive clinical care: providing both stabilizing nursing care and first aid or comfort measures. It is easy to get caught up in the excitement of advanced practice with the discussion of protocols and then to forget foundational nursing care.

Often, in fact, when the appropriate first aid or comfort measures have been rendered, the need for advanced interventions (specifically pain medication) is reduced. Consider a 12-year-old patient who presents with obvious shoulder dislocation from a football injury.

The application of ice with elevation and proper splinting may not only comfort this patient but also decrease his acuity level (as his pain is managed) and prevent the need for some other pain protocol to be initiated.

Such basic nursing care is within the scope of *every* nurse, and yet is often neglected, whereby emergency nurses then give up their high standard of excellence and autonomy of practice. Most emergency nurses cherish this autonomy (that ability to act immediately based upon their keen assessment skills) and love emergency care for this reason, but when there is failure in the basics, that autonomy is undermined and questioned by licensed practitioner colleagues.

Lest you become complacent and think that this is no longer applicable, a study published by McQueen and Gay (2010) found that over 71% of patients presenting over a 1-year period with a confirmed diagnosis of acute traumatic shoulder dislocation did not have a pain score recorded. The study indicates that up to 38% of cases of acute traumatic shoulder dislocation went unrecognized, with associated delays in diagnostic interventions as well as pain interventions. This again confirms that as a triage nurse, you set the trajectory of care throughout the patient's entire stay in the ED.

Advanced Triage Protocols (ATPs)

Beyond initiating basic nursing assessment and care, it's also within your scope to initiate appropriate and collaboratively derived treatment protocols, clinical algorithms, pathways, or standing orders. Combining triage protocols with this practice is referred to as *advanced triage protocols*.

Caution is advised. Nurses practicing advanced triage protocols and interventions must be knowledgeable, clinically current, and experienced in emergency nursing. How do you measure the knowledge base and clinical expertise of a triage nurse? This has proven to be difficult because, although a triage nurse may have many years of experience, the years alone do not quantify expertise. There are nurses with longevity of practice who have not read a journal or attended continuing education in years! Conversely, there are relatively new nurses who yearn for every new learning opportunity. Therefore, the emphasis must be placed upon careful and individual evaluation of the clinical astuteness of each individual nurse.

If nurses could order appropriate diagnostic tests from triage, physicians would have most of the necessary information to make disposition and treatment decisions after obtaining the patient's history and physical. This has the potential to decrease patient time in the ED, decrease overall costs, facilitate patient care, improve patient satisfaction, increase the consistency of care, and improve teamwork.

With all this said, why would any staff member (nurse or physician) oppose the use of advanced triage protocols? Yet we know through direct observation and recent literature that as a group, triage nurses vary significantly in the consistent use of established protocols. A study by Fosnocht (2007, p. 791) analyzed the effect of a triage pain protocol, finding that "individual triage nurse compliance varied between 8% and 96%." And this issue continues: "Despite advanced triage protocol implementation, 37% of triage nurses deviated from practice guidelines" (Wiler, 2010, p. 155). The explanation for noncompliance or opposition may lie in the possibility that a nurse performing triage is not knowledgeable, clinically current, or experienced. The proper use of protocols critically rests on these nursing qualities, as well as the proper development and implementation of advanced triage protocols. Because of staffing constraints, a new or less experienced nurse is often placed in the role of triage nurse. This nurse has less clinical experience and may not easily recognize the less-obvious or atypical clinical presentation.

It should also be noted, however, that the proper use of protocols by nurses can be a tremendous teaching/training tool, and it can even level the playing field for the less-experienced nurse in the treatment area.

Occasionally, the emergency nurse may be encouraged to "do what needs to be done" and get the order later. Unless it is an emergent situation and the action is covered by a protocol (e.g., treating an arrhythmia via an ACLS algorithm), this is unacceptable. For example, an emergency nurse may be asked in reference to administering acetaminophen: "Can't we get an order from a physician at the beginning of the shift to cover the patients we see that day?" And some nurses are told by physicians, "You know what the patient needs—go ahead and do it and I will write the order later." Should a nurse choose to go ahead and perform such an action, that nurse can be held responsible for practicing medicine without a license.

All protocols must be held to this standard. Collaboration between physicians and nurses begins the process. Training of all staff ensures the consistency of usage. But that is not enough. All protocols must be reviewed regularly to evaluate their efficacy and appropriateness. They must also be subjected to ongoing evaluation through some quality assurance (QA) process. And finally, there must be a well-defined process for ensuring that the protocol is properly authenticated (by means of the licensed independent practitioner's signature) and becomes part of the permanent medical record.

First aid and all of the other standards of care and practice become the foundations of emergency triage and nurse-initiated interventions. You must not neglect them as you move toward advanced practice, and you must make certain that they are all permanently recorded in the medical record.

You might believe that advanced triage protocols are facing a slow demise. That would be incorrect. The literature reveals that research to determine best practices regarding the use of advanced triage protocols is ongoing.

You should remain current not only with what is determined by regulatory and governmental agencies in the future but also your professional organization, your state board of nursing, and the Nurse Practice Act.

Patient Disposition

Triage decision-making is based not only on the acuity of the patients and their clinical and nursing needs but also on managing appropriate disposition, order, and safety of the ED as a whole.

Traditional triage has often wrongly been interpreted by ED staff as queuing patients in either a first-come, first-served fashion or making the patient "jump through hoops" by forcing every single patient (other than those needing resuscitation) to follow a rigid process of providing her chief complaint to either a nurse or technician or even to a registration clerk; receiving a comprehensive assessment; full registration; and then, when a specific treatment bed becomes available, the patient is placed in a room to be seen by a physician. However, in the last few decades, much work has been done both in the literature and through various modes of education to establish that highly functional ED triage must be a flexible and dynamic process that incorporates different strategies and elements of point-of-entry assessment and disposition according to particular professional, clinical, and operational judgments.

In order to move from a first-come, first-served mentality, many EDs have employed a "pull-until-full" or "split flow" strategy. Although these initiatives certainly move patients out of the waiting areas, when implemented incorrectly, they may move the bottleneck to the treatment area and cause a nursing nightmare in which patients are in a treatment bed with no nurse available to assess the patient. Therefore, certain process parameters and specific criteria need to be established when making the decision of immediate bedding to avoid these nursing nightmares. And while a comprehensive triage assessment is certainly appropriate for the non-emergent patients, when all beds are full in the ED, the first appropriate action should always be to attempt immediate bedding and bedside registration when possible.

Pull until full—Moving patients from entry directly to an open treatment bed. This strategy may also be known as *immediate bedding*.

Split flow—Patients are split into two categories. Sicker patients are sent to a treatment bed and become horizontal patients (on a stretcher). Those with minor injuries or ailments are provided diagnostic test and treatments but are kept in an area where they are vertical (not placed on a stretcher). This system maintains treatment bays in the ED open and available for sicker patients and improves efficiency of the ED.

Ambulance Triage

Those patients arriving by ambulance should also receive a triage assessment prior to being placed in a treatment room. This may be carried out in locations separate from the traditional triage area, often by the charge nurse or a bed flow coordinator, as long as this nurse is skilled in performing triage. In gravely ill patients, the EMS report may solely indicate a high triage priority and suffice as a rapid triage assessment. However, if a triage assessment proves a lower level acuity, the patient may be placed in the queue with other ambulatory patients. This would be an appropriate disposition because the mode of transportation should not prioritize treatment-area bed assignment.

Critically ill or injured patients get triaged too, whether they arrive by EMS or by private vehicle. Remember: Triage is a process, not a place.

Not all facilities care for trauma patients, but all facilities do at least occasionally care for critically ill patients. And, because triage is a point-of-entry process, this patient population and their initial assessment must be addressed as fully as walk-in patients so that they have the opportunity to be taken smoothly through an ED intake process.

Common Pitfalls in Triage

There are some common pitfalls awaiting every triage nurse. These pitfalls can interfere with the use of critical thinking skills and negatively affect the correct triage decision. The following sections discuss some of those pitfalls.

Concentrating Solely on the Presenting Complaint

Never assume what you see is the whole picture.

Every triage nurse has seen the mystery patients who have come in, been triaged, seen the physician, received treatment, and then have gone home—and the staff never really knows why they came. Was it for almshouse needs? Were they victims of domestic violence but no one picked up on the clues?

All staff must step back and look at the whole picture.

Failing to Elicit the Right Information

It's your job as a triage nurse to be the frontline detective. Often, patients misinterpret their symptoms and fail to communicate well with the nursing staff. After all, they believe you're getting paid to know what is wrong with them.

Utilize open-ended questions. Keep asking questions if the picture is not clear. If you cannot ascertain a clear picture, consider assigning a higher triage level.

Losing Objectivity

Patients seen frequently are at risk for potentially life-threatening illness or injury that may go unrecognized because of the loss of objectivity.

Remember: All patients returning within 72 hours of their last visit and heavy users of the medical system must have a thorough and unbiased assessment.

Becoming Distracted by Too Many Patients

Having to address multiple patients can distract you from focusing appropriately. Staffing may need to be adjusted for better coverage at peak hours; however, there are three steps that can help sort out the crowd at the triage desk:

1. **Focus on the ABCs (airway, breathing, and circulation).**

    Every few seconds, look around the room and confirm that everyone has an intact airway, everyone is breathing, and most everyone is not pale or diaphoretic. Address patients with deficiencies in their ABCs first.

2. **Elicit the chief complaint from each new patient.**

    This includes distinguishing between patients and significant others who have accompanied them. Prioritize those chief complaints.

3. **Decide who gets immediate assessment and treatment and who can wait for a full comprehensive triage.**

Becoming Isolated and Stressed Out

Triage is one of the most geographically isolated spots in most EDs. You have fewer resources (ancillary assistance, supplies, crash cart, snacks, etc.); you may often be forgotten on the list of staff lunches and breaks. The high patient-to-nurse ratio, lack of resources, and little relief spells S-T-R-E-S-S. And stress can take its toll on effective critical thinking.

Quality patient care *demands* that you take breaks. Therefore, don't forget your biological functions. Triage *cannot* be manned by a volunteer or by registration personnel—even to allow you to take a quick bathroom break or grab a snack. Protecting the lobby starts by protecting the triage nurse. (For more information on self-care for emergency nurses, see Chapter 6.)

Improper Use of Equipment

In addition to considering all the clinical possibilities, you must use your equipment properly. Misuse of the most common tools may lead to poor outcomes for your patients. For example, you must use the appropriate-sized blood pressure cuffs. And when taking temperatures, tympanic temperatures are dependent on user technique and are not appropriate for small children and the very elderly, or for anyone who has come in from outside when the weather is hot or cold (McCallum & Higgins, 2012). Pulse oximetry must be viewed carefully. If a patient is cold or alkalotic, the oxyhemoglobin dissociation curve shifts to the left. The result is an oxygen saturation that is higher than normal, but the oxygen cannot easily dissociate from the hemoglobin at the tissue level. This leads to less-effective tissue oxygenation in the face of a high or good oxygen saturation reading. Other factors may decrease the accuracy of pulse oximetry such as the presence of abnormal hemoglobin molecules (i.e., carboxyhemoglobin or methemoglobinemia) (ENA, 2015).

Lack of Excellent Communication Skills

Lengthy waiting times are the greatest source of patient dissatisfaction with an ED visit. But studies reveal the dissatisfaction is more about the psychology surrounding the experience of waiting than about the actual wait times. One study concluded that perceptions regarding waiting time, information delivery, and expressive quality predict overall patient satisfaction, but actual wait times do not. "Therefore, providing information, projecting expressive quality, and managing wait-time perceptions and expectations may be a more effective strategy to achieve improved patient satisfaction in the ED than decreasing actual wait time" (Thompson, Yarnold, Williams, and Adams, 1996, p. 665).

Summary

Emergency departments represent a microcosm of the communities in which we live. Triage is a critical role for any emergency nurse to aspire to—a role in which both autonomy and excellence in holistic nursing care can be practiced with amazing and life-altering results, for you as well as the patient. You have the opportunity and the ability to provide the highest level of nursing care using critical thinking skills, clinical expertise, and compassion.

References

Canadian Association of Emergency Physicians (CAEP). (2008). *Revisions to the Canadian Emergency Department triage and acuity. CTAS guide to implementation.* Retrieved from http://caep.ca/resources/ctas/implementation-guidelines

Canadian Association of Emergency Physicians (CAEP). (2013). *CTAS implementation guidelines, 2013 revisions to CTAS guidelines.* Retrieved from http://caep.ca/resources/ctas#guidelines

Emergency Nurses Association (ENA). (2011a). *Emergency nursing: Scope and standards of practice.* Des Plaines, IL: Emergency Nurses Association.

Emergency Nurses Association (ENA). (2011b). *Triage qualifications position statement.* Des Plaines, IL: Emergency Nurses Association.

Emergency Nurses Association (ENA). (2015, January). *Course in Advanced Trauma Nursing II: A conceptual approach to injury and illness.* Des Plaines, IL: Emergency Nurses Association.

Facione, P. A. (2011). *Critical thinking: What it is and why it counts (2011 update).* Retrieved May 14, 2011, from http://www.insightassessment.com/pdf_files/What&Why2010.pdf

Fernandes, C. G. (2005). Five-level triage: A report from the ACEP/ENA five-level triage task force. *Journal of Emergency Nursing, 31*(1), 39–50.

Fosnocht, D. E. (2007). Use of a triage pain protocol in the ED. *The American Journal of Emergency Medicine, 25*(7), 791–793.

Gilboy, N. T. (2012). *Emergency Severity Index (ESI): A triage tool for emergency department care, Version 4.* Rockville, MD: U.S. Department of Health and Human Services, Agency for Healthcare Research and Quality (AHRQ).

Gurney, D., & Westergard, A. M. (2014). Initial assessment. In E. N. Association, *Trauma nursing core course* (7th ed., pp. 39–54). Des Plaines, IL: Emergency Nurses Association.

Heisenberg, W. (1962). *Physics and philosophy: The revolution in modern science.* New York, NY: Harper & Row Publishers.

McCallum, L., & Higgins, D. (2012). Measuring body temperature. *Nursing Times, 108*(45), 20–22.

McNair, R. (2006). *Patient safety through managing triage and emergency department workflow. Triage First Education; Comprehensive emergency department triage course workbook.* Fairview, NC: Triage First, Inc.

McNair, R. (2012). *ED triage systematics: ED triage comprehensive course.* Fairview, NC: Triage First, Inc.

McQueen, C. G., & Gay, K. J. (2010). Retrospective audit to triage of acute traumatic shoulder dislocation by emergency nurses. *Journal of Emergency Nursing, 36*(1), 21–25.

Thompson, D., Yarnold, P., Williams, D., & Adams, S. (1996). Effects of actual waiting time, information delivery, and expressive quality on patient satisfaction in the emergency department. *Annals of Emergency Medicine, 28,* 657–665.

Thompson, J. D., & Daines, J. E. (1982). *Comprehensive triage.* Reston, VA: Reston Publishing Company, Inc.

Triage. (n.d.). In *Merriam Webster's online dictionary* (11th ed.). Retrieved from http://www.merriam-webster.com/dictionary/triage

Wiler, J. G. (2010). Optimizing emergency department front-end operations. *Annals of Emergency Medicine, 55*(2), 142–160.

11

COMMON CHALLENGES FACED BY EMERGENCY NURSES

–Brian Selig, DNP, RN, CEN, NEA-BC;
Fred Neis, MS, RN, CEN, FACHE, FAEN; and
Jeff Solheim, MSN, RN-BC, CEN, CFRN, FAEN

Emergency departments (EDs), and more specifically hospitals/health systems, are an anchor to communities, much like churches and schools. They form the infrastructure for a population of people, and hospitals are the cornerstone to creating healthy communities. The emergency nurse faces numerous challenges, which can interfere at any given time with the delivery of safe, high-quality emergency care to the ill and injured. Emergency departments are really the only hospital unit that has to be elastic. The ED is unable to truly stop the flow of incoming patients, so beds and staffing can be stretched well past their design. As volumes, acuities, service expectations, operating boundaries (e.g., staffing, space), financial pressures, declining numbers of EDs, and in general the ever-changing landscape of healthcare delivery in total evolve, it's imperative that emergency nurses recognize the challenges and take steps to mitigate them as much as possible. (See Figure 11.1.)

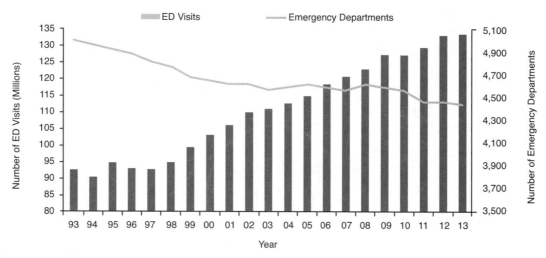

Used with permission of the American Hospital Association

Source: Avalere Health analysis of American Hospital Association Annual Survey data, 2013, for community hospitals. *Trendwatch Chartbook,* 2015. Defined as hospitals reporting ED visits in the AHA Annual Survey of Hospitals.

Figure 11.1   Emergency department volumes versus emergency departments.

Within the first years of the 21st century, changes in financial models and the Patient Protection and Affordable Care Act (2010) have shaped new contours of the definition of emergency care and its place in creating healthy populations. The financial pressures and drivers for quality are constantly on the minds of leaders who are creating the architecture for a more data-driven, transparent, high-quality, and lower-cost delivery system.

> "Having a team thoroughly invested in the outcome of their care is highly effective. The process is endlessly changeable, while the desired outcome the process is designed and continually redesigned to achieve is singular and simple: The best possible outcome for the patient." John Nance (2008, p. 66)

Nurses are indisputably on the front lines of these changes, resurrecting challenges in nursing that have existed for years while creating new challenges. Many, if not all, of the challenges covered herein can be tightly managed and relieved by using best practices in the research and within professional organizations (such as the Emergency Nurses Association and the American College of Healthcare Executives). Another way to overcome many of the challenges is through patient-centric, data-driven process redesign that works to improve standardization and predictability. It's no secret that when asked, emergency nurses will say the busiest day in the department is normally Monday. Why then should we not use data to support this hypothesis and build supporting systems that match this demand? It could aid in everything from staffing to the curve of arrivals, acuity, and length of stay (LOS); to scheduling elective procedures on alternate days to keep inpatient beds available for arriving ED patients; as well as deploying ancillary services in a fashion to keep low turnaround time for tests even with increasing volume.

This chapter focuses on the common workplace challenges facing emergency nursing today. In many ways, each intersects with the others, which can only amplify the issue at hand. The challenges discussed in this chapter have been the perennial focus of workgroups, studies, and research across many professional bodies. Contained within is an attempt to highlight and encapsulate those issues.

Violence in the Emergency Department

In 2014, a hospital security camera captured a patient in an ED in Minnesota chasing and attacking several emergency nurses with a pipe, causing one to suffer a collapsed lung and another a fractured wrist. Although this was certainly not the first act of violence against an emergency nurse, the fact that it was captured on video and was carried on cable news channels brought the issue of violence against nurses to the forefront.

Nurses can be victims of violence in the ED and sometimes the instigators of violence. The common scenarios of violence found include:

- Patient/family/bystander-on-provider violence

- Lateral violence among co-workers

- Occasionally, nurse-on-patient violence

Violence—The "exertion of physical force so as to injure or abuse" or "injure by or as if by distortion, infringement or profanation" (violence, n.d.).

Patient-, Family-, or Bystander-on-Provider Violence

Targeted patient/family/bystander violence toward staff is becoming increasingly common and is a constant threat to the emergency nurse. The ED is steps away from the street, often the literal front door to the hospital. The number of psychiatric patients, a population more prone to violence, has grown in recent decades; incidents of prolonged lengths of stay have also increased, which increase patient and visitor stress. This stress, combined with the fluid nature of the ED, increases the potential for violence. In recent years, nurses have been the victims of spitting, biting, hitting, and even shootings that have raised the national profile of the issue of ED violence. In a study published by the Emergency Nurses Association (ENA) in 2011, more than half the nurses surveyed had been a victim of violence or verbal abuse in the previous 7-day period (ENA, 2011b, p. 16).

Health systems have attempted to respond with additional de-escalation training, increased security and law enforcement presence, rapid response teams, and active shooter drills. During orientation, you may be taught how and where to position yourself in proximity to a route of egress from a patient room, or encouraged to carry a stethoscope in a safer location than around your neck.

In the past, nurses have been reluctant to report violence because they may not have felt they would be supported by either hospital administration or law enforcement. But in recent years, many states have passed legislation making assault on a healthcare worker a felony or misdemeanor, and many health systems have adopted policies that encourage the reporting of violent acts. You need to know and follow both hospital policies as well as state laws in reporting violent events to ensure that the true extent of the problem is documented. This is the best way to ensure that continued efforts to reduce violence in the ED can be implemented.

Lateral Violence

Lateral, also called *horizontal*, violence has become a topic of professional study in recent years. In a review of the literature by Becher and Visovsky in 2012, they found a widespread incidence rate among nurses well above 50% (p. 211). This type of violence can lead to gaps in collaboration and team morale with employees and more importantly affect patient care. Health systems have taken steps to address this, from training to enforcement for both employees and medical staff through disciplinary proceedings. It's also an expectation of The Joint Commission that health-system leaders have policies and processes in place to address this (The Joint Commission, 2008). For more information on lateral violence and how to manage it, see Chapter 6, "Self-Care and the Emergency Nurse."

 Lateral violence—Acts of aggression that occur between colleagues. Other names for lateral violence include bullying, horizontal violence, nurse-to-nurse hostility, or "eating of the young."

Nurse-on-Patient Violence

Nurse-on-patient violence is difficult to understand through the literature. Rates of incidence are unknown, and individual state licensing authorities manage the reports, which, unless they become criminal or civil matters, may not be made public. It can affect licensure as well as be a criminal act and must be strictly dealt with by healthcare leaders. Essentially, a zero-tolerance policy should be adopted. Colleagues and leaders must report these incidents and hold the standard of performance high.

Restraints/Seclusion

A basic tenet of the Constitution of the United States is ensuring freedoms for its citizens. When a patient is restrained or forced against his or her will in seclusion, these basic rights are stripped away. Therefore, you shouldn't take the use of restraints and seclusion lightly.

 Restraint—Anything that impedes on a patient's freedom of movement, including *chemical restraints* (medications given to sedate a patient with the purpose of restraining or reducing movement) or a physical restraint such as soft limb restraints or a chair with a table affixed over it that prevents the patient from leaving that chair against his or her free will.

Seclusion—Involuntary placement of a patient in an isolated area from which the patient is not allowed to leave under his or her own free will.

To protect these rights, The Joint Commission has retrenched to encourage health systems to find alternative care paths for the use of restraints and seclusion. In fact, the mere use of restraint or seclusion is reportable. The use of any modality that's intended to inhibit movement of a patient (for her safety or those around her) has a tremendous amount of accountability placed on the caregivers to document the reason, monitor the patient for effectiveness and safety, and ensure dignity.

Historically, the use of restraints in the ED could have been a combination of medication and a variation of soft and hard limb restraints. The belief was that this was the best way to protect the patient and the caregivers from harm. Alternate therapies/interventions have become more commonplace in the ED to help keep violence to a minimum and support patients in their agitated state. The Centers for Medicare and Medicaid Services (CMS) updated Standard 482.13 to read, "Restraint or seclusion may only be imposed to ensure the immediate physical safety of the patient, a staff member, or others and must be discontinued at the earliest possible time" (CMS, 2008, p. 90). In training programs for emergency nurses, alternate techniques to restraints have included (American Nurses Association [ANA], 2008, p. 10):

- Ensuring correction of underlying pathology (e.g., pain or hypoxia) that may be contributing to harmful behavior

- Talking with the patient

- Physical exercise

- Therapy (e.g., massage, music, or pet)

- Contact with family/friends

- Reduction of environmental stimulation (e.g., light, fall precautions, bed placement)

 The use of a "sitter" may be considered a "restraint" and fall under the guidelines of restraint and seclusion.

Consider the following points when considering or utilizing restraints (Gagnon, 2010):

- Annual training in physical restraints is required for acute care hospitals.

- Least-restrictive methods must be attempted before restraint or seclusion is utilized.

- An order by a medical provider for the use of the restraint must be obtained, which must clearly indicate the reason for the restraint and the time frames for which the restraint can be utilized.

- The reason that a patient is placed in restraints or seclusion must be clearly documented and must demonstrate an immediate threat to life as well as show all other attempts at least-restrictive methods were attempted and why they failed.

- Patients in restraints or seclusion must be assessed every 15 minutes at a minimum for safety and wellbeing, and that assessment must be documented.

▨ Any patient who dies while in restraints or within 24 hours of being released from a restraint must be reported to authorities as a sentinel event.

Each one of these has adaptable components in the emergency care setting to provide for safe and high-quality care. It's incumbent on you to know the laws and regulations as well as institutional policies regarding restraints and seclusion and to implement the use of restraints and seclusion sparingly to protect the rights of patients while at the same time ensuring the safety of patients and others around them.

Service Excellence and Patient Experience

Several nurses and physicians are sitting at the central desk one afternoon during a busy period. A nurse says, while a patient is being escorted back within listening distance, "Why does the triage nurse keep bringing patients back into rooms when we don't have nurses to take care of them?"

It's a near-daily occurrence in EDs. Patients arrive asking for help. While a nurse may have felt under siege from the patient arrivals, two more important things were occurring:

▨ The patient (also known as the customer) believed he was not welcome and that he would not receive good care.

▨ The nurse isn't aware that to meet the needs of the patient and ultimately direct the perception of quality, the triage nurse's evidence-based practice recommends bedding patients as quickly as possible.

Nurses are one of the most trusted professions in the United States, year after year (Gallup, 2014), well ahead of physicians. (See Figure 11.2.) You're in a unique and powerful position of trust with the patients, as well as being the foremost brand ambassador for the health system. This trust exists regardless of whether you're on duty or enjoying time off; you are always representing the health system.

Brands are more and more essential in building patient and community loyalty. This has become an exceptionally hot topic in recent years as hospitals have had their Hospital Consumer Assessment of Healthcare Providers and Systems (HCAHPS) publicly released on the federal hospital registry (http://www.medicare.gov/hospitalcompare). Patient satisfaction is part of the scores published on this registry, and reimbursement is being tied to these scores.

U.S. Views on Honesty and Ethical Standards in Professions

Please tell me how you would rate the honesty and ethical standards of people in these different fields – very high, high, average, low, or very low?

	% Very high or high	% Average	% Very low or low
Nurses	80	17	2
Medical doctors	65	29	7
Pharmacists	65	28	7
Police officers	48	31	20
Clergy	46	35	13
Bankers	23	49	26
Lawyers	21	45	34
Business executives	17	50	32
Advertising practitioners	10	44	42
Car salespeople	8	46	45
Members of Congress	7	30	61

Dec. 8-11, 2014
Rated in order of % Very high or high

GALLUP

Figure 11.2   People inherently trust nurses.

Increasingly, emerging research shows that patients' perception of quality in the delivery of care, including quality of care, is tied directly to their satisfaction with their experience in the ED. The top drivers normally include how quickly they see a provider, a short overall length of stay, and staff communication, both with the patient and among each other. Interestingly, there is an unexpected absence of any mention of a correct diagnosis. Patients assume outright that their nurses and physicians are clinically exceptional. There is also a precipitous decline in patient satisfaction scores the longer patients are in the ED for their episode of care, especially past the 2-hour mark (Press Ganey, 2011). Press Ganey found that hospitals with exceptional service have the best financial outcomes, further solidifying the argument that customer service must be one of the cornerstones to good ED care.

With patient experience rocketing to the top of priorities for leaders in healthcare, and patient satisfaction now being tied to reimbursement strategies, ED staff are being asked to take a greater role in ensuring harmony between clinical performance and patient satisfaction. Investments have been made in using best-practice initiatives to set accountability in behaviors and exceptional service. As patient satisfaction increases, other ED metrics tend to improve. For example, "left without being seen" rates tend to drop, revenues increase, and risk decreases, all further contributing to increased patient satisfaction.

Strategies to improve patient satisfaction have included:

- **Strong leadership:** Leadership sets the tone and accountability for a culture of safety, quality, and service (Mayer & Jensen, 2009). It's paramount for leaders to model expected behaviors.

- **Service standards:** Create policies or practices that reflect the culture and behavioral expectations when at work. This may include a dress code and scripting of written or verbal communication, as well as performance expectations to improve key metrics (e.g., satisfaction, peer reviews).

- **Empty waiting rooms:** Evidence shows that perception can help to accelerate the sense of lower length of stays in the ED. One way to achieve this perception is to bring patients back to a bed as soon as it is empty, keeping the patient feeling as if she is moving closer to seeing a provider. For more information on immediate bedding and the triage experience for patients, see Chapter 10, "The Emergency Nurse in the Role of Triage."

- **Key words/scripting:** The use of discreet and intentional language to influence the patient relationship is an important part of improving patient satisfaction. The power of language AIDET (acknowledge, introduce, duration, explanation, thank you) has become a commonly used framework to verbally communicate with patients and families (Studer, 2003, p. 94). It can be a powerful influence on strengthening relationships and engaging a patient.

- **Rounding:** Rounding is a customer-service technique in which identified individuals visit each patient and family member at regular intervals to determine that their needs are being met and they have no questions. The interval of rounding is set by the institution. Rounding may be carried out by management, charge nurses, staff nurses, customer service representatives, or any combination of these as determined by department policy. Staff may view rounding as an interruption in the delivery of care, which can pull at the very heart of safety and quality as well as serve as an employee dissatisfier. However, setting a regular cadence for interacting with a patient and setting the expectation of when the nurse will return can dramatically decrease interruptions between interactions.

- **Patient satisfaction representatives in the waiting rooms and clinical areas:** When beds are not available and patients must wait in the waiting room, some hospitals have deployed either specially trained volunteers or paid greeters to provide comfort during the wait. Greeters may provide magazines, updates on the wait, or access to food and drink for family members.

- **Improvement in the physical environment:** Brighter colors, comfortable stretchers, televisions, and Wi-Fi are all used as elements of creature comfort to improve the patient experience and pass the time.

■ **Provider in triage (PIT):** Various models of PIT exist in the literature. One model has a provider screening patients for a medical emergency in the triage area. This provider may treat-and-street low acuity patients, meaning they never need to occupy a bed. The overarching objective of PIT is to ensure timely door-to-provider times that exceed a patient's expectation. These practices normally result in increased patient satisfaction and decreased left-without-being-seen (LWBS) metrics.

■ **Discharge phone calls:** The discharge process from the ED can be rushed at times, and often the patient is still absorbing his diagnosis and the environment. This lends itself to an opportunity for the staff to circle back with the patient 48 to 72 hours later in a phone call. This has been an increasingly popular practice for nurses. It has been found in the literature that approximately 30% of patients do not understand various aspects of their discharge instructions (Zavala & Shaffer, 2011). Additionally, some patients may be expecting follow-up on a test that was performed while in the ED for which the results were not yet available at the time of discharge. Calling patients back a couple of days post-discharge can ensure they understand instructions and have an opportunity to ask clarifying questions. Call-back programs following discharge from the ED may be done for 100% of patients discharged, or they may be targeted at a certain population of discharged patients. Sometimes the call-backs are done by members of the management team, such as the charge nurse, and other times they may be done by the emergency nurse. Regardless of how the ED chooses to establish the program, it has been shown to improve patient satisfaction.

Taken in isolation, these strategies are not normally found to be successful. A transformational shift in culture is required for the entire staff with strict accountability in order to have the desired outcomes. Much like the steps of cardiopulmonary resuscitation or the process of trauma care, adding structure to patient care such as scripting and rounding provides the framework for maximal customer service performance. It's the clinician who uses critical judgment to adapt to each situation based on the assessment of needs. Collaterally, research has found that organizations with strong service ethics tend to be the employer of choice, leading to an improved work environment overall.

Recidivism (Frequent ED Utilizers)

With bed capacity in EDs normally constrained, financial reimbursement marginal, and the need to engage patients to be participants in their healthcare plan constantly emphasized, frequent utilizers can place a tremendous burden on the department. Frequent utilizers tend to be defined as having four visits or more annually. Interestingly, while the actual number of patients who meet this definition of a frequent ED utilizer is surprisingly low, they represent nearly 25% of the entire ED volume (The Advisory Board Company, 2010).

Reasons for being a frequent utilizer of emergency services vary. Commonly, these patients have addictions, lower coping skills, or factors that decrease their ability to access other care options (e.g., transportation, work, socioeconomic status, substance abuse, or psychiatric issues). As value-based purchasing and a greater emphasis on quality have emerged, health systems have become even more aggressive in identifying these high-risk patients and attempting to develop alternatives to decrease ED usage. Strategies include:

- **ED case management:** Deploying a case manager directly in the ED whose responsibilities include identifying and then helping to manage patients who use the ED frequently. Interventions usually include ensuring primary care physician (PCP) connection, prompt PCP visit following the ED episode, and close coordination with the inpatient team to set up supportive discharge planning when the patient is admitted.

- **Care management:** This role has had increasing importance as health systems have assumed risk or been penalized financially for quality outcomes. A care manager is assigned to patients identified as high risk to overuse the ED. A partnership of sorts is formed in which the care manager is the primary point of contact to evaluate the patient as a whole and work to elevate the patient's engagement and participation in staying healthy, whatever that baseline may look like.

- **Community EMS:** As the efforts to improve population health and provide the right care, at the right time, in the right setting have taken hold, innovation is required. Emergency Medical Services (EMS) is really the tip of the spear to help intervene and connect patients to the right care settings and services. Community EMS agencies have been setting up partnerships with health systems to deliver care to a home and also attach patients to support services to improve health; Figure 11.3 shows one example of a community EMS.

Ethics in the ED

A nurse's adult stepson comes to the ED seeking care in the "fast track" area. The nurse happens to be assigned to that area and takes the assignment to care for the man, initially saying nothing to her colleagues about the relationship. Shortly before discharge, the nurse alerts the physician to the relationship, only for the purposes of making sure he gets a prescription. Another nurse discharges the patient.

In many health systems, this scenario could be a violation of a conduct policy. Not all policies have this level of specificity, nor is it always found to be a violation of a practice act. But could the fact that the nurse cared for her own family member and requested a specific prescription be construed as an ethical challenge?

Spokane
FIRE DEPARTMENT
CARES
Community Assistance Response Team

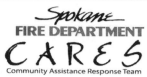

What is the CARES Team?

The CARES Team is a program within the Spokane Fire Department that is in place to interface with citizens who have received a response from fire personnel and are identified as needing social service or other support system assistance. Generally the citizen needs help that is available through existing social services programs, but the individual was not able to access them through traditional means. In most cases, FD responders find these individuals feeling isolated or are in some type of crisis and don't know where to turn for help. Often, these citizens generate many 9-1-1 calls for aid.

CARES was founded in 2008 by the Spokane Fire Department in conjunction with Eastern Washington University. The team is composed of Eastern Washington University students who are majoring in the Social Work degree programs. These students meet their academic practicum requirements by serving the CARES Team as student Interns. The Interns are overseen by the Social Response Manager, who is an employee of the City, hired in cooperation with EWU.

EASTERN
WASHINGTON UNIVERSITY
start something big

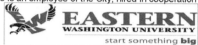

CARES Team members normally serve academically an entire school year (September through June) to meet their educational learning requirements. However, each member also volunteers many hours between the academic quarters and throughout the summer as well. Educational requirements focus on engagement, assessment, intervention within the scope of mental health issues and crisis intervention. Students undergo orientation and training that helps them to become knowledgeable about local community agencies, diversity issues, and vicarious trauma. Team members also experience ride along time with FD response units to experience firsthand the circumstances faced in the field. The educational training that social workers are required through the social work program emphasizes a strict code of ethics that mirrors the Fire Department's mission.

What Does the CARES Team Do?

CARES works in collaboration with the Spokane Fire Department to assist vulnerable populations who face barriers in identifying and utilizing appropriate community resources. The CARES Team visits individuals in their home, works with them to identify their needs, advocates with them and connects them to appropriate resources.

CARES' Responsibilities Include:

- In-home visits and client assessments
- Contacting and brokering with other Spokane agencies
- Advocating, brokering and empowering on behalf of the client
- Program development
- Internal and external marketing
- Participate in local coalitions
- Grant writing

Why CARES?

CARES was implemented in order to strengthen community relationships, decrease 9-1-1 over-users or abusers, decrease 'on-scene' time for FD response units for 'social service' calls, decrease level of frustration for front line crews, provide an expanded scope of care and a higher level of service to customers of the FD. Each EMS incident can tie up a FD unit and ambulance resulting in a call cost to the City of approximately **$750.** CARES impacts the Spokane FD in a positive and professional manner while assisting customers and community services.

To learn more about CARES, contact the Spokane Fire Department at: SFDCARES@spokanefire.org or call CARES at 509-625-7042 or 509-625-7166.

Figure 11.3 Example of a community EMS program in Spokane, Washington.

Nurses are presented with a labyrinth of ethical challenges in the ED (access to care, end-of-life, etc.), often on a daily basis. In the majority of situations, experience provides nurses with the ethical framework in which to navigate these scenarios. Other times, you may realize the presence of an ethical dilemma but be unsure what steps to take. Having the ability to identify and ask for assistance is a sign of a mature nurse.

Table 11.1 reviews basic ethical principles that you should consciously or unconsciously apply to the care that you provide.

Table 11.1 Ethical Principles for Nurses	
Ethical Principle	*Definition*
Autonomy	Patients who are of sound mind have the ethical right to make decisions about what will and will not be done to their person. Most ethical dilemmas end when autonomy is applied, because if the patient can legally make an autonomous decision, you should honor that decision.
Beneficence	Not all patients in the ED can make an autonomous decision, possibly because they lack developmental maturity, or perhaps they have an altered mental status from the use of illicit substances or a medical condition. In these cases, autonomy cannot be employed and you must apply beneficence to the care given. Beneficence means to "promote good" or "be of benefit to." When a patient cannot make an autonomous decision, ask yourself when providing care to a patient, "Does the care I am giving promote good and benefit my patient?" If the answer is "yes," the care is likely ethically right and should be carried out. If the answer is "no" or "uncertain," seek further counsel from others or the ethics committee.
Nonmaleficence	This is based on the concept "do no harm." When caring for a patient who cannot make an autonomous decision, ask yourself, "If I provide this care (or if I do not provide this care) will harm come to the patient?" If the answer is "no," the care is likely ethically correct and should be carried out. If the answer is "yes," seek further counsel from others or the ethics committee.
Justice	This ethical principle is based on fairness and demonstrates humanity and professionalism. When this principle is applied, it ensures equal care to all people who present to the ED. It is the principle on which the Emergency Medical Treatment and Active Labor Act (EMTALA) is based.
Veracity	Always be truthful to your patients. In doing so, you meet the ethical principle of veracity. This may include revealing information needed by decision-makers to provide informed consent, supplying information that allows patients to decide whether to take a particular medication or treatment, or disclosing a medical error honestly when it occurs.
Fidelity	You have a responsibility to your patients to keep promises and be loyal, also known as *fidelity*. Being a patient advocate and questioning treatments or behaviors that are believed to be outside of the patient's best interest is one way to invoke the principle of fidelity.

Source: Heilicser, 2013.

Although ethical principles are clear in the abstract, exercising them in some situations is far from easy. One ethical principle may clash with another, creating an ethical dilemma. You bring a different ethical framework to work than a different nurse, so what may be right for you may create an ethical dilemma for another. Whenever you feel something is ethically wrong, bring the situation to the attention of a supervisor. If resolution cannot be reached this way, then utilize the hospital's ethics policy to activate the ethics committee. The patient should always be the primary concern, and you must always remember your role as a patient advocate. At the same time, you must be cognizant that not every person has the same ethical beliefs, and there are times when actions may be carried out that seem ethically wrong to you but are not viewed as ethically wrong by other decisions-makers.

Patient Consent and Refusal of Care

The same freedoms that allow a patient to be free from restraint and seclusion also allow a patient to decide what is and is not done to his or her person. Violating these freedoms is considered battery. Therefore, it's incumbent on you to ensure that a patient has consented to care before undertaking that care.

 Battery—Harmful or offensive touching by one individual to another.

There are four main types of consents that are recognized to allow care in the ED. Table 11.2 provides an overview of these types of consent.

Table 11.2 Types of Consent

Type of Consent	Definition
Express consent	This is the general consent that is frequently obtained by the staff member who registers the patient. Express consent typically covers all non-invasive low-risk procedures that may be carried out. The only person who can provide express consent is an individual who is capable of making independent decisions, or someone who can legally consent on behalf of the patient who is incapable of making an independent decision (such as a minor or an unconscious patient). Express consent may be more informal than a signature on a form obtained during arrival to the ED. If you approach a patient with a vacutainer and the patient extends his or her arm (and the patient is capable of making an independent decision), then express consent is being given by the patient.

Informed consent	Express consent does not cover invasive or high-risk procedures. Hospital policy determines what procedures require consent beyond express consent. As the name implies, the individual providing informed consent must be informed about the procedure to be performed, the risks and benefits of that procedure, and the likelihood that those risks or benefits will occur. The person providing this information must be a licensed independent provider. If anyone else, including an emergency nurse, provides the information, true informed consent has not occurred. The patient or legal representative must consent to the procedure after he or she is informed in order for true informed consent to have occurred.
Implied consent	There are many times in the ED when a patient is unable to provide either express or informed consent because he or she lacks the legal capacity to do so. A patient in cardiac arrest, for example, cannot consent to life-saving treatment, nor can a patient unconscious after suffering a stroke. Showalter (2014) writes that in a medical/surgical emergency, consent is not required (p. 367); instead, care is provided under implied consent. It is important to note that implied consent ends when express consent is available. If a legal representative arrives and does not consent to the treatment that is being carried out under implied consent, the medical team must reconsider continuation of care.
Involuntary consent	Psychiatric patients may lack the mental capacity to consent to treatment, yet they are not in a medical or surgical emergency; therefore, treatment cannot be rendered under implied consent. In these cases, involuntary consent may be utilized to provide care. Involuntary consent is generally utilized for patients who are at risk of harming themselves or others but lack the mental capacity to provide express or informed consent. In most jurisdictions, the only person who can provide involuntary consent on behalf of another person is a physician, a law enforcement officer, or a judge.

Sometimes a patient refuses to provide consent for treatment, even when the medical team feels it would be advantageous for the patient to receive that treatment. If the patient is capable of making an independent decision and refuses to provide consent, then care cannot be given without risking a charge of battery by the patient.

Refusal of care carries with it significant risk. The Emergency Medical Treatment and Active Labor Act (EMTALA) requires that all patients who come to the ED receive a medical screening exam and appropriate stabilizing care. If the patient leaves without those elements being carried out, it could be construed as an EMTALA violation, resulting in fines to the institution. You have to avoid communicating with anyone in such a way that could be construed as encouraging the person to leave without being seen. In fact, you should always encourage the patient to remain for the complete medical screening exam and appropriate treatment. When the patient still refuses that care, document the discussion and the patient's understanding of the conversation(s) to protect yourself as well as the institution. For further discussion of EMTALA, see Chapter 12, "Risk Management and Quality Issues Affecting the Emergency Nurse."

Aside from EMTALA, patients who refuse care are at risk for a deterioration of their condition, which not only has implications for the patients but also carries significant risk for the institution to which they initially reported. Clear documentation of the discussion with the patient and the patient's understanding of the conversation before refusing care provides a layer of protection for you and the institution.

When it comes to refusal of care, the best course of action is to involve the physician whenever possible. The physician should share the risks of refusing care with the patient. It is not an all-or-nothing equation, either. A competent patient may choose to refuse elements of the treatment plan without refusing the care entirely. For example, the patient may choose not to have a computerized tomography (CT) scan of her head, yet agree to an intravenous line and laboratory tests. Remember to document the discussion and the patient's understanding of the conversation(s).

Patient Throughput

The ED is often referred to as the front door to the hospital. This means the ED takes all comers, leaving them with a superior first impression and ensuring patients all move through their stay as quickly as possible. The ability to pull a patient through the ED from the time of arrival to time of discharge has been discussed heavily in literature and conferences nationwide. It's a key driver of patient satisfaction. Additionally, as crowding in the ED increases, threats to safety, quality, and timeliness of care mount (Institute of Medicine [IOM], 2006, p. 131). You're an essential participant in creating a system that efficiently manages the patient's time in the department. Mayer and Jensen (2009) write that a key to breaking the code to ensure optimal flow is to match capacity to demand, doing so in one of two approaches: smoothing patient demand or matching service to capacity (p. 27).

In examining the subcomponents of a patient's stay in the department, your role affects the length of time a patient is present. (See Figure 11.4.) Having agreed-upon definitions for steps and intervals is important in order to assess performance. Wiler et al. (2015) published a consensus-driven article that provided guidance on standardized metrics and intervals for EDs to assess both throughput and overall performance. These intervals include arrival to provider, provider to disposition, and disposition to discharge.

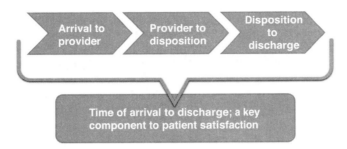

Figure 11.4   Nurses affect a patient's length of time in an ED.

Time of Arrival to Discharge

Time of arrival to discharge refers to the length of time between the first moment of contact with a staff member to the time when the patient leaves the ED. This overall time is a key driver of patient satisfaction. Typically, the lower this time, the more satisfied a patient (see Figure 11.5).

Arrival to Provider

Also referred to as "door-to-doc," *arrival to provider* is the time from the first moment of contact with a staff member to the time when a provider (normally a physician, advanced practice nurse, or physician assistant) arrives at the patient's side. EDs have various definitions of the time of arrival. For some, it's when patients sign in at the registration desk; for others, it's when patients are first seen by the triage nurse or when the medical record is initiated. Most processes have the patient coming in contact with several staff members and moving multiple times before a provider is seen. In any of the scenarios, the patient is expecting to see a provider as quickly as possible. Hospital leaders, recognizing arrival to provider time as paramount to success, have developed strategies to compress this time frame. Putting the patient at the center of any process is critical to service improvement. There have been various strategies (e.g., pull-to-full, immediate bedding, provider in triage, pre-emptive test guidelines) with the underlying principle being to meet the patient's expectations of seeing a provider most expeditiously to begin care. Marino, Mays, and Thompson (2015) reported improved door-to-physician time as well as collateral improvement in patient satisfaction after a process was implemented to immediately bed a patient until the ED was full. A challenge encountered at times when redesigning the process is the cultural shift required to limit the information needed upfront, distilling out what you need to know from what you want to know (in other words, eliminating non-value information or steps). Many times, you should enter only what is necessary for assigning the appropriate triage level and bed assignment.

One at a Time

Patient Forced Through a Succession of Steps

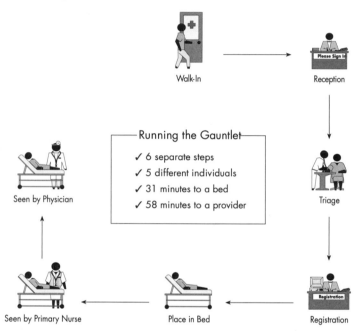

Running the Gauntlet

✓ 6 separate steps
✓ 5 different individuals
✓ 31 minutes to a bed
✓ 58 minutes to a provider

Improving Emergency Department Throughput (2008). Published by The Advisory Board Company. ©2008 The Advisory Board Company. All rights reserved.

Source: The Advisory Board Company, 2008, p. 3.

Figure 11.5   The process a patient goes through from arrival to discharge.

Provider to Disposition

Provider to disposition is the period of time that begins after seeing a provider when a care plan has been established and executed and ends when the provider makes the decision to admit or discharge the patient. During this time, tests are run, some with fixed processing (e.g, lab work) and others that involve the patient moving (e.g, radiology exams). Successful EDs are those where the nursing staff have helped to organize the course and speed of the patient to parallel processes and order tests early in the visit.

Disposition to Discharge

Disposition to discharge is the time between the provider making a decision to admit or discharge and the actual departure of the patient from the department. You have the best opportunity to affect those patients being discharged.

Boarders in the Emergency Department

Once the decision is reached to admit a patient from the ED, but the inpatient bed is not available, the patient becomes a *boarder* (Wiler et al., 2015, p. 548). Boarding supports the broader idea that ED throughput is dependent less on the functioning of the ED and more on the hospital as a whole. In the early part of this century, regulatory agencies and health systems took a keen interest in the issue of overcrowding in EDs. It was a large dissatisfier of patients and was stressing EDs. As capacity surges more and more, patients are forced to wait for care. Headlines in newspapers and television (Castillo, 2014; Cox, 2008) announced the latest deaths believed to be a result, in part, of long wait times. Singer, Thode, Viccellio, and Pines (2011) found a correlation between boarding in the ED and a rise in mortality.

The IOM (2006), in its report *Future of Emergency Care,* recommends abolishing the practice of ED boarders. Alternatives include developing an enterprise-wide response to managing inpatient flow on a system level, using data and best practices in throughput to pull admissions from the ED up to the right bed at the right time.

The American College of Emergency Physicians (2011) makes the following recommendations regarding the boarding of admitted patients in the ED:

- Patients should be transferred to an inpatient unit as soon as the decision to admit is made. If that cannot be immediately facilitated, the hospital should provide supplemental staff to care for the patients so that emergency nurses can continue to care for ED (as opposed to admitted) patients.

- If boarding patients impede on the ability to care for ED patients, boarded patients should be distributed to inpatients units even if inpatient beds are unavailable (patients may need to be cared for in hallways or other non-traditional areas of the inpatient unit until a room becomes available).

- Staffing patterns on inpatient units should be utilized by the ED to care for boarded patients. If, for example, the staffing ratio for patients in the intensive care unit is two patients for each nurse, then one nurse should care for no more than two boarded intensive care unit patients in the ED.

■ Hospitals must utilize every measure possible to facilitate the availability of inpatient beds.

Ambulance Diversion

The subject of ambulance diversion touches at the heart of the core mission and "can lead to catastrophic delays in treatment for the seriously ill and injured patients" (IOM, 2006, p. 21). Ambulance diversion has mainly occurred in more urban areas as a method to decompress already busy EDs. Yet, diversion is typically a response to a symptom of more downstream hospital capacity issues, rather than the inability of the ED to care for incoming patients. It was thought to help give breathing room for those already in the ED to provide optimal care and improve throughput. Research has shown just the opposite.

Ambulance diversion—Occurs when a hospital worker notifies pre-hospital personnel that the hospital is not available to take ambulance patients. This requires the ambulance to bypass that hospital and take the patient to a hospital that's not on diversion. This can prolong transport times, especially if multiple hospitals are on diversion and the ambulance must travel long distances to find a hospital available to accept the patient.

In 2009, the state of Maryland became the first to ban diversion. Burke et al. (2013) reviewed the effects of this ban on key metrics including ED length of stay and ambulance turnaround time, finding no significant negative impact on EDs around the state. Other communities have worked to eliminate diversion with the increasing pressures of population health and keeping patients within the system. Figure 11.6 shows that hospitals don't have enough beds to accommodate ambulance patients in the ED, which is why they choose to go on diversion.

Research has shown that more patients who arrive via ambulance will require admission than those who walk into the ED. When a hospital goes on diversion, ambulatory patients continue to arrive, while ambulance patients will be taken elsewhere. Because admitted patients bring significantly more revenue to the hospital than patients seen and discharged from the ED, ambulance diversion may actually cause a loss of revenue to the hospital, especially if diversion is frequently utilized or utilized for long periods of time (Augustine, 2013). One study concluded that a hospital lost $5,845 per hour of ambulance diversion (Litzenburg & Dorsey, 2011).

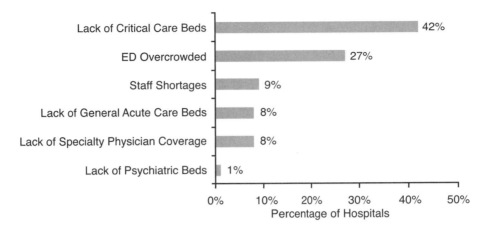

Lack of Critical Care Beds — 42%
ED Overcrowded — 27%
Staff Shortages — 9%
Lack of General Acute Care Beds — 8%
Lack of Specialty Physician Coverage — 8%
Lack of Psychiatric Beds — 1%

Percentage of Hospitals
0%   10%   20%   30%   40%   50%

Source: American Hospital Association (AHA), 2010. Used with permission of the American Hospital Association.

Figure 11.6   Common reasons for hospitals to initiate ambulance diversion.

Aside from loss of revenue, other pitfalls of ambulance diversion must be considered. If ambulances are forced to bypass the closest ED on diversion, definitive care for that patient will be delayed in prolonged transport times, increasing the potential for negative medical outcomes. Ambulance diversion also consumes community pre-hospital resources. The longer an ambulance is on the road transporting patients, the less available that vehicle is to pick up another patient, potentially causing further delays in treatment.

One may successfully argue that there are times when an ED is so full or the acuity is temporarily so high that the arrival of more patients would truly create an unsafe situation. But those times should be rare and should be carefully orchestrated with pre-hospital personnel, other local facilities, and the community as a whole to minimize the impact on patient safety. If a hospital finds itself on diversion frequently, this should create a level of concern about the hospital's ability to manage its flow of patients and precipitate a critical review of processes from the ED through to the inpatient units to minimize or eliminate ambulance diversion. You can be pivotal in raising concerns about frequent diversion and developing solutions to the problem.

Communicable Disease Management

In October 2014, a patient arrived at a Dallas, Texas, hospital after a recent visit to Liberia. He was quickly diagnosed with Ebola virus disease (EVD) and died a few days later (ENA, 2015). This patient represents the first case of Ebola in the United States, and signaled yet another significant event in communicable disease management.

For the emergency nurse, communicable diseases pose a significant risk because the patients are often not aware of their risk for these types of conditions, and because the patient's final diagnoses are almost always undefined upon arrival to the department. This puts the healthcare workers in ED settings at high risk and underscores the importance of extensive planning and preparation for these types of situations.

EDs and their parent organizations are responsible for ensuring that all staff members are properly prepared to deal with patients with communicable diseases. The ENA (2010b) believes that nurses must be trained to detect patients at risk for communicable diseases, isolate those patients, initiate treatment, and report the issue to the appropriate departments and agencies.

While working in the ED, you have no idea which patient has Ebola, SARS, H1N1, HIV, hepatitis C, or any number of other communicable diseases. You can take several steps to minimize the risk of transmission to yourself and others should these patients present for care:

- **Use standard precautions as a basic barrier to spreading disease.** Standard precautions mandate the use of barrier devices such as gloves, eye protection, masks, and gowns to protect healthcare workers from exposure to bloodborne and airborne pathogens (Liang, Theodoro, Schuur, & Marschall, 2014). You should have these products readily available and be familiar with how to use them. Avoid shortcuts such as pulling off the tips of gloves while starting an IV.

- **Practice good hand hygiene.** Standards for hand hygiene in the hospital setting mandate the use of alcohol-based gel or foam before and after each patient contact. This method has demonstrated superior reduction in bacterial counts when compared to soap and water handwashing (Liang et al., 2014). Despite this, though, hand hygiene compliance in the ED has been demonstrated to be only between 10% to 90% (Liang et al., 2014).

Regardless of the precautions you take, patients with communicable diseases still enter the doors or EDs with little or no warning. When these patients arrive, take the following steps to improve safety levels for everyone involved (Delaney & Reed, 2015):

Ebola virus disease (EVD)—Ebola is a form of hemorrhagic fever of the Filovirus family. In 2014, the largest and most complex outbreak in history affected West Africa and spilled over into other areas of the world (ENA, 2015). Patients present with high fever, headache, vomiting, abdominal pain, hemorrhage, diarrhea, and weakness, and the disease has a mortality rate above 50% (ENA, 2015). Treatment for the disease is largely palliative and focuses on aggressive hydration, blood replacement therapy, and limiting the effects of sepsis.

1. Ask screening questions to help identify patients at risk.

2. Move patients at higher risk away from others.

   This may be into a designated, segregated waiting area, or even into a negative air-flow room.

3. Provide the appropriate personal protective equipment (PPE) for all staff and encourage its use.

4. Engage the infection control department immediately.

5. Heavily sanitize potentially infected areas.

Patient care for this population is highly specialized because all bodily fluids are highly contagious (Feistritzer, Hill, Vanairsdale, & Gentry, 2014). Staff members must wear biocontainment-unit-level PPE, transport of the patient outside of the containment unit is not recommended unless absolutely necessary, laboratory testing is highly scrutinized and controlled for exposures, and liquid and solid waste have very specific disposal requirements (Wadman et al., 2015). For a patient with a positive diagnosis of Ebola virus disease, chest compressions are an absolute contraindication, and resuscitative measures after a cardiac arrest are almost always futile (Wadman et al., 2015).

Disaster Preparedness and Response

Very ironically, the day before one of the greatest tragedies occurred in the United States (September 11, 2001), *U.S. News and World Report* ran a cover story featuring EDs at capacity and the entire system at the breaking point (IOM, 2006, p. 259–260). It essentially laid out in detail how EDs were stretched on a daily basis to handle what had become the normal operating capacity.

Disasters are typically understood to be an event (man-made or natural) that occurs with low probability and yet yields a large number of ill or injured individuals (IOM, 2006). Both the Emergency Nurses Association and the federal government encourage health systems to take an all-hazards approach to assessing potential threats to the community and even internally to the health system (e.g., power failure, loss of water). Through this process, providers can identify the most likely disasters and set plans in place.

 Disaster—"Disasters are serious disruptions of the functioning of a community or a society involving widespread human, material, economic, or environmental losses and impacts, which exceeds the ability of the affected community or society to cope using its own resources" (Hammad, Arbon, Gebbie, & Hutton, 2012, p. 236).

Preparation for a Disaster

Hospitals should have a well-established disaster plan. The organization needs to work out details ahead of time so that it can remain self-sufficient for a period of 72 hours. This might include storage of supplies, availability of food and water, and establishing contracts with local vendors that could help them out. The hospital should establish alternate care locations, or locations within the hospital other than the ED, that could handle a large influx of patients should the ED find itself at capacity. For instance, an organization could designate the hospital cafeteria as the location for stable patients and its GI lab as the location for the moderately injured. The ED should be reserved for the most acutely ill. Supply carts should be available at a moment's notice for these areas. Other considerations during disaster planning might include communications in the event cellular and landline communication is unavailable, documentation methods if computers are down, and the availability of emergency bins with flashlights, extension cords, and other necessities.

The organization also needs to be prepared for a chemical or biological disaster that could require decontamination. Decontamination facilities should be available in all EDs, and all future construction plans should include decontamination services. If decontamination facilities are not available, organizations can purchase commercial decontamination trailers or even portable decontamination facilities. In addition to this, appropriate personal protective equipment (PPE) needs to be available to protect staff members during this type of disaster. For more information on decontamination areas, see Chapter 8, "Common Areas Within the Emergency Department."

Perhaps the most critical part of disaster management in the ED is frequent personnel training. Key employees in both the ED and the hospital's incident command center should participate in National Incident Management System (NIMS) training. This training is a nationally driven approach to incident command that is applicable to all types of disasters regardless of size, duration, or location (NIMS, 2015). Courses are available online or in person and teach participants a coordinated approach to disaster management that can be applied to government and community officials, EMS providers, and healthcare workers, among others. Additional information on training is available at the Federal Emergency Management Administration (http://www.fema.gov/training-0/). In addition to this training, you should know how to activate the disaster system, what your role is in a disaster, where to take patients, and where to get resources.

Role of the Emergency Nurse

Your role in a disaster situation can depend on the type of the disaster, how the disaster has affected the operations capacity of the organization, the number of victims, and other factors. One such role is triage nurse. Appropriate triage of patients takes on a new importance during a disaster situation and differs from the role that the emergency nurse plays when sitting at the triage desk during a routine shift. In a disaster situation, the triage nurse must quickly determine the patient's triage category and move the patient to the care area designated by the hospital for the patient's triage category (Howard & Foley, 2015). The triage nurse performs a quick assessment of each patient and places the patient into one of the following triage categories shown in Table 11.3.

Table 11.3 Triage Categorization Using Disaster Triage

Color	Triage Category	Description
White	Dismiss	Minor injury that does not require the care of a physician
Green	Wait	"Walking wounded"
Yellow	Observation	Injured but stable, does not have life-threatening injuries
Red	Immediate	Critically ill
Black	Expectant	Dead on arrival or unlikely to survive even with treatment

Source: Stoppler, 2014.

The nurse then places a triage tag of the appropriate color around the patient's neck if local EMS providers have not already done so. This ensures that all providers know the status of the patient at a glance.

Other roles you may assume during a disaster situation can include general patient care, team leadership, or patient resuscitation (Hammad et al., 2012). Studies have shown that during disaster situations, nurses who are well versed in these roles on a daily basis suddenly do not understand what they should be doing (Hammad et al., 2012), which reinforces the need for both a strong incident command structure within the organization and also for extensive and frequent training for ED and hospital personnel.

Hospital Emergency Response

> An individual runs up to the triage window and reports a "man down" in the hospital's parking garage. Do you respond? If so, how?

This scenario occurs frequently for ED personnel. Showalter (2014) writes about the requirement of 250 yards of responsibility imposed by the U.S. Health and Human Services department (p. 342). This can be interpreted as in any direction from the ED. In some cases, this can include a parking garage or stand-alone structure. Stepping away from the literalness of this measure, it is still a daunting responsibility for ED staff to be able to respond outside the department.

ED and hospital staff tend to take a conservative approach to hospital response. There may even be a division of response based on patient location. For example, if the patient is on a nursing unit (such as a family member who experiences chest pain), the hospital's rapid response team may come from the ICU. If that same patient is located in a public space (such as a lobby or waiting room), then the ED may assemble a team to respond. The dynamics of responding outside of the department is nothing short of the pre-hospital environment found in EMS. There is the issue of scene safety that is always paramount, not to mention medical equipment and the ability to stabilize and transport the patient back to the ED. A response team may consist of a senior nurse and a physician or tech. Much of this may depend on staffing levels in the department. EMS may need to be called to assist. Security should always be part of the team to ensure a safe working environment.

Telephone Advice or Release of Patient Information

The release of patient information has had a change in calculus in large part because of the passing of the Health Insurance Portability and Accountability Act (1996). Patients have the right, generally speaking, to have access to, and control of, their medical records (Showalter, 2014, p. 299). Hospital policy determines the correct course of action to satisfy the request for records. Customarily, the patient needs to work through the health information management (HIM) office of the system to get access to records, rather than the ED. Patients also have the legal right to know who has gained access to their records.

- **Scenario 1:** The patient normally must sign a release form to authorize the transmission of his or her medical record to a payer and other entities. In the customary course of registration, this authorization is signed and filed.

- **Scenario 2:** The patient's brother calls for an update on the patient's status. In this case, the health system would have a process in place to verify authorization to release the information over the phone. It may require a password to ensure authentication.

- **Scenario 3:** A patient is being discharged and requests a copy of his or her records. In many cases, the patient is referred to the HIM department to get the copy. ED staff normally aren't asked to distribute copies of healthcare records.

- **Scenario 4:** Upon discharge from the ED, the patient is to follow up with his or her physician, who is not connected to the health system's medical record. In most cases, the patient has signed an authorization that includes release of records to his or her provider of record. The records are transmitted to the physician without incident.

For more information on the Health Insurance Portability and Accountability Act (HIPAA), see Chapter 12, "Risk Management and Quality Issues Affecting the Emergency Nurse."

Family Presence During Resuscitation

The bedside of a patient whose condition is declining, who is being resuscitated, or even one who is in cardiac arrest can be a chaotic place. Multiple providers and lots of equipment, combined with a sense of urgency, can create a scenario that can be less than optimal. The addition of family members to this situation therefore becomes a hotly debated topic. Opponents of family presence during resuscitation (FPDR) claim that family members should not see their loved ones in the state of resuscitation and that they would want to remember them as they were in life, that FPDR exposes the hospital to legal risk, or that the family could obstruct the efforts of the medical team (Bradley, Lensky, & Brasel, 2011). Proponents believe that when family members are present, they are more likely to find comfort witnessing the team work so hard to care for their loved one that it promotes a more professional atmosphere among the healthcare team, and that family presence comforts patients if they are successfully resuscitated (Bradley et al., 2011).

Trends in the literature support involving the patient's family members in the resuscitation process. One study demonstrated that 72% of patients would want their family members present during their own cardiac arrest, and most stated that they would want to witness their own loved one's resuscitation (Lederman, Garasic, & Piperberg, 2014). Seventy-five percent of parents indicated that they would insist on being present for the resuscitation of their child, and individuals who had been present for a previous resuscitation were one and a half times more likely to want to be present for subsequent interventions (Dwyer, 2015). In addition, men were less likely to fear witnessing the resuscitative process than women but were more concerned about being a distraction to the healthcare team (Dwyer, 2015). Finally, post-traumatic stress disorder (PTSD) related symptoms are more likely to be present in those family members who are *not* present for a loved one's resuscitation (Jabre et al., 2013).

As an increasing number of professional organizations, including the Emergency Nurses Association, publish position papers supporting FPDR, more and more hospitals are also implementing policies that encourage this practice. As such, you should help your employer implement the practice as well. When family members are present, you should ensure that:

- A staff member is dedicated to supporting the family. The staff member's role should be to provide comfort measures as well as to explain what is happening to their loved one in terms that they can understand.

- An appropriate number of family are allowed to be present based on the physical space in the room.

- The family is educated on what they can and cannot touch; encourage them to touch and talk to their loved one when appropriate.

- A private area is designated that can be used by the family that includes plenty of seating and a phone so that the family can call other members of their support system.

- The family can spend time with the patient for an extensive duration after the resuscitation has ended. Many organizations have family viewing rooms available where the patient and their family can be together after an unsuccessful resuscitation that does not tie up the valuable resource of the major resuscitation or trauma room.

Organ and Tissue Donation

You work tirelessly to save lives each and every day. However, for patients with catastrophic illnesses or injuries, your role must often shift to supporting family members and friends through the end of life process. In 2015, over 120,000 people in the United States were waiting on a life-saving organ transplant (Health Resources and Services Administration [HRSA], 2015). Unfortunately, a significant mismatch exists between the number of organs available for transplant and the number of patients waiting, with 21 people dying each day while waiting for an organ (HRSA, 2015), as shown in Figure 11.7.

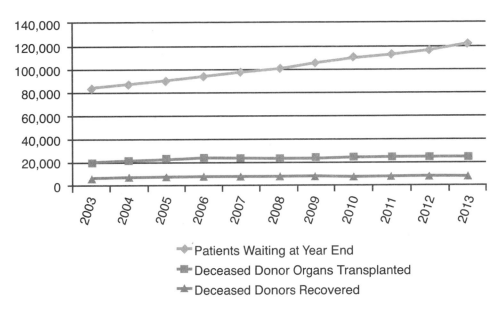

Source: UNOS. Based on OPTN data as of January 1, 2013. Retrieved from http://optn.transplant.hrsa.gov/. Permission to reprint from UNOS.

Figure 11.7 The number of people waiting for an organ donation.

Though organs from one donor can save up to eight lives (United Network for Organ Sharing [UNOS], 2015) and the average donor is able to donate 4.87 organs (Phillips, 2013), this gap exists for several reasons (Gilligan, Sanson-Fisher, & Turon, 2012):

- In the United States, African Americans, Hispanics, and Catholics are less likely to be registered as organ donors.

- Surviving family members are often not aware of a patient's wishes regarding organ donation.

- How and when family members are approached regarding donation is key to their likeliness to consent to donation.

The Organ and Tissue Donation Process

Patients in need of an organ transplant are first placed on a national registry list that is maintained by the United Network for Organ Sharing (UNOS). The ranking of the patient within that list is dependent on a variety of measures, including the patient's need for the organ to both live and sustain an appropriate standard of life (UNOS, 2015). Organ procurement organizations (OPOs) in 11 geographical regions then partner with UNOS when organs become available to determine the best possible match based on an extensive list of criteria. Determinants of an available organ's allocation might include (among others) the recipient's waiting time on the UNOS list, medical acuity, degree of biological match, and distance from the available organ (HRSA, 2015).

Timing in the organ and tissue donation process is critical. Organs are only viable outside of the body for a limited time (HRSA, 2015), reinforcing the need for all emergency nurses to be well versed in the organ and tissue donation process in order to maximize the impact of such a generous gift. Maximum organ preservation times are:

- Heart & Lung: 4 to 6 hours

- Liver: 8 to 12 hours

- Pancreas: 12 to 18 hours

- Kidney: 24 to 36 hours

Role of the Emergency Nurse in Organ Donation

You're normally on the front lines of recognizing potential donors, and as such, you play a significant role as patient advocate, family liaison, and clinical expert to initiate any organ or tissue donation process. The first step in the process is to notify the regional OPO of any patient whose death has occurred or might be imminent. These clinical triggers may vary by region, by OPO, or even by hospital policy (Phillips, 2013), so it's important to be well educated on these criteria. Then your role moves to supporting the family. It's important not to offer donation to the family at this point, because the OPO still needs to determine if the patient is a candidate to donate (Phillips, 2013). Once the OPO determines the patient is a candidate for donation, the family can be approached about the donation process. It's imperative that someone trained as a designated requestor (which can be the emergency nurse) have this conversation with the family because consent rates increase dramatically based on the qualifications of this individual (Gilligan et al., 2012).

There are two types of organ donors. Donation after brain death donors (DBD) are those patients who have sustained a catastrophic brain injury and have been declared brain dead from both a clinical and legal standpoint (Phillips, 2013). These patients remain on life support until the time that the organs are procured. Donation after cardiac death donors (DCD) are those patients who have a life-threatening injury or illness that requires life support measures and who are unlikely to survive should they be removed. You can be called to care for both types of patients.

First Person Authorization and Donation

First person authorization legislation makes a patient's pre-death declaration of his or her intent to donate organs legally binding (Traino & Siminoff, 2013). These declarations are most often in the form of a living will or are noted on the patient's driver's license. In these cases, though the family can legally challenge the declaration, studies have found that in 66% of deaths in which the patient had a first person authorization, the family was aware of the patient's intent prior to the patient's death (Traino & Siminoff, 2013). In addition, in a review of legal cases involving first person authorization, over 99% of judgments favored the wishes of the patient (Kristopher, 2015).

Impaired Co-Workers

Nurses who practice while impaired pose a significant risk to themselves, their co-workers, and their employer, but most importantly to their patients. It's estimated that 10% of nurses have substance abuse problems (Burton, 2014), and 6% to 8% of substance abusing nurses consume enough alcohol or medication to impair their practice and jeopardize the care they deliver to patients (ENA, 2010a). All emergency nurses are responsible for monitoring for impaired practice.

Although impaired practice can manifest itself in many ways, easy access to controlled substances and the busy environment of the ED provide unique opportunities for emergency nurses to divert medications. Nurses may steal prescription pads and write their own prescriptions, take all or part of a patient's prescribed medications for their own use, ask co-workers to dispose of (*waste*) medications with them without properly disposing of the medication, or even sift through sharps containers looking for partially used vials. Most commonly, opioids are the drug of choice for nurses who divert medications (Berge, Dillon, Sikkink, Taylor, & Lanier, 2012).

Keep an eye out for warning signs that might indicate that a peer is impaired. These could include staff members who start to lose interest in their personal appearance and come to work with little regard for their personal hygiene, nurses that are frequently late or difficult to locate on the unit, or those who more obviously show signs such as slurred speech and an unsteady gait (Starr, 2015).

Nurses who divert medications, however, do not always consume the medications themselves and may therefore not appeared impaired. The intent of their diversion may be to sell the medications to others. As such, pay close attention to patients who complain that their pain is not well controlled or that they have not received their scheduled dosages (Starr, 2015), because this might be an indicator that the patient's nurse might be diverting medications.

The most important thing that you can do when you suspect that a peer is working impaired is to immediately notify your supervisor and protect the patient from any potential harm. It's essential for managers and supervisors to be educated on organizational policy as well as their State Board of Nursing practices regarding impaired practice so that when concerns are brought forward, they can respond appropriately. Actions vary by state, but a nurse who has been determined to be impaired can face significant repercussions including monetary penalties, loss of license, or even imprisonment (Clark, 2011). However, in many states, a nurse who self-reports his or her substance abuse to the State Board of Nursing can often receive leniency if he or she completes mandated counseling and rehabilitation programs (Starr, 2015). Healthcare organizations are also at risk if they fail to report diversion incidents and could incur fines of up to $10,000 per occurrence (Clark, 2011).

There are several things that you can do to minimize the risk of diversion and impaired practice in your department. Some of these might include:

- Implement high-level security features such as biometrics for controlled-substance dispensing machines.

- Run frequent reports looking for variances in use among members of the same team.

- Document medication administrations quickly and accurately.

- Pay attention. If you are asked to waste medications, make sure you watch the entire process.

- When wasting, draw up and dispense medications into the sharps container rather than disposing of medications still in the vial.

- Always log off after completing activities at the dispensing machine.

- Provide continuing education on impaired practice and diversion in the workplace.

Social Media

A nurse helps a physician remove a cockroach from a patient's ear. The bug is placed into a specimen cup. The nurse takes a picture of the bug and posts the picture and comment on her Instagram page.

A patient in the waiting room takes a photo of a nurse reading a magazine while working in triage and posts it to her Facebook page with the caption "Why doesn't she help me?" along with the name of the hospital.

The rapid trajectory of utilization and innovation of social media means that health systems must adapt policies and practices quickly. The changing landscape shows the power of social media to raise awareness of the health system, advocating, and educating. There are three sides to this issue in the ED, discussed in the following sections.

Staff and Social Media

Seventy-one percent of adults with Internet access have a Facebook account and 63% use it daily (Langenfeld, Cook, Sudbeck, Luers, & Schenarts, 2014). Although privacy settings are available on most social media sites, many people do not use them appropriately, making anything posted there potentially open for public scrutiny. The two pitfalls of social media that you may fall into are posting information that may violate a patient's privacy or posting information that may not even be associated with work but casts you in a less-than-professional light.

Patient privacy issues must always be considered, both from a legal standpoint (HIPAA, for example) and an ethical standpoint. The guiding principle when deciding what to post on social media should be institutional policy. A good rule, however, is to go one step further and avoid posting anything related to the workplace on a social media site.

You must also realize that even if you don't post something to social media, anyone else can, including patients and their visitors. Displaying a professional demeanor at all times while in the workplace minimizes the risk of being cast in a negative light by someone else via social media.

As much as you'd like to think that your personal life outside of work and your professional life are completely separate, social media blurs that line. Registered nurses are considered professionals 24 hours a day. If a registered nurse commits a felony, even when not at work, she will lose her nursing license. Posting pictures or comments on social media sites that may be considered by others to lack professionalism, such as consuming alcohol or illicit drugs or posting polarizing political or religious comments, even outside of the workplace, may reflect negatively on the emergency nurse. This information could be used by an employer or the nursing board for disciplinary action and can be used by potential future employers to deny employment. In one study performed by Langenfeld et al. (2014), 26.3% of residents had either potentially unprofessional or clearly unprofessional information posted on a Facebook page.

Institutions and Social Media

Although social media can negatively impact you when not used appropriately, it can be used by health systems in a very positive manner. Institutions are using technology to raise their brand awareness. This may include posting interviews with physicians, ads for upcoming events, and even showing actual surgeries; the possibilities are hampered almost only by the imagination. Pew Research Center states that one-third of Americans use the Internet as a major resource when they have a medical issue, and 41% of Americans use social media when choosing a healthcare provider (Trader, 2013).

Patients

Patients are talking about their healthcare on social media—an important reason why the delivery of exceptional service is so important when a patient comes to the ED. The best marketing is done by word-of-mouth. Once posted on social media, it's always on social media.

Summary

While emergency nursing can be an extremely rewarding career, especially for those who enjoy the variety and excitement it brings, it can also be fraught with challenges that can cause the emergency nurse undue stress, legal difficulties, and other hurdles that must be dealt with. Being able to recognize these challenges in advance and knowing the resources available to help meet the challenges is an important part of ensuring success as an emergency nurse.

References

Advisory Board Company. (2010). *Managing frequent flyers* [webconference]. Retrieved from https://www.advisory.com/technology/emergency-compass/members/events/webconferences/2010/managing-frequent-flyers

American College of Emergency Physicians. (2011). *Boarding of admitted and intensive care patients in the emergency department.* Irving, TX: American College of Emergency Physicians.

American Hospital Association (AHA). (2010). *Annual survey.* Retrieved from http://www.aha.org/research/reports/tw/chartbook/2010chartbook.shtml

American Hospital Association (AHA). (2015). *Annual survey.* Retrieved from http://www.aha.org/research/reports/tw/chartbook/ch3.shtml

American Nurses Association (ANA). (2008). *Reduction of patient restraint and seclusion in healthcare settings* [Position statement]. Retrieved from http://www.nursingworld.org/MainMenuCategories/EthicsStandards/Ethics-Position-Statements/Reduction-of-Patient-Restraint-and-Seclusion-in-Health-Care-Settings.pdf

Augustine, J. J. (2013, November 24). The true cost of ambulance diversion. *Emergency Physicians Monthly.* Retrieved from http://epmonthly.com/article/the-true-cost-of-ambulance-diversion/

Becher, J., & Visovsky, C. (2012). Horizontal violence in nursing. *MEDSURG Nursing 21*(4), 210–214.

Berge, K., Dillon, K., Sikkink, K., Taylor, T., & Lanier, W. (2012). Diversion of drugs within health care facilities, a multiple-victim crime: Patterns of diversion, scope, consequences, detection, and prevention. *Mayo Clinic Proceedings, 87*(7), 674–82.

Bradley, C., Lensky, M., & Brasel, K. (2011). Family presence during resuscitation. *Journal of Palliative Medicine, 14*(1), 97–98.

Burke, L. G., Joyce, N., Baker, W. E., Biddinger, P. D., Dyer, S., Friedman, F. D., & Epstein, S. K. (2013). The effect on an ambulance diversion ban on emergency department length of stay and ambulance turnaround time. *Annals of Emergency Medicine, 61*(3), 303–311.

Burton, K. (2014). Emerging from the darkness and stepping into the light: Implementing an understanding of the experience of nurse addiction into nursing education. *Journal of Nursing Education and Practice, 4*(4), 151–164.

Castillo, M. (2014, January 27). Man found dead in NYC hospital waiting room more than 8 hours after entering. *CBS News*. Retrieved from http://www.cbsnews.com/news/man-found-dead-in-st-barnabas-hospital-waiting-room-8-hours/

Centers for Medicare and Medicaid Services (CMS). (2008, October 17). *CMS manual system.* Retrieved from https://www.cms.gov/Regulations-and-Guidance/Guidance/Transmittals/downloads/R37SOMA.pdf

Clark, J. (2011). Mother's little helper: The problem of narcotic diversion. *Air Medical Journal, 30*(6), 294–296.

Cox, L. (2008, September 25). ER death points to growing wait-time problem. *ABC News*. Retrieved from http://abcnews.go.com/Health/story?id=5884487

Delaney, M., & Reed, L. (2015). Recognizing and responding to a new era of infectious and communicable diseases. *Journal of Emergency Nursing, 41*(2), 138–40.

Dwyer, T. (2015). Predictors of public support for family presence during cardiopulmonary resuscitation: A population based study. *International Journal of Nursing Studies, 52,* 1064–1070.

Emergency Nurses Association (ENA). (2010a). *Chemical impairment of emergency nurses.* Retrieved from https://www.ena.org/SiteCollectionDocuments/Position%20Statements/CHEMICALIMPAIRMENT.pdf

Emergency Nurses Association (ENA). (2010b). *Communicable diseases in the emergency department.* Retrieved from www.ena.org

Emergency Nurses Association (ENA). (2011a). *Definitions for consistent emergency department metrics* [Consensus statement]. Retrieved from https://www.ena.org/about/media/PressReleases/Documents/07-13-11_DefinitionsED_Metrics.pdf

Emergency Nurses Association (ENA). (2011b). *Emergency department violence surveillance study.* Retrieved from https://www.ena.org/practice-research/research/Documents/ENAEDVSReportNovember2011.pdf

Emergency Nurses Association (ENA). (2015). *Ebola virus disease (EVD).* Retrieved from https://www.ena.org/practice-research/Practice/Documents/EbolaTopicBrief.pdf

Feistritzer, N., Hill, C., Vanairsdale, S., & Gentry, J. (2014). Care of patients with Ebola virus disease. *The Journal of Continuing Education in Nursing, 45*(11), 479–81.

Gagnon, L. (2010). Behavioral health emergencies. In R. Steinman & P. Howard (Eds.), *Sheehy's manual of emergency care: Principles and practice* (pp. 677–688). Philadelphia, PA: Mosby-Elsevier.

Gallup. (2014, December 18). *U.S. views on honest and ethical standards in professions.* Retrieved from http://www.gallup.com/poll/180260/americans-rate-nurses-highest-honesty-ethical-standards.aspx

Gilligan, C., Sanson-Fisher, R., & Turon, R. (2012). The organ donation conundrum. *Progress in Transplantation, 22*(3), 312–16.

Hammad, K., Arbon, P., Gebbie, K., & Hutton, A. (2012). Nursing in the emergency department (ED) during a disaster: A review of the current literature. *Australasian Emergency Nursing Journal, 15,* 235–44.

Health Resources and Services Administration (HRSA). (2015). *How organ allocation works.* Retrieved from www.optn.transplant.hrsa.gov

Heilicser, B. (2013). Ethical dilemmas in emergency nursing. In M. Hammond, & P. Gerber-Zimmerman (Eds.), *Sheehy's manual of emergency care* (pp. 43–48). Philadelphia, PA: Mosby-Elsevier.

Howard, P., & Foley, A. (2015). Disaster triage—Are you ready? *Journal of Emergency Nursing, 40*(5), 515–17.

Institute of Medicine (IOM). (2006). *Future of emergency care: Hospital-based emergency care, at the breaking point.* Washington, DC: The National Academies Press.

Jabre, P., Belpomme, V., Bertrand, L., Jacob, L., Broche, C., Normand, D., & Adnet, F. (2013). Family presence during cardiopulmonary resuscitation. *Archives of Cardiovascular Disease Supplements, 5*, 105–110.

The Joint Commission. (2008). *Sentinel event alert: Behaviors that undermine a culture of safety.* Retrieved from http://www.jointcommission.org/assets/1/18/SEA_40.PDF

Kristopher, S. (2015). Can the family block organ donation? *Nursing, 45*(5), 16–17.

Langenfeld, S. J., Cook, G., Sudbeck, C., Luers, T., & Schenarts, P. J. (2014). An assessment of unprofessional behavior among surgical residents on Facebook: A warning of the dangers of social media. *Journal of Surgical Education, 71*(6), e28–e32.

Lederman, Z., Garasic, M., & Piperberg, M. (2014). Family presence during cardiopulmonary resuscitation: Who should decide? *Journal of Medical Ethics, 40*(5), 315–19.

Liang, S., Theodoro, D., Schuur, J., & Marschall, J. (2014). Infection prevention in the emergency department. *Annals of Emergency Medicine, 64*(3), 299–313.

Litzenburg, T. A., & Dorsey, N. B. (2011, March 1). Ambulance diversion: Solution or problem? *AHC Media.* Retrieved from http://www.ahcmedia.com/articles/129787-ambulance-diversion-solution-or-problem

Marino, P. A., Mays, C. M., & Thompson, E. J. (2015). Bypass rapid Assessment Triage: How culture change improved one emergency department's safety, throughput and patient satisfaction. *Journal of Emergency Nursing, 41*(3), pp 213–220.

Mayer, T., & Jensen, K. (2009). *Hardwiring flow: Systems and processes for seamless patient care.* Gulf Breeze, FL: Fire Starter Publishing.

Nance, J. J. (2008). *Why hospitals should fly: The ultimate flight plan to patient safety and quality care.* Bozeman, MT: Second River Healthcare.

National Incident Management System (NIMS). (2015). *NIMS frequently asked questions.* Retrieved from http://www.fema.gov/pdf/emergency/nims/NIMSFAQs.pdf

Phillips, D. (2013). Organ and tissue donation basics. *Nursing Made Incredibly Easy, 11*(1), 30–36.

Press Ganey. (2010). *Emergency department pulse report.* Press Ganey. Retrieved from http://www.pressganey.com/Documents_secure/Pulse%20Reports/2010_ED_Pulse_Report.pdf

Showalter, J. S. (2014). *The law of healthcare administration* (7th ed.). Chicago, IL: Health Administration Press.

Singer, A. J., Thode, H. C., Viccellio, P., & Pines, J. M. (2011). The association between length of emergency department boarding and mortality. *Academic Emergency Medicine, 18*(12), pp. 1324–1329.

Spokane Fire Department. (n.d.). *CARES.* Retrieved from https://my.spokanecity.org/fire/operations/cares/

Starr, K. (2015). The sneaky prevalence of substance abuse in nursing. *Nursing, 45*(3), 16–17.

Stoppler, M. C. (2014, December 1). Medical triage: Code tags and triage terminology. *MedicineNet.com.* Retrieved from http://www.medicinenet.com/script/main/art.asp?articlekey=79529

Studer, Q. (2003). *Hardwiring excellence: Purpose, worthwhile work, making a difference.* Gulf Breeze, FL: Fire Starter Publishing.

Trader, J. (2013, June 24). Social media and healthcare: Navigating the new communications landscape. *Healthcare IT News.* Retrieved from http://www.healthcareitnews.com/blog/social-media-and-healthcare-navigating-new-communications-landscape

Traino, H., & Siminoff, L. (2013). Attitudes and acceptance of First Person Authorization: A national comparison of donor and nondonor families. *Journal of Trauma Acute Care Surgery, 74*(1), 294–300.

United Network for Organ Sharing (UNOS). (2015). *Organ allocation.* Retrieved from https://www.unos.org/data/

violence. (n.d.). In *Merriam-Webster's online dictionary* (11th ed.). Retrieved from http://www.merriam-webster.com/dictionary/violence

Wadman, M., Schwedhelm, S., Watson, S., Swanhorst, J., Gibbs, S., Lowe, J., ... Muelleman, R. (2015). Emergency department processes for the evaluation and management of persons under investigation for Ebola virus disease. *Annals of Emergency Medicine, 66*(3), 306–314.

Wiler, J. L., Welch, S., Pines, J., Schuur, J., Jouriles, N., & Stone-Griffith, S., (2015). Emergency department performance measures updates: Proceedings of the 2014 Emergency Department Benchmarking Alliance Consensus Summit. *Academic Emergency Medicine, 22*(5), 542–553.

Zavala, S., & Shaffer, C. (2011). Do patients understand discharge instructions? *Journal of Emergency Nursing, 37*(2), 138–140.

12

RISK MANAGEMENT AND QUALITY ISSUES AFFECTING THE EMERGENCY NURSE

–Laurel Grisbach, BSN, RN, CPHRM

The emergency department (ED) is perhaps the area of the hospital with the broadest array of uncertainties and risks over which providers have limited control. No other department in the hospital is open 24 hours a day, required to evaluate and stabilize acute and chronic patients of every age, gender, and acuity without any control over the number of patients or timing of arrival. As a result, emergency nurses must be flexible, adaptable, and able to anticipate conditions that are contrary to patient safety so that mitigating measures may be implemented before patient harm occurs. To this end, you need to understand the principles of professional liability as they affect the delivery of patient care and use all available tools to mitigate risks to patient safety. Having knowledge and awareness of hospital and departmental policies and procedures, state and federal laws and regulations directing the care and treatment of patients, and published literature and research identifying patient safety concerns and evidence-based recommendations for best practices enhances the quality of patient care while minimizing professional liability risk exposure.

Acceptable Standard of Care

In 2000, the Institute of Medicine (IOM) published *To Err Is Human: Building a Safer Health System.* This report estimated that between 44,000 and 98,000 people die in hospitals each year as a result of preventable medical errors. Through this report, the IOM issued a call to action for healthcare facilities to set a minimum goal of a 50% reduction of preventable medical errors over the subsequent 5 years (Kohn, Corrigan, & Donaldson, 2000).

Just prior to the IOM report's publication, The Joint Commission on accreditation of healthcare published its first *Sentinel Event Alert* in 1998, encouraging facilities to conduct a root cause analysis to drill down and identify primary and contributing factors for events resulting in serious patient harm, disability, or death (referred to as *sentinel events*). The primary goal was to encourage hospitals to report sentinel events and share the lessons learned from root cause analyses. Data was tracked and trends were identified. The data was and continues to be monitored for frequent events with commonalities in the primary and contributing factors. This chapter discusses sentinel events more in-depth in the "Risk Identification" section.

This information is shared publicly through the use of *Sentinel Event Alerts* so that all healthcare organizations may review and implement the lessons learned to reduce the likelihood of these events ever occurring again. In 2002, The Joint Commission established the first set of National Patient Safety Goals, several of which have become the acceptable standard of care (The Joint Commission, 2015).

The IOM and The Joint Commission are not alone in their research to improve patient safety. Many organizations drive research and development of best practices to heighten healthcare quality and are excellent resources when updating departmental policies and procedures:.

- Lucian Leape Institute of the National Patient Safety Foundation, 2007

- Center for Patient Safety, 2005

- Pennsylvania Patient Safety Authority (PPSA), 2002

- Joint Commission Resources (JCR), 1998

▦ Institute for Healthcare Improvement (IHI), 1991

▦ Agency for Healthcare Research and Quality (AHRQ), 1989

▦ CRICO Risk Management Foundation (CRICO/RMF), 1979

▦ Emergency Care Research Institute (ECRI), 1968

Risk Management

In the broad sense, risk management involves protecting the assets of an organization. When applied to the clinical setting, this requires consideration of legal and regulatory requirements, clinical operations, effects on the workforce, and the impact of interventions upon the risks and workflow of others. Today's clinical risk-management plan focuses on protecting the organization's assets by promoting patient safety to reduce the risk of patient harm, and by increasing focus on workplace safety (Carroll & Nakamura, 2011a).

A recent report by the American Hospital Association (AHA, 2015) indicates that between 1991 and 2013, ED visits grew by 45 million while the number of hospital EDs was reduced by 668. Many of the closures were due to costs of operations surpassing reimbursement for services. Some of the revenue loss was triggered by the shift of patients seeking care in ambulatory surgery centers and physician offices, where the cost of providing care was less. Unfortunately, this shift did not reduce overhead expenses for the remaining hospitals with EDs that must maintain operations around the clock to provide a safety net for patients with nowhere else to go. Sustaining an adequate safety net requires sufficient numbers of healthcare professionals to meet the community's needs.

Over the next decade, the U.S. Bureau of Labor Statistics estimates that hospitals will need an additional 900,000 healthcare staff members and projects a shortage of between 46,000 and 90,000 specialist and generalist physicians (AHA, 2015). In addition to the projected shortage of healthcare staff, a study by the Centers for Disease Control and Prevention (CDC, 2011) indicated that it is unlikely patient volumes will be on the decrease. Instead, the study showed that the vast majority of patients seen in the ED have urgent or emergent needs and therefore require the level of care provided in the ED setting (see Figure 12.1). It also states that numerous patients initially seen in a physician's office or urgent care are sent to the ED for a higher level of laboratory and radiology services not available in the alternative setting (CRICO Strategies, 2015).

Proponents of the Affordable Care Act (ACA) hope that the provided health insurance will increase the number of people being seen by a primary care provider and reduce the number of patients using the ED for routine healthcare. A fact sheet issued by the American

College of Emergency Physicians (ACEP) addressing the anticipated effects of the ACA on EDs said that the ACA provides insurance coverage but doesn't guarantee access to medical care (American College of Emergency Physicians, 2013). For these reasons, it's difficult to project if there will be a significant decrease in the number of ED visits in the next several years to offset the reduction of needed healthcare staff. What is known is that heavy patient volumes, an aging population with multiple comorbidities, and a reduction of healthcare providers create a complex environment ripe for human errors and patient harm.

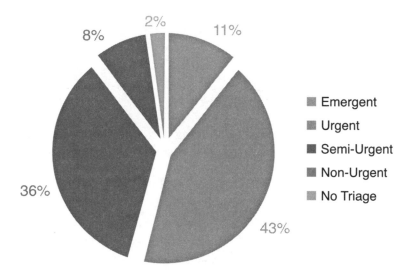

Source: Centers for Disease Control and Prevention; National Hospital Ambulatory Medical Care Survey, 2011.

Figure 12.1   ED visits by level of urgency.

Legal implications in the ED may include both general and professional liability. *General liability* occurs when there are hazards in the environment of which employees have knowledge but fail to act on in a timely manner, resulting in personal injury or other damages. The most common examples of general liability issues in the ED are loss of patient valuables or belongings and slips and falls due to trip hazards or wet floors. Less common but also considered within the definition of general liability are allegations of defamation or slander. *Professional liability* involves an allegation of negligent care or omissions. Care provided by the nurse will be scrutinized to establish if the nurse remained within the scope of practice and met the current standard of care.

Negligence, Malpractice, and Litigation

According to CRICO Strategies (2015), one in eleven malpractice defendants is a nurse (National Practitioner Data Bank [NPDP], 2015). Considering there are currently close to 4 million actively practicing nurses in the United States (Henry J. Kaiser Family Foundation, 2015), this is a significant number. Involvement in a professional liability case, even if you are eventually released from the lawsuit, can be a life-changing event. Many lawsuits are not filed for close to 2 years and may be active lawsuits for several years depending upon any appeals filed by either party. The good news is that only 5% of professional liability claims go to trial, and of those, close to 80% receive a defense verdict with no payout to the plaintiff (Pennsylvania Patient Safety Authority [PPSA], 2011a).

Negligence—Requires the presence of four elements:

- Duty to the patient
- Breach of the duty
- Breach resulted in patient injury or damages
- The injury or damages were a direct result of the breach

Allegation—Statement of fact upon which the plaintiff (person filing the suit) is basing the claim that the defendant violated the standard of care or operated outside of the scope of practice.

Notice of Intent—Filed by the plaintiff prior to officially filing the claim with the court. This letter serves to let the defendant know a lawsuit is pending.

Summons & Complaint—The official court filing for the lawsuit with the assignment of a case number.

Statute of Limitations—An established period from either the event or awareness within which the plaintiff must file a claim. The statute of limitations may differ between states. Failure to meet the time limit may nullify the claim.

Appeal—Occurs when an individual does not accept the court's verdict. Appealing a decision involves filing a request for the judge to take another look at the case and rule on it again. It may also involve the case going before a higher court to review the facts and make a ruling on it.

Claims are made by issuing a demand for payment, sending a *Notice of Intent,* or serving the individual with a *Summons and Complaint.* If you are on the receiving end of any of these three methods for triggering a claim, immediately notify your department supervisor and facility risk manager.

Anatomy of a Lawsuit

Sometimes nurses get lucky and know that an error was made resulting in injury. Perhaps the nurse is aware of an unanticipated event that upsets a patient or family member; this is the best time to notify department leadership and work with the risk management department to conduct an investigation to determine whether there is justification for making an early settlement. All negotiations are made through the risk management or legal department; you should never make any promises that a bill will be waived or ongoing care provided free of charge. This is all a part of settlement negotiations and requires insight into *causation* (i.e., if the event or omission directly caused the injury) and special knowledge of the value of damages.

Once the claim is made, the litigation process begins in a series of steps:

1. **Notification of the claim or impending litigation** *(service).*

2. **Each party gathers information and requests the opposing party to produce information** *(discovery).*

   This may include depositions in which those involved in the event, witnesses, and experts are questioned by the opposing attorney while under oath. You may be requested to respond to a set of *interrogatories* (specific questions) frequently answered with the counsel of your attorney with a sworn attestation as to your truthfulness. This step can also include acquiring copies of policies and procedures in effect at the time of the event, as well as copies of the medical record from multiple sources, such as hospital, emergency physician's billing copy, primary care physician, and transfer paperwork sent to a receiving facility.

3. **Either party may ask the court to take a look at the undisputed facts to determine whether the remaining information is sufficient to warrant a trial** *(summary judgment).*

4. **If the plaintiff's case has merit and direct causation, the attorneys from all sides will get together and negotiate a fair financial settlement so that a costly trial can be avoided** *(settlement conference).*

5. **Your time in court before a judge and jury** *(trial).*

   This may not be the ultimate end, because appeals by either side can go on for many years.

Professional Liability Insurance

The healthcare facility provides professional liability insurance coverage for the care provided by licensed staff while on duty. The coverage is in effect as long as you're practicing within the scope of practice and not engaging in criminal acts. A question frequently asked is whether you should purchase individual coverage in addition to the hospital's policy. In most cases, the hospital's coverage is sufficient; however, there may be situations when the hospital desires to settle against your wishes, or perhaps there is a conflict of interest and you prefer independent representation. Another consideration for additional coverage is if the policy will cover legal representation while under review by licensing or regulatory agencies. These investigations are not always part of the hospital's policy.

If you participate as a volunteer at a hospital-sponsored event hosted by your employer, the hospital provides professional liability coverage for you at that event. If, however, you participate in patient care activities outside of the scope of employment, such as volunteering at high school football games or community events, you need to verify that the organization hosting the event is providing professional liability coverage for any alleged negligent act occurring at the event. Ultimately the decision as to whether you should purchase additional coverage is a personal one.

Over the course of a career, it's likely that you'll come across an emergent situation while off duty and feel compelled to help, with whatever resources are available. In today's litigious society, you may hesitate to get involved due to fear of not being covered by a professional liability policy in the event of a poor outcome. Most states have regulations or laws to protect those engaging in a rescue from liability. These laws are commonly referred to as *Good Samaritan* laws and protect you as long as there is no expectation of compensation, and no gross medical errors are made (Widgery, 2014). The laws usually allow for human factors such as making a reasonable mistake. Every state has different nuances within its Good Samaritan coverage. Some states only offer Good Samaritan protection to trained rescuers who come across a situation, while others allow coverage for members of the general public as well. And then there are those states restricting Good Samaritan protection to members of the general public only when trying to control active bleeding or perform CPR. You should be familiar with your state's specific parameters for Good Samaritan protections (California Health and Safety Code §1799.102).

Care for the Caregiver Involved in Litigation

The effects of being named in a lawsuit are very stressful and far-reaching. When involved or named in a lawsuit, you may feel isolated when advised by your attorney not to discuss the facts of the case with anyone. If other colleagues are also involved, the tension on the unit can become hostile, hinder team communication, and create an environment contrary to enhancing patient safety. Individuals going through these difficult times are often referred to as *second victims* (Brenner, 2010). You're considered a second victim if you:

- Witnessed an event

- Made an entry in a patient's medical record

- Were involved in the care of the patient when the event occurred

- Personally made the error

Signs that you're under stress from being a second victim are:

- You relive the event.

- You feel anger, frustration, shame, or guilt.

- You have difficulty concentrating.

- Your sleep is disturbed and you feel fatigued and depressed.

- Your heart rate and blood pressure are elevated.

- You experience shaking tremors.

Some things you can do to relieve the stress are:

- Participate in social interactions.

- Share your feelings with someone you trust.

- Exercise, get plenty of rest, and eat healthy.

- Avoid alcohol or self-medicating.

- Seek professional help.

 Even providers not directly involved, but named in the suit because their initials are somewhere in the medical record, can experience the stress and frustration of being listed as a "Doe 1-100" on the Summons and Complaint.

Common Allegations in Emergency Medicine Litigation

By recognizing the common causes leading to patient harm in the ED, you can implement evidence-based approaches to reduce the likelihood of the events reoccurring. As a patient advocate, you're in a prime position to use this information to enhance a culture of safety within the department. In a 2011 report from Physician Insurers Association of America (PIAA), *diagnostic error* was present in 49% of its emergency medicine closed claims (claims that have settled or otherwise been finalized) and 60% of the indemnity paid between 1985 and 2010. Additional causes for professional liability claims were cases involving improper performance of a procedure and medication errors (PIAA, 2011):

- **Failure to diagnose:** Acute myocardial infarction, appendicitis (surgical abdomen or pelvis), meningitis

- **Improper performance of procedure:** Assessment and patient interview, physical exam

- **Medication errors:** Dosage error (including an overdose), drug omission, wrong drug

Standard of Care

You have a duty to treat patients with a certain level of care (*Young v. Cerniak,* 1984). The measure to determine that level is "what a reasonable nurse, of like or similar training and experience, would do under like or similar circumstances" (*Cline v. William H. Friedman & Assoc.,* 1994). *Standards of care* are determined in several different ways:

- **A community standard of care or locality rule** may be used to determine that the nurse is functioning at the same level as other emergency nurses at surrounding hospitals (*Logan v. Greenwich Hosp. Assoc.,* 1993).

- **A state-wide standard of care** prevents clinicians in small communities from being called to testify about the standard of care provided by their colleagues (*Shilkret v. Annapolis Emergency Hosp. Association,* 1975).

- **A national standard of care** is driven by regulatory bodies and accreditation agencies (*Sheeley v. Memorial Hosp.,* 1998).

Occasionally, the standard of care is established through court rulings creating case law (Carroll & Nakamura, 2011a). To keep abreast of current standards of care, you must complete continuing education as a requirement of maintaining licensure and specialty credentials.

Hospital policies and procedures are one of the first documents sought during the discovery period of the litigation process. Plaintiff attorneys frequently begin their case evaluation by looking to see if the nurse abided by the hospital's policies and if the policies reflect the current standard of care. It's vitally important that the policies are current and that staff are aware of their content. Some hospitals have well-orchestrated processes in place for policy review and revision, including rolling out any substantive changes to frontline staff; others find themselves in a daily survival mode, resulting in policies becoming obsolete and without revision. It's important that you know how to access current policies and procedures and periodically take the time to review them for any changes that could affect current practice.

Laws—Enforceable rules made through legislation, executive decree, or by binding precedents established through legal proceedings.

Statute—Law passed by the supreme state or federal legislature. Statutes may be designated to be retroactive once the law is passed.

Regulation—Established by a regulatory agency within the powers given to it by the government. Regulations may be used to add clarity and precision to statutes, and although adoption by the agency is required, they do not need to go through legislative channels.

Regulatory Bodies

Regulatory bodies may be state or federal agencies granted certain power and oversight responsibilities by statute or legislative rule. These agencies may establish criteria by which those under their authority must abide, called *regulations*. The regulations may not exceed the scope of authority granted to the agency by the legislature. At times, state regulatory bodies may enact regulations that are more restrictive than federal law. When this occurs, it's best to abide by the most restrictive standard to ensure compliance. Examples of oversight provided by federal regulatory bodies follow:

■ **Centers for Medicare & Medicaid Services (CMS)** provides oversight to facilities receiving payment through a Medicare contract to ensure that cost-effective, quality care is provided to their members. They require documentation of medical necessity and appropriateness for diagnostic tests and treatment for which they are being billed. CMS developed the billing codes used throughout the industry and reimburses hospitals for the care provided to their members based upon the quality of the care provided, as reflected in mandatory data reporting and the patient's experience during the hospital visit.

■ **Centers for Disease Control & Prevention (CDC)** monitors infectious diseases and works collaboratively with other agencies around the world to control the spread of disease. The CDC maintains statistics of infectious disease rates, provides treatment guidelines during outbreaks, and conducts research to develop ways to eradicate the threat of an outbreak. Under its regulatory powers, the CDC requires healthcare providers to report specific diseases and genetic conditions and shares information regarding hospital-acquired infections with CMS.

- **Food and Drug Administration (FDA)** establishes rules and requirements for testing and clinical trials prior to approving drugs, medical devices, vaccines, and other biologics for use. The FDA watches for safety issues, adverse reactions, and medical errors involving items previously approved and issues alerts or recalls.

- **Agency for Healthcare Research and Quality (AHRQ)** is a federal agency operating under the Department of Health and Human Services with a focus on the improvement of quality in healthcare. The agency provides grants for research used to establish evidence-based practice guidelines. In 2007, the Hospital Consumer Assessment of Healthcare Providers and Systems (HCAHPS) survey tool developed by the agency began being used nationally to provide standardized feedback of the patient's experience while hospitalized. HCAHPS scores are publicly reported to provide transparency and comparisons of patient experiences at different hospitals. The scores are also used by CMS to determine the rate of reimbursement for care. Effective January 2015, CMS may raise or lower a facility's reimbursement by 1.5% and by 2% starting in 2016 (Centers for Medicare & Medicaid Services [CMS], 2014). Although the percentages appear small, their impact on the hospital's bottom line is significant.

Medicare reimbursement is tied to the hospital's HCAHPS scores. These scores measure the patients' perception of their experience while hospitalized.

- **Occupational Safety and Health Administration (OSHA)** establishes and monitors health and safety regulations for use in the workplace. Some of its regulations affecting the healthcare industry are the requirement for respirator fit testing, handling hazardous materials and gases, and dealing with bloodborne pathogens. OSHA inspectors perform evaluations for hazards and plan approval prior to beginning construction. OSHA also responds to investigate serious accidents involving the death or dismemberment of a worker. Employers found to be out of compliance with providing a safe and healthy work environment may face significant fines.

Accreditation Agencies

The American College of Surgeons (ACS) was the first organization to establish a minimum standard for care in hospitals and began conducting onsite visits to verify compliance in the early 1900s. In 1951, several medical and hospital associations joined together to create a non-profit organization called the *Joint Commission on Accreditation of Hospitals* (JCAH), later to become *The Joint Commission,* and the ACS eventually transferred its standardization program over to The Joint Commission. By the mid-1960s, Congress passed the Social Security Act of 1965, indicating that any hospitals accredited by JCAH were deemed to be compliant with most of the Medicare Conditions of Participation for hospitals. Over the years the focus of the surveys changed, placing greater emphasis on the organization's actual performance through the use of quality indicators. In 2008, Congress enacted a new law requiring any accreditation body seeking to obtain deeming authority to apply through CMS. Three accreditation bodies were granted deeming authority: The Joint Commission, Det Norske Veritas Healthcare, Inc. (DNV-GL), and Healthcare Facilities Accreditation Program (HFAP). Each accreditation organization takes a different approach toward meeting the CMS Conditions of Participation, some less prescriptive than others, making them more attractive to potential members (The Joint Commission, 2015).

Risk Identification

Risk identification is one of the primary tools used to boost patient safety and reduce opportunities for harm. The delivery of healthcare requires a complex and ever-changing environment. New technologies and treatment methods are introduced at a rapid pace, challenging nurse educators and department directors to keep up with staff education and competencies. Recognition of risk factors may come from a plethora of sources including patients and visitors, licensed and unlicensed staff, and vendors. Ideally, risks should be identified *proactively* so that processes can be enhanced to address the vulnerabilities before harm occurs. *Reactive* identification is less desirable because by definition it means an adverse or unexpected event has already occurred before action is taken.

Proactive Approaches

Unfortunately, steps to improve patient safety and patient care are usually taken after a negative outcome. An analysis of the outcome identifies weaknesses and allows strategies to be developed to reduce the likelihood of recurrence. The problem with this approach is that a negative outcome had to occur for the process to be initiated. In an ideal world, risk identification would be undertaken proactively before a negative event occurs. Numerous processes are in place to assist with proactive risk identification.

Failure Mode and Effects Analysis

Engineers developed the failure mode and effects analysis (FMEA) technique to explore possible mishaps and malfunctions of military systems. The process was adopted by the healthcare industry because it provides a systematic approach to identify process failures and their relative impact in the event of an occurrence. This same tool may be used to prioritize multiple performance improvement activities. The tool consists of four areas of focus:

1. List the various steps in the process.

2. Evaluate each step to identify what could possibly go wrong in that process.

3. Look into each of the possible process failures to identify what would cause that failure to occur.

4. Assess the consequences of each possible failure.

Each section is assigned a score that is then calculated to determine the ultimate degree of risk if the process failure occurs. Once prioritized, each causative factor is reviewed and measures implemented to prevent that factor from occurring, thus preventing the process failure (Department of Veterans Affairs, 2011).

 A nurse administers 50 mg of a medication and is surprised to find the physician only ordered 25 mg. The nurse mentions the situation to the physician, who modifies the order to match the dose administered. This is still a medication error and should be reported.

Event Reporting, Near Misses, and Good Catches

Reporting unexpected events is necessary for several reasons. The information helps organizational leadership become aware of trends in errors and areas of vulnerability, heightens awareness of processes in need of improvement, alerts the risk manager to issues that may result in litigation or trigger the need for disclosure, and notifies administration of situations triggering an obligation for reporting to an outside agency. Event reports are underused in many institutions due to fear of disciplinary actions or retaliation. At times, underreporting may occur because of a reporting structure that is too cumbersome and time-consuming. To maximize the positive effects of event reporting, leadership must be trustworthy and provide closed-loop communications to reassure the reporting party to the extent possible that something is being done about the issue (Carroll & Nakamura, 2011b). Administrators who recognize human beings as fallible understand that there will be times when employees will make mistakes. Those seeking to identify a process failure before blaming the individual will be more apt to develop a healthy culture of safety within the institution. Facilities with strong safety cultures may show a higher number of events reported, including those of near misses or good catches (Carroll & Nakamura, 2011b).

Every state has statutes and case law establishing protection of *privileged information* from discovery. Information that is *protected* means that in the event of litigation, the plaintiff would not be entitled to receive a copy of the information. The protection may be granted through peer-review, quality-assurance, and risk-management laws, or it may rely on attorney-client privilege. Even when a document is protected, it's possible for an inadvertent act (e.g., telling your friend about the event while discussing your day at work) to remove that privilege. Hospital policy on event reporting and participation in investigations dealing with adverse events provides guidance for maintaining privilege (Carroll & Nakamura, 2011a).

Reactive Approaches

Because proactive risk identification has not been historically embraced in healthcare, risks and actions taken to reduce those risks are often reactive. While it's essential to carefully analyze negative events after they occur, this does not prevent the event from occurring in the first place. Therefore, healthcare facilities should use proactive approaches to reduce negative events but also be prepared to enact reactive approaches when appropriate. Numerous reactive processes can be used to identify and reduce risks in the delivery of healthcare.

Sentinel Events

Sentinel events have a profound effect on patients, family, and friends, as well as healthcare workers and the community. A phrase frequently stated by the victims and family is that they don't want the event to ever happen to anyone again. One of the ways that healthcare organizations can help to make sure it doesn't happen again is prompt notification of the event so that a designated group can determine if the event is serious enough to require an evaluation team to conduct a *root cause analysis* (RCA).

Similar to the failure mode and effects analysis, a root cause analysis is conducted after the fact, and:

1. Steps in the processes leading to the occurrence are listed.

2. Another list is developed demonstrating how the process should have worked according to any policies or procedures.

3. If it is discovered that staff developed a work-around to a step in the process, the team drills down a bit further to discover why staff believed it necessary to create a work-around.

For instance, if nurses are supposed to scan medication bar codes while at the patient's bedside but instead are scanning all medications with the scanner connected to the computer on wheels in the hallway, it's important to discover why nurses are not using the portable scanners. It's likely not because of a lack of awareness of what they are supposed to do; rather, it's due to an equipment or process issue.

4. **After all of the process, human, and environmental factors are evaluated, an action plan is developed to address each of the contributing factors leading to the event.**

    A single cause seldom leads to an event. For example, a medication error happened because the nurse pulled the wrong medication out of the drawer of the medication dispensing machine. Some RCAs might stop there and say the action plan is to educate the nurse to be more careful when removing medications from the machine. But if the drill-down continued, they may find that the nurse pulled the wrong medication because the wrong medication was in the specified slot where the other medication should be. The drill-down would then continue to try to determine why the wrong medication was in the designated slot.

It's necessary to continue to drill down so that the real issue is identified and modified if necessary to prevent a reoccurrence. Of equal importance is for hospital administrators to understand that a lack of knowledge or understanding is usually not the cause of the event, yet when errors occur, one of the first action items listed is to educate the staff.

Sentinel event—An unexpected occurrence involving death or serious physical or psychological injury, or the risk thereof. Serious injury specifically includes loss of limb or function (The Joint Commission, 2015).

In its efforts to obtain data for evaluation of possible trends, The Joint Commission strongly encourages its members to self-report when a sentinel event occurs and provide a copy of the root cause analysis for review. Many hospitals choose not to self-report due to a fear that the information would become public and place them at greater risk of litigation, with the RCA being used as evidence against them. This may be true; however, with the push toward transparency and disclosure, much of the information will be common knowledge to the patient and family, so those protections were voluntarily forfeited. One of the benefits of self-reporting is the ability of The Joint Commission to identify trends and alert other healthcare providers throughout the world of the events and contributing factors as well as issue recommendations for preventing the events at other institutions. The Joint Commission provides two great quality-improvement tools using the self-reported data: Sentinel Event Alerts and an annual report of the leading root causes to sentinel events. The report is frequently used as a foundation for discussion of the upcoming year's patient safety and risk management plans (The Joint Commission, 2014) (see Figure 12.2).

Top Five Root Causes of Sentinel Events Reviewed by
the Joint Commission in 2014

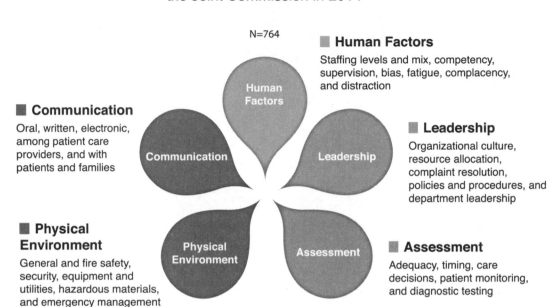

Figure 12.2 An example of the root causes of sentinel events in 2014.

Mandatory Reporting

Many regulatory and accreditation agencies require hospitals to report on quality measures. Additionally, federal and state laws require patients presenting with certain conditions, such as victims of abuse or injury by a firearm, to be reported to a law enforcement agency. This information helps track risk of harm to society so that mitigating actions can be taken to minimize harm. Failure to report the required information may result in fines and, in some instances, incarceration. It's important to recognize that the federal Health Insurance Portability and Accountability Act of 1996 (HIPAA) makes allowances for some mandatory reporting and authorizes the release of *personal health information* (PHI) when necessary to comply with federal and state reporting laws, coordinating a patient's treatment, and healthcare operations, such as billing, peer review, and quality-improvement activities (45 CFR §164.506, 2002).

Duty to Warn Third Parties

You're frequently exposed to situations prompting consideration of the necessity to warn a third party of possible impending harm. States vary in their approaches for determining the *duty to warn a non-patient third party*. The duty may be triggered for many different reasons, such as to protect the public's health, warn an individual of medication precautions, or notify an identifiable intended victim of the threat.

Most states recognize the importance of protecting public health by requiring hospitals to report certain diseases to the CDC for monitoring and follow-up. Once reported, the CDC or health department follows up with those who may have been exposed to the disease to ensure they are alerted of the need to seek medical attention (45 CFR §164.506, 2002). For instance, if an individual was diagnosed with severe acute respiratory syndrome (SARS), the physician diagnosing the patient would have the duty to report the virus so that individuals recently exposed to the patient could be contacted and advised to observe for early signs and symptoms of SARS and when to seek treatment. Several states have limited the duty to warn requirement to only those times when the patient poses harm to a known individual (*Tarasoff v. Regents of the University of California*, 1976). An example of this is when a patient is identified as having a sexually transmitted disease. The healthcare provider would have a duty to report so that the sexual partners could receive notification of their exposure and receive treatment. Similar to the duty to warn unnamed but predictable third parties is the requirement to notify the Department of Motor Vehicles of patients experiencing a lapse of consciousness. This allows the department to restrict the individual's license until the condition leading to the lapses can be stabilized to the point where the individual has gone a specified period of time without a reoccurrence.

Another type of a duty to warn is the requirement to warn a patient of the dangers or risks associated with taking certain medications (*Watkins v. U.S.*, 1979). Patients taking sedatives, narcotics, or anti-anxiety medications are frequently advised not to operate heavy machinery or drive while under the effects of the medication. Failure to warn the patient of potential harmful activities prior to discharge may result in liability exposure for the healthcare provider and hospital. As an ED nurse and patient advocate, you should verify that the patient understands the medication warnings during aftercare instructions. Note any warnings given to patients in the documentation.

Across the country, mental health professionals have a duty to warn intended victims of violent crimes when a patient makes a specific threat. Some states extend or permit other physicians to warn intended victims. The seminal case regarding duty to warn third parties is *Tarasoff v. Regents of the University of California*. In this case, a psychiatric outpatient informed his therapist that he intended to kill a young lady matching Tatiana Tarasoff's description. Although the patient did not identify Tatiana by name, the allegation was that the therapist had enough information to figure it out. Two months after making the threat, the patient did indeed murder Tatiana Tarasoff. The California Supreme Court found that no one owes any duty to protect an individual who is endangered by a third person unless he has some special relationship with either the dangerous person or the potential victim. It was decided that the psychiatrist qualified as having such a relationship with his patient (*Tarasoff v. Regents of the University of California*, 1976). Another California case, *Thompson v. County of Alameda*, resulted in a ruling that even though a specific victim does not need to be named by the dangerous person, the intended victim must be readily identifiable to trigger a duty to warn (*Thompson v. County of Alameda,* 1980). Because there is no standard approach to laws requiring a duty to warn, you need to seek out the laws in the state where you practice.

Periodically, you might be faced with a patient's condition falling outside of the state's authorized duty to warn, yet it pulls at your moral, ethical, and professional values. The discrepancy generates an internal struggle resulting in strong feelings of a duty to warn society. An example of such a situation is when an airline pilot is brought in by paramedics, found in an altered state. The patient has a strong alcohol-like odor and several bottles of hard liquor. A nurse overhears the patient's visitor tell someone over the phone that she hopes he sobers up in the next 4 hours because he is scheduled to be the captain on a transcontinental flight, but knows he will sign out against medical advice if necessary. The nurse is concerned that something could go horribly wrong if the intoxicated pilot is allowed to get on that flight and fears for the safety of the hundreds of people on the flight. The nurse wonders if an anonymous call should be made to the airline administrators recommending that they conduct a fitness for duty check on the pilot when he arrives. This is a very tough call and not one that should be made in isolation. The nurse should consider available resources such as notifying the department supervisor and facility risk manager so that legal guidance can be obtained.

Primary Causes of Unexpected Events

Healthcare is a complex process. It involves numerous individuals, working either together or independently to carry out an activity. Consider, for example, something as simple as getting a chest X-ray. Generally, this is initiated by a physician or other licensed independent practitioner. A unit secretary on the patient unit requests the X-ray, and different support staff in radiology process it. The patient's nurse needs to ready the patient for the exam. Arrangements need to be made to transport the patient. A radiology technician performs the exam. A radiologist reads the chest X-ray. But behind the scenes, a plethora of other individuals are involved. Multiple biomedical engineers likely ensured all the equipment used was in correct working order, numerous housekeeping personnel ensured that all the areas were appropriately maintained, information technology worked to ensure that order entry in the computer system was seamless, and the list goes on.

Unfortunately, complex systems sometimes fail or had inadequacies built into them that doomed the process from the outset. It's essential that you understand how they function within the complex process known as healthcare to reduce unexpected events.

Process Failures

According to the findings of the Institute of Medicine's report, *To Err Is Human: Building a Safer Health System*, the majority of medical errors do not result from individual reckless-ness or the actions of a particular group—this is not a "bad apple" problem. More com-monly, errors are caused by faulty systems, processes, and conditions that lead people to make mistakes or fail to prevent them (Kohn et al., 2000). The ultimate goal of patient safety programs is to improve the reliability of the processes to accomplish the desired result, thereby improving safety. There are many reasons why processes can fail: lack of redundancy, communication failures, lack of access to information, and human error are just a few (Carayon & Wood, 2010).

Patient handoffs should include a list of outstanding tests awaiting results. Tests ordered in the ED may get overlooked if the inpatient unit is unaware that a result is pending. Contributing fac-tors are:

-   Physicians are generally responsible for following up on results for tests they order. When test results for an admitted patient return after the patient is already taken to the floor, the ED staff may fax the results to the floor believing that the patient is no longer their responsibility. Unfortunately, the floor nurse may not be aware that the ordering (ED) phy-sician did not review the results and may presume that any abnormal findings were already reported to the admitting physician during the handoff. Adding to the error poten-tial is the fact that the admitting physician may not be aware that there was a pending test result ordered by the ED physician so may not know to look for it.

-   Policies and procedures should include a clearly defined process for follow-up on positive culture results and diagnostic discrepancies. There should be a clear delegation of responsibilities as to time frames for notifying the ordering physician as well as who is responsible for following up with the patient.

One example of a process failure is the failure to address discrepancies of labs and X-rays. According to a 2014 report by CRICO Strategies, diagnostic errors accounted for 16% of ED claims occurring from 2008 to 2012 (Hoffman, 2014). CRICO further noted that 1 in every 1,000 diagnostic encounters in the ambulatory setting will result in patient harm due to a diagnostic error. These numbers imply that an average-sized hospital may have 5 to 10 patient deaths annually due to a diagnostic error (Graber, 2014). Failure to contact the patient to provide culture results or resolve discrepancies between the initial read conducted by the ED provider and the findings by the radiologist conducting the over-read accounted for 46% of those claims. The primary reasons for the failure to follow up with the patient were due to the failure to obtain specialty consultations when indicated and various communication glitches (Hoffman, 2014). ED patients discharged or admitted from the department before the return of all test results are at greater risk of falling prey to this vulnerability.

Human Factors

Many studies examine human factors and the role they play with medical errors. One of the foundational theories by Rasmussen (1990) and Reason (2000) distinguishes between two types of failures leading to human error: *latent conditions,* those that are embedded into the process, creating an inevitability of an error due to poor design; and *active failures,* resulting from an individual's actions or behaviors, and therefore difficult to foresee.

Slips, Lapses, and Mistakes

James Reason spoke of slips, lapses, and mistakes as three active failures playing a significant role in errors. We are all exposed to these three conditions by the very nature of our humanity.

- A *slip* is an accidental or unintentional act. An example of a slip is when a nurse reaches for one medication and inadvertently picks up a different one without realizing it.

- A *lapse* occurs when something is overlooked or missed, such as when the nurse intended to call to check on culture results but forgot.

- A *mistake* happens when a nurse does something thinking it was the right thing but was wrong. An example of a mistake is when a nurse deliberately administers a medication to a patient believing there is a physician order for it.

These three active failures are much different from a *violation,* in which an individual knows the right thing to do and makes a conscious decision not to do it (Carayon & Wood, 2010).

 Violation—An active failure different from slips, lapses, and mistakes. It involves knowing the right thing to do and making a conscious decision not to do it (Campbell, Croskerry, & Bond, 2007). Examples are silencing clinical alarms, taking shortcuts to procedural timeouts, not truly ensuring a patient's understanding of aftercare instructions, or not following policies regarding double-checks on high-risk medications.

Script Concordance and Cognitive Bias

Clinical decision-making requires a process of assessment and development of a working diagnosis along with a list of differential diagnoses for consideration. Additional data is evaluated as it becomes available in order to reach a final clinical impression. Information gathered through serial assessments and test results will either support or be contrary to the working diagnosis (Reason, 2000). Much like putting together the pieces of a puzzle, the data will either fit the diagnosis or it won't. When time allows, a slower, *analytic approach* to decision-making may be used to deliberately test the working diagnosis through deductive thinking. Other times may call for a more rapid *nonanalytic* approach. The nonanalytic approach uses the recognition of complex associated patterns developed over time to make quick judgments (Lubarsky, Dory, Duggan, Gagnon, & Charlin, 2013). A veteran clinician may recognize this as an indescribable sense or "gut feeling" about what is likely going on with the patient.

The ED presents a rapid-paced, at times chaotic environment in which decisions must be made quickly. To meet this need, the decision-making process must frequently be shortened such that there is no time to use an analytic approach. Instead, the clinician accesses these networks of organized knowledge, called *scripts,* as a mental shortcut for reasoning. Scripts help the clinician to reach a conclusion more rapidly. Scripts form over time as a nurse applies the knowledge learned in school to the clinical setting. Eventually, the nurse observes patterns with patient presentations that are consistent with specific diagnoses (Campbell et al., 2007). An example of this dynamic is when a patient arrives pale and diaphoretic with complaints of chest pain and shortness of breath. The nurse will likely begin thinking of possible cardiac causes. When more data becomes available, such as discovering that the chest pain is sharp and worsens with perspiration, the nurse may shift from thinking about cardiac causes to those that are pulmonary in nature. As the nurse becomes more expert, his or her scripts become more refined.

The use of scripts may be more expedient but is not without risk (Lubarsky et al., 2013). At times, scripts may draw the nurse's attention down a specific path of familiarity while ignoring other likely considerations. In these instances, the scripts are creating a bias. Possessing an awareness of your biases may empower you to use caution when triaging, assessing, and relaying information to the physician.

There are many types of cognitive bias that may lead you down the wrong path, resulting in a missed or delayed diagnosis and subsequent delay of treatment:

■ *Triage cueing:* Occurs when a clinician allows the judgment made by someone else early in the diagnostic process to sway thoughts toward potential clinical pathways (Campbell et al., 2007). This can happen when the triage nurse writes down a diagnosis instead of objective symptoms as a chief complaint. For example, writing that a patient has a chief complaint of constipation for 2 weeks instead of using the patient's words ("patient states she has not had a bowel movement in 2 weeks despite use of magnesium citrate, GoLytely, Fleets, and soapsuds enemas; pain 10/10") paints an entirely different picture of the patient's risks and acuity. The approach taken by the triage nurse could make the difference between the ED physician telling the patient to take a laxative and follow up in 5 to 7 days with her primary care provider and conducting an abdominal workup to assess for risk of impending perforated bowel. To avoid triage cueing, you should document patients' complaints in their own words using quotes and then provide objective information to justify the triage acuity assigned. Because the triage assessment is conducted objectively, the findings may or may not support the patient's stated chief complaint.

- *Visceral bias:* Arises when either positive or negative feelings toward patients influence decisions made. When this bias is blended with the *framing effect* (decision being influenced by the way in which the scenario is presented), the results can be catastrophic (Campbell et al., 2007). This risk is apparent in any ED where staff refers to chronic pain patients as "drug seekers" or "frequent flyers." The negative labeling of patients should be your first alert that a visceral bias is having an influence, and therefore, special care must be taken to ensure that bias does not result in inadvertently framing the patient's complaint. Diagnoses are missed when providers see chronic pain patients as nuisances wasting beds rather than exploring further to determine if this pain is different than usual and completing an objective medical screening exam. Epidural abscess is just one of many diagnoses missed in this high-risk patient population, and when treatment is delayed, may result in paralysis or death.

- *Anchoring bias:* The tendency to fixate on certain features of the patient's presentation too early in the process and then fail to adjust as more information becomes available (Campbell et al., 2007). An example of this bias at work is seen when a middle-aged woman presents to the ED with a chief complaint of feeling fatigued, lightheaded, and having difficulty breathing. Her vital signs upon arrival show an elevated blood pressure, heart, and respiratory rate, so the physician orders a repeat set of vital signs prior to discharge; they were unchanged. The physician decided early on that the patient was having an anxiety attack and kept that diagnosis despite the abnormal repeat vital signs and "borderline" EKG. The patient was discharged with a prescription for Xanax and told to follow up with her primary care physician in 2 days. The patient had a missed myocardial infarction that may have been diagnosed had the physician not immediately fixated on the diagnosis of anxiety and failed to consider the serial assessment findings and test results that may have drawn that diagnosis into question. Failure to address abnormal vital signs is a common allegation in missed diagnosis claims. Patients with abnormal vital signs upon discharge should also have a note in the record indicating the physician was advised and acknowledged the information and was comfortable moving forward with the original discharge plan.

> ▪ *Confirmation bias:* Occurs when the clinician develops a hypothesis of the patient's diagnosis and then seeks evidence to support it, rather than looking for evidence that might lead down a different decision pathway (Campbell et al., 2007). An illustration of this is a 46-year-old male who arrives in the ED complaining of shortness of breath increasing over the past few weeks. Breath sounds were diminished, and the physician orders a chest X-ray seeking to confirm the suspected diagnosis of pneumonia. The chest X-ray shows bilateral lower lobe infiltrates, and the diagnosis of pneumonia is confirmed. Because it appears to be a mild case and the patient seems to be doing well, the patient is discharged home with a prescription for antibiotics and direction to follow up with his primary care physician this week, sooner if not feeling better within the next 2 days. What the physician failed to acknowledge were the multiple small lesions throughout all of the patient's lung fields. They were missed because the physician was looking strictly for infiltrates to confirm the suspected diagnosis, so the incidental findings were overlooked. Failure to follow up on incidental findings is one of the primary issues with delay of diagnosis and treatment claims and is frequently an avoidable exposure.

Compassion Fatigue

The ED is more than just a fast-paced environment where acute and chronic patients of all ages, illnesses, and injuries come to seek immediate care. It's a physically, spiritually, and emotionally draining setting for patients and caregivers alike. For the ED nurse, exposure to human tragedy and suffering is routine, yet each exposure to loss takes a little piece of the nurse with it. Najjar, Davis, Beck-Coon, & Doebbeling (2009) stated that compassion fatigue usually occurs in caring professionals who absorb the traumatic stress of those they help. When significantly outnumbered by patients in need of their care, emergency nurses may become frustrated or disheartened, feeling that they failed the patient that needed them most. Some will reach the point where they question whether or not they can provide quality care and if this profession is the right fit (Buckley, 2014).

To reduce the impact of compassion fatigue:

- Develop a healthy work/life balance
- Exercise and maintain a healthy diet
- Set aside play time
- Take time to care for yourself physically and spiritually

Compassion fatigue is described as a "combination of physical, emotional, and spiritual depletion associated with caring for patients in significant emotional pain and physical distress" (Lombardo & Eyre, 2011, p. 1). According to Charles Figley, symptoms can include a lack of joyfulness at work, reduced empathy, headaches, muscle tension, fatigue, mood swings, irritability, depression, and difficulty sleeping (Figley, 1995). The nurse with compassion fatigue will have a negative impact on the entire department and lack that caring connection needed by so many patients during their time of crisis. The therapeutic relationship between a nurse with compassion fatigue and the patient is one in which the patient is less likely to open up and share important information with the nurse and may even become adversarial. The resentment the nurse develops toward the patient may result in a lack of attentiveness to patient requests and avoidance of the patient, which could ultimately result in patient harm. Nurses with compassion fatigue may require intervention to help them recover and restore the culture of safety within the department. Interventions may include debriefing, onsite counseling, or bereavement interventions (Sanchez, Valdez, & Johnson, 2014). To learn more about compassion fatigue and how to avoid it, see Chapter 6, "Self-Care and the Emergency Nurse."

Communication Failures

Communication failure ranked in the top three sentinel event root causes reported to The Joint Commission in 2014 and is the number one cause for delays in treatment (Sentinel Event Statistics Data, 2015). Breakdowns in communication may be oral, written, or electronic and may take place between healthcare providers, administrators, patients, and families. Issues can present at any point throughout the patient's stay, between the time of arrival until the time of disposition. While in the ED, there are certain points in time when the risk of communication failure is greater than others, such as during transitions of care (handoffs), when working as a team, documenting in the medical record or on special forms, and when providing patients with aftercare instructions.

Handoffs

Whether the nurse is receiving a report from a paramedic or handing off the patient to another clinician, the quality of the report has a direct influence on the quality of the ongoing care provided to the patient. Failure to receive a quality report from paramedics in the field can make the difference between the ED being prepared to receive the critical patient upon arrival or being caught flat-footed when the patient rolls in, in full arrest. Handoffs occurring within the ED may be especially vulnerable to communication failure due to the many visual and auditory distractions in the ED environment. The distractions also increase the possibility of confusing elements of one patient's report with another's when giving a report from memory. It's unlikely that the handoff report will be complete or thorough when both the sender and receiver are hurried and trying to multitask. Because clinicians have little control over the environment within the department, they may need to draw upon tools designed to trigger discussion about critical elements of care. Many handoff tools are available; however, those most widely accepted are Situation-Background-Assessment-Recommendation (SBAR), I PASS the BATON, Ticket to Ride, and Safer Sign Out (see Table 12.1).

Table 12.1 Tools to Use for Patient Handoffs

Tool	When to Use It	Description
SBAR*	General handoffs	**S**ituation **B**ackground **A**ssessment findings **R**ecommendations
I PASS the BATON**	General handoffs	**I**ntroduce self **P**atient identified **A**ssessment **S**ituation **S**afety issues The **B**ackground **A**ctions taken **T**iming for priorities **O**wnership **N**ext steps in plan
Ticket to Ride***	Transportation handoffs	Written report stays with patient when leaving unit 1. Identifies if patient will be returning to unit or if this is a one-way trip 2. Specifies information about allergies, risks, special needs/precautions, pain management and monitoring 3. Patient status is updated prior to returning patient to unit
Safer Sign Out****	Physician turn-over of care	1. Review general information about patient including tests and results 2. Introduce physician taking over care and provide the physician with report in front of the patient 3. Update the patient on the current plan and establish expectations 4. Allow accepting physician and patient to ask questions

*Developed by Michael Leonard, Doug Bonacum, and Suzanne Graham of Kaiser Permanente of Colorado

** Developed by U.S. Department of Defense Safety Program

*** Developed at St. Joseph's Health System in Orange County, California

****Developed by Emergency Medicine Associates, PA, PC, located in Germantown, Maryland

No matter the approach, the patient should be included at some point in the handoff process. When the patient is included, it allows the patient to bring up any changes that may have occurred or new complaints not already covered during the report. It also encourages patients to take an active role in developing their plans of care, which ultimately improves their compliance with the plan after discharge. Another good practice when receiving a report is to write down the information provided. This not only helps maintain continuity of care but also helps to ensure that all information is passed forward when time comes for another transition of care. An additional benefit of writing down the information is that it helps increase memory when the receiver is listening to, writing, and reading the information. Although making errors is unavoidable, they can be reduced through the use of memory triggers and tools prompting the clinician to give a brief, clear, complete, and structured report.

Team Communication

A 1994 study conducted by the National Transportation Safety Board found that 73% of all of the major aviation accidents occurring between 1978 and 1990 transpired on the first day that a crew flew together. It went on to show that 48% of those occurred on the first flight of the day. The causative factor was that the team had not spent enough time together to develop a team dynamic. Fatigue was a factor contributing to procedural and judgment errors in many of the accidents investigated in this study; however, in 90% of those incidents, other crewmembers had an awareness but failed to challenge the team member making the error (National Transportation Safety Board, 1994).

Reliance on teamwork is readily seen in the ED. Every emergency nurse will at some point in time develop a special bond when working with a certain team so that each of the team members can almost anticipate what will happen next. This dynamic leaves the team feeling like they can take on anything the shift may throw their way. But what about all of those other times when that dynamic doesn't exist? It is at those times when the team leader and members of the team must use extra caution. Some techniques are:

- Audibly communicate thoughts by using *callouts*.

- Acknowledge receipt of information through *closed-loop communications*.

- Use *team huddles* at the beginning of the shift to establish role assignments so that everyone is clear as to who will lead the team and maintain situational awareness during times of increased activity, respond to inpatient codes, work specific areas, relieve for breaks, perform triage, and back up the nurse assigned to the critical or trauma beds.

Excellent teamwork has been found to reduce and prevent medical errors, increase efficiencies, and help increase the timeliness of responding to patients' needs and expectations (Kipnis, Rhodes, Burchill, & Datner, 2012).

Situational awareness—Being aware of what is going on around you.

Shared mental model—A shared understanding of the team's purpose, what they are trying to accomplish.

Callouts—Verbally and clearly stating information to others. For example, loudly stating findings that are uncovered during the assessment of a trauma patient during a trauma resuscitation.

Closed-loop communication—A sender gives a message that is then repeated by the recipient. The sender then confirms that the message has been correctly understood.

One of the key components found in high-functioning teams is excellent communication. For communication to remain effective during times of chaos, the leader must direct the team in such a way that all are in agreement about the team's purpose and have a shared mental model. Tasks must be assigned to individuals rather than just calling out orders into the air and hoping someone is implementing them, and all team members, regardless of their roles, must feel comfortable speaking up when concerned about a patient or unsafe condition.

Documentation

Documentation plays a crucial role in communicating information between healthcare providers to promote continuity of care. When the ED gets busy, documenting procedures performed, medications administered, and the patient's responses may get set aside until the end of the shift. The delay can increase the opportunity for error due to missing pieces of the patient's experience while in the ED. It's during these same busy periods when documentation has an increased likelihood of being entered in the wrong patient's record and containing incomplete or inaccurate information. When possible, attempt to review the patient's record prior to the end of the shift to verify that it is accurate and complete.

Aftercare Instructions

Aftercare instructions are provided to patients as a means of continuing the plan of care started in the ED until the patient can follow up with the primary care physician. The patient's compliance with the plan may be the difference between feeling better or experiencing a deterioration of condition, triggering a return visit to the ED. Several factors may affect the patient's ability to understand the instructions, which will directly affect the patient's compliance with the plan:

- The patient may be distracted by pain, hunger, fatigue, malaise, or just the thought of being discharged when given the instructions.

■ Language barriers, visual impairments, and literacy and educational level may prohibit the patient from fully understanding the information.

■ The patient may be experiencing the effects of adrenalin due to the acute, episodic nature of the visit and may lack the ability to process all of the information provided.

In fact, studies show that ED patients forget up to 80% of the information provided to them during the discharge process by the time they reach their cars. It's important for the ED team to recognize the patient's limitations and take steps to counteract them:

■ The patient should receive a legible, written or printed copy of all of the instructions for reference at a later time.

■ Font size should be large enough for the elderly or visually impaired patient's review.

■ Content should be written at somewhere between a third and fifth grade reading level.

■ Include an invitation written in bold font at the top of the form to return to the ED with any worsening of condition or new concerns.

■ Use interpreters as necessary when there is a language barrier. One study showed that when a family member is used as the interpreter, 23% to 52% of the words and phrases are interpreted incorrectly (Wilson, 2013). When using hospital personnel as interpreters, be sure they have been authenticated and credentialed to do so.

Many electronic aftercare instruction programs print several pages of information, not all specific to the patient's needs. When instructions are printed for more than one diagnosis, information between the various sets may contain conflicting information. Review all printed sheets for consistency and clarify for the patient which measures he or she should follow. Consider using a highlighter or underlining the information important for the patient to review.

Because aftercare instructions contain critical information such as when the patient should follow up with the primary care provider and signs for when he should return immediately to the nearest ED or call 911, it's important for the patient and/or family to understand the instructions. You shouldn't ask, "Do you have any questions?" and assume if the answer is "no" that the patient fully understands the plan. A better approach is to say, "What is your understanding of when you need to return to the nearest emergency department immediately?" When you take those extra few minutes to determine the patient's understanding of the treatment plan, you increase the likelihood of compliance with the plan.

Mitigating Risk

An important concept in providing quality care is recognizing, either proactively or reactively, potential risks that could have negative outcomes. But quality care is more than just recognizing potential risks; it's working on a plan that can be used to minimize or eliminate those risks.

Providing Quality Care

Continuing to strive for the delivery of excellent quality of care is an ongoing process. Healthcare workers must identify clinical challenges, collect data, review evidence, and pilot plans made specifically to address those challenges. As more evidence becomes available, current practices are evaluated and modifications made when necessary to ensure that the quality of the care provided affords the patient with the best opportunity for a positive outcome. Although individual facilities conduct some independent quality studies through the hospital's quality improvement committee, many of the quality improvement indicators are driven by outside agencies and incorporated into the facility-specific plan.

In the 2001 report on "Crossing the Quality Chasm," the Institute of Medicine (IOM) proposed six aims to improve healthcare systems: safe, effective, patient-centered, timely, efficient, and equitable care (IOM, 2001). Building on this effort, in 2007, the Institute for Healthcare Improvement launched the *Triple Aim* campaign calling for hospitals to pursue three simultaneous goals: provide a better patient care experience, improve population health, and lower healthcare costs. All of these efforts are supported by CMS, as reflected in its guidelines indicating that providing quality care goes beyond whether the patient received competent care but rather rises to the level of whether the patient *perceived* the experience to be good.

Quality Improvement Program

The activities of hospital quality improvement committees in most states are protected from discovery under the peer review protection granted by the Health Care Quality Improvement Act of 1986 (HCQIA, 42 USC §11101); nevertheless, there is a broad range of additional protections across the nation. The Patient Safety and Quality Improvement Act of 2005 is a federal statute developed by the Agency for Healthcare Research and Quality to establish a structure for hospitals, doctors, and other healthcare providers to voluntarily report information to patient safety organizations (PSOs) and maintain privilege against discovery so that patient safety events can be aggregated and analyzed. By providing a mechanism to engage in quality improvement activities with more robust protections, the agency hoped there would be greater participation. Based upon the collected data, PSOs provide feedback and develop and disseminate recommendations, protocols, and best practices to their members. This information may then be used by healthcare facilities to determine quality improvement goals and utilize the tools provided to reach those goals. In addition to quality considerations issued by PSOs, a portion of each hospital's quality improvement program includes monitoring The Joint Commission and CMS core measures and implementing processes designed to reduce the likelihood of experiencing a never event.

 Privilege against discovery—Documents that are a product of formal peer review activities conducted according to a specific set of requirements may be kept confidential by the peer review body.

Core Measures

Core measures were initially developed by The Joint Commission to measure the quality of care provided for patients with certain high-risk presentations. The quality indicators reflect an evidence-based approach to the standard of care and strive to increase the timeliness in which the care is delivered. Core measures include:

- Time from arrival to departure for admitted ED patients

- Admit decision time to ED departure time for admitted patients

- Blood cultures prior to first dose of antibiotic

- Antibiotic within 6 hours for diagnosis of pneumonia

- Assessing pain and effectiveness of treatment

The Joint Commission members are required to submit data specific to each measure they have agreed to monitor (The Joint Commission, 2010). Recognizing the cumbersome nature of data collection and use of valuable resources, The Joint Commission and CMS have merged several of their initiatives, reducing data collection efforts and allowing more time to focus on using the data to improve the quality of patient care (Peasah, McKay, Harman, Al-Amin, & Cook, 2013).

Accountability Measures

In an effort to maximize health benefits to patients, in 2011, The Joint Commission developed a new categorization of measures referred to as *accountability measures*. Twenty-two of these measures came from The Joint Commission (2010) 28 item core measure set; however, they were required to meet four criteria before receiving consideration for inclusion into the new category.

Criteria include:

- **Research:** There is strong scientific evidence demonstrating that performing the process will improve patient outcomes.

- **Proximity:** The measure has been determined to have a close connection between performing the process and a better outcome for the patient.

- **Accuracy:** The measure has been demonstrated to accurately assess whether or not the process was used.

- **Adverse effects:** The process has little to no chance of inducing an unintended adverse response.

Because of the strong connection with supporting evidence, The Joint Commission believes these measures should be mandated for accreditation, public reporting, and pay-for-performance. All measures that are not part of the accountability set *(non-accountability measures)* should just become recommendations (Chassin, Loeb, Schmaltz, & Wachter, 2010). Core measures sets that are now part of the accountability measures affecting the ED are those addressing heart attack, heart failure, pneumonia, stroke, immunization, tobacco treatment, and substance abuse.

Never Events

The concept of *never events*, also known as *serious reportable events,* was first developed by the National Quality Forum (a nonprofit membership organization created to promote patient protections, healthcare quality measurement, and public reporting) in 2001. These events are rare but devastating when they occur, so the goal of the program is to implement quality improvement measures to drive the number of these events to zero. As of 2011, the list was comprised of 29 never events with mandatory reporting required in 11 states, and reporting of several of the listed items required in an additional 16 states.

Examples of never events are when a patient death or serious injury is associated with:

- Patient falls

- Pressure ulcers

- Hospital-acquired infections

- Patient suicide, attempted suicide

- Failure to follow up or communicate test results (laboratory, pathology, or radiology)

In 2008, CMS issued notice that it would no longer pay for "non-reimbursable serious hospital-acquired conditions" (Lembitz & Clarke, 2009). Included in the list are many of the never events, any of which could occur in the ED setting. Some of the more common events are wrong-site surgeries or procedures, retained foreign object following a procedure, hospital-acquired infections, administration of incompatible blood, and development of a stage III or IV pressure ulcer (National Patient Safety Forum, 2011).

In an attempt to introduce a more positive approach toward these patient safety risks, the Institute for Healthcare Improvement (IHI) introduced the concept of *always events* focused on what is important to the patient and families (Lembitz & Clarke, 2009). Examples of always events are:

- Introduce yourself and wear a name badge.

- Treat patients and people with respect.

- Wash your hands when entering and exiting a room.

- Allow the patient and family to ask questions.

- Conduct a handoff at the patient's bedside and include the patient in the report.

Clinical Practice Guidelines

Clinical practices guidelines are the bridge between the results of nursing research and applying the information to clinical practice. The Clinical Practice Guidelines Committee of the Emergency Nurses Association reviews new and existing evidence-based research to develop recommendations or guidelines believed to be most effective to address a clinical need. Once implemented, the guidelines are reviewed and revised as new research becomes available to ensure they continue to meet the standard of care.

Examples of some important clinical issues currently being researched to identify ways to reduce associated risks and increase the quality of patient care in the ED are the use of and reliance on clinical alarms, addressing abnormal vital signs, reducing patient throughput times, improving quality of care provided to boarded patients, and the effectiveness of checklist assessments to identify incidental patient risks while in the ED. These are just a few of the current areas of research but reflect serious clinical issues in the ED that lead to an increased risk of patient harm. Nursing research is a vital component for improving quality care and enhancing patient safety.

Regulations and Laws

Some federal laws and regulations fundamentally affect the quality of care provided in the ED. The Emergency Medical Treatment and Active Labor Act is perhaps the most far-reaching of those laws. The Health Insurance Portability and Accountability Act (HIPAA) is another robust law established to protect a patient's privacy while still allowing the information sharing for quality improvement and care coordination activities.

COBRA/EMTALA and Patient Transfers

The Emergency Medical Treatment and Active Labor Act (EMTALA) is a federal statute enacted by Congress in 1986 as part of the Consolidated Omnibus Budget Reconciliation Act (COBRA). The statute was established in response to the practice of patient dumping by the hospital where the patient first presented to another hospital. This practice was generally as a result of a patient's inability to pay or for discriminatory reasons. Congress believed that patients (such as women in active labor or those requiring emergent care) should receive emergency care at any ED regardless of the ability to pay, rather than being sent to county hospitals or those providing charitable care. Despite being in effect for close to 30 years, emergency personnel continue to struggle with compliance. Section 1867 [42 U.S.C. 1395dd] (a) of the Social Security Act requires that:

> If an individual comes to the emergency department (at any Medicare-participating hospital offering emergency services), and a request is made on the individual's behalf for examination or treatment for a medical condition, the hospital must provide for an appropriate medical screening examination (MSE) within the capability of the hospital's emergency department, including ancillary services routinely available to the emergency department, to determine whether or not an emergency medical condition (EMC) exists. (U.S. Commission on Civil Rights, 2014, p. 1)

Figure 12.3 outlines the steps emergency personnel should take when a patient comes to the ED.

In recent years, EMTALA investigators found an increased trend of discharging patients with psychiatric conditions without an appropriate discharge plan; at times the patients were discharged to street corners or bus stations. These findings served to bring EMTALA back into the public eye as hospitals were once again being held under close scrutiny for ongoing EMTALA compliance. The Centers for Medicare & Medicaid Services (CMS) as well as the Office of the Inspector General (OIG) are the two organizations primarily accountable for conducting investigations of alleged violations. On average, approximately 500 EMTALA complaints are received annually with close to 40% resulting in citations. In addition to monetary penalties, facilities and providers found in violation of EMTALA may be excluded from participation in federal healthcare programs. This could result in hospitals becoming financially unviable and providers ineligible for credentialing (U.S. Commission on Civil Rights, 2014).

Once the emergency medical condition is ruled out or stabalized, EMTALA is no longer in play and patients may be transferred or discharged to follow-up for post-stabilization care.

- **Patient Comes to ED**

  Seeking treatment for a medical condition

- **Conduct MSE**

  Evaluate patient using all resources available to facility without regard to ability to pay

- **Rule Out or Stabilize EMC**

  Rule out stabilize to the best of your capability, the patient's emergency medical condition

- **Discharge**

  Discharge home, transfer to higher level of care, or admit

Figure 12.3 The basic principles of EMTALA.

The rules for engagement and compliance with EMTALA are quite simple. When a patient comes to the ED seeking evaluation and treatment for a medical condition, the patient is triaged and seen by the medical provider in accordance with acuity at presentation. A qualified medical provider (QMP) then conducts a medical screening examination to determine whether the patient has an emergency medical condition. There will be times when the MSE is as simple as looking at a rash, or it may be complex, requiring obtaining a culture, serial labs, diagnostic imaging, and specialty consultation. Ultimately, if a diagnostic test is important for developing a clinical impression and would be performed on an insured patient, it also needs to be performed on the uninsured. Providing disparate care based upon a patient's insurance status or ability to pay is an excellent way to find the hospital and providers on the receiving end of an EMTALA investigation. If the patient is found to have an EMC, every effort must be made to stabilize that condition utilizing all of the appropriate resources available at the facility. If a higher level of care is needed to stabilize the patient, a transfer must be initiated to another facility possessing the capacity to manage the patient's condition.

 Capacity—Possessing adequate numbers and availability of qualified staff, beds, and equipment, taking into account any past practices by the hospital to accommodate additional patients in excess of its occupancy limits. For example, if the stated capacity of a hospital is 200, but it is known to stretch the limits to 205, 205 is its true capacity.

You need to realize that triage is not a medical screening examination. Triage is the process used to determine a patient's acuity and the order in which the medical provider evaluates patients. Only a qualified medical provider can conduct a medical screen examination. Individuals may be deemed as *qualified* to conduct an MSE when they meet the requirements as written in the medical staff rules and regulations approved by the governing body. Emergency physicians are generally deemed qualified to conduct an MSE, but other physicians with privileges at the facility may not be and therefore would not be able to meet their patients in the ED without receiving an MSE by the emergency physician. Perinatal nurses are frequently deemed qualified to rule out the presence of labor in pregnant women; however, those nurses must use extreme caution not to exceed the scope of their delegated authority. Any chief complaints that are not labor-related should be evaluated by the obstetrician or emergency physician. Acceptance of ED nurses as qualified to conduct medical screening exams through the use of standardized protocols varies significantly from state to state. Each hospital's EMTALA policies and procedures will reflect any limitations or nuances found within the state's practice.

Triage nurses are frequently responsible not only for triaging patients upon arrival but also for collecting demographic information, medications lists, medical history, and completing all social and risk assessments. The extra data collection can greatly increase the amount of time it takes the triage nurse to complete a triage examination. These delays may result in avoidable exposure to an EMTALA citation, some of which include:

Delay of medical screening exam (MSE)	Failure to conduct a complete MSE for a patient with psychiatric complaints
Using triage as an MSE	Lack of physician certification
Incomplete or failure to conduct an MSE	No serial assessments
Failure to stabilize prior to transfer	Reasons, risks, and benefits not written
No vital signs or assessment at time of transfer	Failure to provide ongoing stabilizing treatment throughout ED stay
Failure of on-call physician to respond	Missing times, dates, and signatures
Failure to arrange a safe transport	Discharge without reasonable follow-up plan

The delay of triage may also expose the nurse to allegations that had it not been for the triage delay, there would not have been a delay of diagnosis and treatment leading to the patient's injury. Hospital administrations must carefully weigh the risks and benefits of assigning additional tasks to the triage nurse against the risk of patient harm due to any resulting delay of triage. For more information on the triage nurse and the process of triage, see Chapter 10, "The Emergency Nurse in the Role of Triage."

EMTALA is also known as the *patient dumping law*. It is therefore no surprise that the law strictly regulates acceptable reasons for a patient's transfer to another facility. When EMTALA is in effect, there are only two acceptable reasons for transferring a patient:

- The patient requests a transfer.

- The patient requires transfer to a higher level of care for stabilization of an emergency medical condition.

Transferring for any other reason, such as physician preference or a request by a payor such as a health maintenance organization (HMO), serves as red flags to EMTALA investigators in the event your facility is the recipient of an EMTALA complaint. Steps to transfer a patient:

1. **Advise the patient or patient's representative of the reason for the transfer, the expected benefit, and any risks involved with the transfer.**

   The discussion involves the process of obtaining an informed consent and therefore is a non-delegable practice of medicine. This discussion must be held between the patient and physician or advanced practice provider.

2. **Provide information in layman's terms and thoroughly document it on the transfer paperwork.**

   When documenting the benefit of the transfer, indicate the specific service, expertise, or equipment that the receiving facility has that makes it a higher level of care (e.g., "Patient needs a CT scan to rule out a bleed in the brain. Our CT scanner is down.").

3. **Review the transfer paperwork for completion, making sure the documentation of the consent discussion is thorough, reflects the patient's unique risks and benefits, and is signed, dated, and timed by the patient or patient's representative.**

   Facilities have been cited for checking off a box indicating "deterioration of condition." That phrase would not be helpful for many patients or their family members who are unfamiliar with what that could mean. It's best to consider the clinical impression for the patient and think about what the provider would expect to see if the condition worsened (e.g., increased pain, loss of airway, damage to the heart muscle, damage to the nerves). The patient has a right to refuse the transfer to a specific facility or an ambulance transport.

There are *only two* acceptable reasons for an EMTALA transfer: patient request and to provide a higher level of care.

Verify that the physician has documented the patient's capacity to make that decision and have the patient or authorized individual sign a "Refusal of Medical Screening Exam," "Refusal of Transfer," or "Refusal of Ambulance Transport" form to evidence that risks of refusal, benefits of acceptance, and any alternatives were discussed.

One important component of the patient's transfer assessment and paperwork is the physician's certification of the patient's stability for transfer. For a patient with an emergency medical condition, EMTALA defines the term *stabilized* as (within reasonable medical probability) "no material deterioration of the condition is likely to result from or occur during the transfer of the individual from a facility. With regard to a pregnant woman, she is stabilized when she has delivered the child and the placenta" (U.S. Commission on Civil Rights, 2014, p. 77). Many emergency physicians complete the certification of the patient's stability when they first determine the need for transfer to a higher level of care.

Caution should be used because it can sometimes be several hours between the time a transfer is requested and the time of the transport team's arrival. It's wise to document the patient's vital signs and (at minimum) a focused assessment of the presenting complaint at time of transfer. This serial assessment will help to evidence the patient's stability for transfer at the time of departure from the ED. Regardless of the patient's stability for transfer, it's the responsibility of the ED physician to affect a safe transport to the receiving facility by writing a transport order to ensure the patient is transported by the proper mode and accompanied by qualified personnel and equipment to address any issues arising during transport.

 Some patients will be unstable at time of transfer because they cannot be stabilized until they receive specialized treatment at the receiving facility. The ED physician should indicate these patients are *unstable* on the Physician's Certification.

You should be aware of several key points. If the facility is a higher level of care operating under CMS Conditions of Participation and has the capacity and capability to accept the patient, it must do so. Failure to do so may result in the sending facility reporting a suspected EMTALA violation, thus sparking an investigation by government enforcement agencies. EMTALA does not require any facility to self-report its own suspected violations, but when another facility is suspected to have breached EMTALA, the facility has 72 hours to report. It's important to notify the unit supervisor and facility risk manager as soon as possible. EMTALA violations you should report are:

- **Sending facility:** Sending patients without acceptance by receiving, patient not sent by appropriate mode or level of care, or sending patient without completed transfer documents.

- **Receiving facility:** Demanding face sheet with insurance information, requiring insurance authorization prior to acceptance, or refusing to take patient because it's saving the only available bed.

- **On-call physician:** Admitting patient to avoid coming in, failing to come in resulting in patient transfer, or ordering more tests to delay need to respond.

There may be times when a situation triggers a potential for an allegation of an EMTALA violation, such as when a law enforcement officer does not wish to wait in the ED while a transfer is arranged for a patient requiring admission in a locked psychiatric facility. Law enforcement officers are not bound by EMTALA and may have other pressing duties. If the officer wishes to leave and take the patient directly to a psychiatric facility and refuses to wait until an EMTALA compliant transfer can be arranged, ask where he is taking the patient and then notify the receiving facility of the situation. Without providing the patient's name, the receiving facility should be advised of the situation and invited to contact the originating hospital upon the patient's arrival so that any labs, assessments, or diagnostic testing already completed can be faxed. A facility event report should be completed to allow hospital administrators to monitor these events and utilize the data when meeting with law enforcement to develop a mutually agreeable process for dealing with these patients in the future.

Evidence of compliance with EMTALA falls largely upon the quality of the documentation. Best practice is to utilize a checklist to verify all required documents are complete and present; however, a checklist alone will not ensure the quality of the content. Take a moment to review the reason, risks, and benefits of the transfer. Make sure the names of the accepting physician and facility representative are listed with dates and times of the patient's acceptance. Never delay transporting the patient due to incomplete charting. Send the available documentation with a note at the top indicating "Documentation Incomplete," and advise the receiving facility that the final record will be faxed upon completion. When dealing with an electronic record set, make sure that all components of the designated record set are printed and enclosed with the transfer packet.

Health Insurance Portability and Accountability Act (HIPAA)

The Health Insurance Portability and Accountability Act of 1996 was enacted to secure certain patient information, called protected health information (PHI). *Protected health information* consists of demographic information as well as anything else that might further identify the patient, such as a diagnosis. Violations of HIPAA result in fines that range from $100 per violation to $50,000 per violation if there was willful neglect (conscious, intentional failure to comply). Despite the best of intentions of ED staff, issues in the ED are complex, resulting in confusion over the requirements and inadvertent breaches.

Patients entering the treatment area may be accompanied by a guest. When hurried, the nurse may assume that because the patient is allowing the individual to come into the treatment area during the initial examination, it implies consent for that individual to be privy to any information disclosed during that exam. This type of assumption may lead to violating the patient's privacy rights. When first introducing yourself to the patient, turn to the guest and ask how they are related. Advise that there may be some sensitive information discussed and ask if the patient prefers the guest to step out for a few minutes. Other situations creating confusion for emergency nurses are when law enforcement requests patient information, when a VIP or high security patient is present, or when the media seeks information about a patient involved in a major media event. The golden rule for releasing PHI to any source regardless of the reason is to provide the minimum necessary to accomplish the task.

Remember that very important people aren't only celebrities, athletes, or politicians. Sometimes a member of the hospital board of directors or a wealthy hospital donor may be viewed as a VIP.

Information requested by law enforcement doesn't require a patient's authorization for release when complying with a court order such as a warrant, subpoena, or summons. It's also allowable when necessary for identifying or locating a suspect, fugitive, material witness, or missing person. An officer may need to receive PHI when conducting an investigation responsive to a mandated reporting requirement such as child or adult abuse. When the patient is in custody and returning to a correctional institution, a copy of the record may be provided to the officer for the purpose of continuity of care. When information contained in the record is necessary to prevent or lessen a serious and imminent threat to the health or safety of an individual or the public, a copy may be released to an officer. The amount of information permissible for release under these circumstances should be outlined in the administration's HIPAA policy.

VIP patients may pose a temptation for staff to access the record to find out the patient's status; if staff is not directly involved in the patient's care, this would be a HIPAA violation. If providing care to the patient, information reviewed in the record is restricted to only that set of information necessary for the provider to know. Anyone accessing the record must be directly involved in the patient's care or accessing for quality, peer review, or auditing purposes. All patients, not just VIPs, should be given the option to opt out of the hospital's list of admitted patients.

Patient care provided in hallway beds is another opportunity for inadvertent HIPAA breaches. HIPAA allows for treatment in semi-private rooms, wards, or hall beds if necessary to effectively care for patients. It also requires the hospital staff to take reasonable precautions to limit the information that may be overheard by others. Examples of safeguards include speaking in a low volume, talking away from others when possible, and having white noise in the area to make it more difficult for others to understand what is being said.

Information about a patient may be shared as necessary to identify, locate, and notify family or those responsible for the patient's care, of the patient's location, general condition, or death.

As necessary, this may include providing information to family members, police, the press, or the public at large (45 CFR 164.510(b), 2002).

Information about the patient's condition and the location of the patient may be released when the media requests the information and specifically mentions the patient's name. The patient's condition should be restricted to general terms like "undetermined," "good," "fair," "serious," or "critical." Disclosure of the nature of the patient's accident or injuries is not allowable without the patient's permission. HIPAA protections remain in effect even after a patient's death, so no information may be released without the media inquiry including the patient's name.

The HIPAA privacy law provides for many opportunities of inadvertent release of patient information. When in doubt, seek clarification before releasing any PHI.

Implementing Best Practices

As the age-old adage goes, there is no reason to reinvent the wheel. The same can be said of providing quality care. Some hospitals have developed excellent systems in which to provide quality care with little risk, known as *best practices*. When best practices are shared, they can be adopted by other institutions. This decreases the need for each hospital to waste resources to determine a best practice that has already been implemented elsewhere. This section reviews some best practices currently utilized in the healthcare industry.

Staffing Ratios in the Emergency Department

It has long been believed that there must be a direct correlation between nurse staffing ratios and improved patient outcomes. In 2004, California became the first state to enact legislation mandating minimum nurse-to-patient ratios and being prescriptive as to what those specific ratios should be. The focus was based upon patient acuities generally found on specific types of units rather than the actual acuity of the patients on the unit at any given time. Congress then passed the Registered Nurse Safe Staffing Act of 2013, requiring each Medicare participating hospital to establish a hospital nurse staffing committee to implement staffing plans addressing the unique characteristics of their patients and hospital units, attaching civil monetary penalties for those in violation. There are currently 13 states with laws and regulations addressing nurse staffing ratios; however, California remains the only state that mandates minimum staffing levels that must be maintained at all times regardless of the number of patients (e.g., the ED must have a minimum of two nurses present) (American Nurses Association [ANA], 2014).

Few studies look specifically at the effects of increased nurse-patient ratios in the ED setting and direct effects on patient outcomes. One California study looked at specific indicators the year prior to the enactment of the mandatory nurse-patient ratios and monitored the same indicators for a 1-year period after the implementation of the new ratios. The baseline ratios consisted of one nurse for every three patients in the resuscitation areas of the ED and, depending on the activity in the department, one nurse for every 8 to 12 patients in the less acute areas.

The non-flexible mandated ratios became one nurse to two patients in the resuscitation area and one nurse to four patients in the less acute area. Study results showed an increase in time from registration to time to treatment area bed of approximately 40 minutes. This number then increased the total throughput time from registration to discharge by 30-plus minutes. The primary reason for the increase was due to patients remaining in the lobby to avoid exceeding the nurse-to-patient ratios in the treatment area, even when nurses had the capacity to care for the additional patients. Quality indicators such as number of medication errors and acute coronary syndrome patients receiving aspirin were unchanged, and while there was an improvement in time of antibiotic administration for patients with pneumonia, this was also a new measure introduced in 2004 when the study was taking place, so it cannot be distinguished if the staffing ratios had any affect or if the improvement occurred due to other factors (Weichenthal & Hendey, 2011).

Other nurse ratio studies focus on the education and experience of the staff (staff mix) in the department rather than numbers. These studies are consistent with the Emergency Nurses Association position statement on staffing and productivity in the ED (ENA, 2011). The solution still remains unclear but what is clear is the importance of continued nursing research to ensure that guidelines and recommended practices actually achieve the desired results.

Risk Assessments

In an effort to identify high-risk patient conditions before harm occurs, nursing assessments conducted in the ED focus on early identification of the exposures through the use of checklist trigger tools. The checklists are frequently embedded in the electronic medical record and may be created as hard stops, forcing the assessments to be complete prior to advancing forward to other screens (see the upcoming section about electronic medical records). Risk assessments frequently found as part of the primary or secondary triage assessment address risks related to falls and suicide. The assessments may help to identify these risks; however, they are of little value unless the information is acted upon and measures taken to reduce the risk.

For more information on the unique needs of patients that pose a risk in the ED, see Chapter 14, "Challenging Patient Populations Encountered by the Emergency Nurse."

Fall Risks

The aging geriatric population is prone to falls. Even relatively minor falls can lead to more significant morbidity and mortality than that seen in younger populations (American College of Emergency Physicians et al., 2014). Although the elderly present a high-risk group for falls, a wide array of patients presenting to the ED are also at significant risk of falling. Early recognition of fall risk, with appropriate interventions addressing the risks, helps protect the safety of these vulnerable patient populations. Fall-risk assessment tools used for inpatients may not adequately capture the causative factors resulting in patient falls occurring in the ED such as alcohol intoxication, syncope/near syncope, use of sedating medications or illicit drugs, altered mental status, and seizures. Another area not covered by the inpatient assessment tools is the differentiation of the types of falls reflected in the patient's fall history. Distinguishing between a single incident of a mechanical fall, one caused by physiological factors, or a patient who is fall-prone helps the ED provider determine the degree of fall risk exposure. Once the care team recognizes causative factors, they can implement interventions addressing any specific needs to enhance plan effectiveness (Flarity, Pate, & Finch, 2013).

Suicide Risks

Suicidal patients are often brought to the ED for evaluation and frequently require holding for observation pending admission or transfer to an inpatient psychiatric facility. One in ten suicides are by individuals seen in an ED within 2 months prior to dying. Keeping these patients safe in the chaotic environment of the ED can be difficult. Providing a safe environment for these patients goes beyond placement in a "safe" room; it requires an assessment of the patient's current suicidal ideation and elopement risk as well as placement in a gown to allow for searching the patient's possessions for weapons, medications, or other contraband that may provide an opportunity to follow through with the plan (Bagley, 2013). Triage nurses should pay attention for the presence of potential predictors for suicidal risks, such as patients with previous and/or multiple suicide attempts, feelings of depression or hopelessness, diagnosis of post-traumatic stress disorder, substance and alcohol abuse, chronic illness, and significant negative life events. Several suicidal risk scales are appropriate for use in the ED and can be incorporated as part of the patient assessment process for patients found to be suicide risks.

Evidence-Based Protocols

Evidence-based protocols, once thought to be pushing physicians into the practice of cookbook medicine, are gaining acceptance as studies begin to reflect their effectiveness with reducing morbidity and mortality. Three presentations for which evidence-based protocols are commonly used are with patients presenting to the ED with acute ST-segment elevation myocardial infarction, stroke, and sepsis. Each of these presentations requires rapid identification and treatment to minimize the likelihood of death or serious disability. The protocols help the ED team to quickly establish a shared mental model so that all are working together toward one common goal and can anticipate next steps. As with other research-dependent recommendations, the practice protocols are being reviewed and revised on an ongoing basis to ensure they continue to reflect the latest research recommendations.

Simulation

Simulation affords healthcare providers the opportunity to develop and maintain competency when dealing with low-frequency, high-acuity scenarios. This approach to interactive learning allows the participant to make mistakes and receive feedback in a safe environment as well as develop team communication skills and self-confidence as competency increases. Simulation can be as simple as giving an injection into an orange or as complex as using computers and high-fidelity manikins to practice invasive techniques and implement algorithms. The learner develops muscle memory by actually performing the procedure, using the equipment, and interacting with others on the team. Engaging in simulation activities to promote competency is a best practice.

Documentation

Documentation is the primary source of continued communication between healthcare providers and offers a snapshot in time of the patient's condition and response to interventions. When reviewed from beginning to end, the documentation should provide a clear and accurate timeline reflecting when information was first known, orders provided and carried out, the patient's response, and any further actions taken throughout the patient's stay in the ED. You must remember that documentation in the medical record is used for many different purposes, such as:

- Continuity of care, patient instruction, and key discussions

- Billing

- Confirmation provider remained within scope of practice and met standard of care

- Best memory of care provided or deliberately omitted

- Evidence in litigation

Additionally, the record must contain elements necessary to comply with regulatory compliance. In 2006, PricewaterhouseCoopers conducted a survey at the request of the American Hospital Association. Findings determined that documentation mandates add 30 minutes of paperwork to every 1 hour of patient care and in some cases add 1 hour of paperwork to every 1 hour of patient care (PricewaterhouseCoopers, 2006). Because the ED is often the gateway into the hospital, responsibility for obtaining the additional information gets placed upon the shoulders of providers in the ED—frequently the triage nurse. Approximately 16% of hospital EDs continue to use a paper record set; the vast majority utilize an electronic medical record (EMR).

Paper Charting

Many hospitals continue to use a hybrid medical record in which certain forms are scanned into the electronic record set. These are generally forms requiring a patient's signature or those used during computer downtime. For others, the paper record may be required due to the incompatibility of the hospital's EMR for use in an acute outpatient setting such as the ED. Regardless of the reasons, there are pros and cons to using hardcopy medical records.

Pros: Paper records allow you to quickly flip through the pages to locate a specific entry or verify an order while en route to the patient's bedside. The narrative entries found in a paper record serve to communicate the patient's story. Understanding the story helps the nurse provide more compassionate care because he or she sees the patient as an individual and not just a diagnosis. Another plus for using a paper chart is that special logs or forms can be placed on a clipboard for quick access, making them conducive to contemporaneous documentation.

Cons: Compliance with CMS documentation requirements is difficult. Legibility and failure to document times, dates, and signatures are frequent issues found with a paper record. Pages can be misplaced, misfiled, or unfile-able due to a lack of patient information such as name, date of birth, and medical record number. Management of paper charts requires large amounts of storage space and manpower to compile, review, and file.

Electronic Medical Records

Eighty-four percent of hospital EDs use an electronic medical record for documentation. Some are products designed with the needs of EDs in mind but may not be able to interface with the EMR used for inpatients. When this is the case, primary care physicians with access to the inpatient's EMR may not be able to access the patient's ED record. One of the concerns with using an EMR is that many of the systems purchased by the hospital for use throughout the facility are not designed with the needs of the ED in mind. They can be difficult to use and may be limited in the amount of modifications that can be made to make it more functional for the acute ambulatory setting. Even the best electronic medical records have pros and cons for usage.

Pros: Records can potentially be accessed from anywhere and through several different devices such as a smartphone, tablet, or computer. Entries are immediately available, legible, automatically dated and timed when the entries are made, and contain an electronic signature based on the user's password. Previous visit histories can be accessed in moments, 24 hours a day. Templates can be embedded in the electronic record set to offer differential diagnoses for the physician's consideration, and offer documentation cues for high-risk assessments, some of which include:

- Wounds

- Restraints

- Procedural sedation

- Physician orders for life-sustaining treatment (POLST)

- Standardized protocols (sepsis, STEMI, stroke)

- Informed consent

- Aftercare instructions

Alerts and hard-stops can be added to require completion of certain data fields before you are allowed to move forward. Electronic medical records are excellent for data collection and reporting, and many of the EMR programs gather specific data components needed to enhance billing and increase revenues.

Cons: EMRs are used to collect and sort data. In order for this to take place, checkbox fields and dropdown selections must be used, and narrative notes discouraged unless absolutely necessary. In the absence of a narrative note, the chart is sanitized and lacks unique information that could help distinguish one patient from another. The nurse may develop tunnel vision and become driven by the need to complete the checkboxes such that the patient becomes lost in the process. Relying strictly on the use of checkboxes may result in the medical record providing an incomplete picture of the patient's presentation when read by others.

Using an EMR can be time-consuming, requiring multiple clicks and passwords just to access the section of the record needed to make an entry. Data displays may appear disjointed, requiring a lot of navigating through several screens to review documentation from the previous shift. The more difficult the information is to access or read, the less likely others are to make an attempt to access it. One concern unique to electronic records is when making a single data entry error, the record may auto-populate multiple areas of the record with that information, thus spreading the misinformation throughout the entire record. If the error is not caught, the patient may be at risk of harm. One study found documentation of patient's medication lists to be a significant issue, with only 22% of the records being accurate. Approximately 79% of audited records listed medications that the patient was no longer taking, and 76% of nonprescription medications were not listed at all (Monte et al., 2015). Data entry errors may occur due to many causes: distractions, human error such as clicking the wrong box, entering information on the wrong patient's record, or making mouse roller errors when using dropdown menus. Some medication dropdown menus contain large numbers of medication selections, many of which are not necessary, increasing the opportunity for an incorrect selection. Perhaps one of the biggest negatives of EMRs is that when printed, many are disjointed, making it very difficult to get an idea of the patient's course of care.

Minimum Documentation Standards

Minimum documentation standards are determined by CMS, state law, accreditation agencies, professional associations, and hospital policies. Compliance with CMS requirements has a direct effect on Medicare reimbursement. The minimum data set requirements from CMS are found in CMS Conditions of Participation §482.24(c), which states, "The medical record must contain information to justify admission and continue hospitalization, support the diagnosis, and describe the patient's progress and response to medications and services" (CMS, 1986).

Do's and Don'ts of Documentation

Always remember to document key communications in the record. Information should include the method used for communication, participants in the discussion, facts presented, recommendations provided, and decisions made. Table 12.2 gives examples of items that should always be included in your notes and behaviors that you should avoid.

Table 12.2 Documentation Tips

Always	*Avoid*
Document serial assessments focused on presenting complaint	Using subjective comments such as "pain improved"
Acknowledge and address discrepancies	Using the copy/paste feature of the EMR
Acknowledge and address abnormal vital signs	Keeping copies of your shift notes
Use objective observations such as "patient states pain is 7 on scale of 0–10"	Adding addendum comments long after the patient leaves
Record patient's response to treatments and medications; and next steps taken	Keeping a copy of the note because you fear it may become a lawsuit in the future
Indicate changes in condition	Having more than one open record at a time
Enter the time of the event if documenting at a later time	Using EMR with default settings on "normal" or "within normal limits"

Other High Risk Considerations for the ED Nurse

The chaotic nature of the ED creates many risks for patients as well as for nurses, both physically and legally. Some risks are inherent in the job. Some risks are unknown and may catch the emergency nurse unaware. But some legal risks are well known, and being aware of these risks as well as ways to minimize them will serve the emergency nurse well.

Informed Consent

In the landmark case *Schloendorff vs. Society of NY Hospital,* 1914, the court ruled that "Every human being of adult years and sound mind has a right to determine what shall be done with his own body; a surgeon who performs an operation without his patient's consent commits an assault for which he is liable for damages." Assault could be alleged if there is a failure to obtain evidence of informed consent or if the practitioner exceeds the scope of the consent or performs a different procedure than the one listed on the consent form.

There are four primary types of consent:

- *Consent for services* is generally covered on the Conditions of Admission form. This consent allows the healthcare provider to perform tasks such as conduct an examination, draw blood for lab work, suture wounds, and take X-rays.

- *Implied consent* operates from the principle that assumes an unconscious patient (reasonable person) would consent to emergency care if the patient were conscious and able to consent. The definition of what constitutes an emergency differs from state to state; however, the most restrictive definition requires the threat of loss of "life or limb" if medical care is withheld. The exception to implied consent occurs if the patient has previously indicated that he would not want treatment.

- *Informed consent* is a process involving a discussion between the medical provider and the patient addressing risks, benefits, and alternatives of a given procedure or treatment. Because the informed consent discussion involves the practice of medicine, it's non-delegable to registered nurses. CMS requires that each hospital medical staff create a list of procedures requiring an informed consent. To be considered a properly executed consent, it must include the following minimum elements: name of the hospital where the procedure or treatment is taking place, specific name of the procedure/treatment, name of the responsible practitioner performing the procedure, and a statement attesting that the procedure/treatment, including anticipated benefits, material risks, and alternative therapies, was explained to the patient and/or the patient's representative. The form must be signed, timed, and dated by the patient or representative.

  It's important for the healthcare provider to use layman's terms when explaining a procedure to the patient and not rely exclusively on written materials to provide education about the procedure. A detailed, well-written informed consent form for a specific procedure doesn't take the place of the informed consent discussion. Because informed consent depends on the patient's capacity to understand the information and make a decision about whether to proceed with the recommended procedure, the physician should make a note in the patient's record evidencing the patient's decision-making capacity. As the patient's advocate, you should verify that the patient received informed consent and had the opportunity to ask questions. Ask the patient what procedure he is having and his understanding of risks, benefits, and any alternatives. If the patient is at all unclear, ask the physician to return for further discussion.

- *Informed refusal* is the process by which a patient may decide to refuse a specific treatment, medication, or diagnostic test. The discussion is much the same as that for the informed consent and should be documented in the same manner. A best practice is to seek to understand the reason the patient wishes to refuse the procedure and make an effort when possible to meet that patient's need.

Affordable Care Act

Effective January 1, 2014, the Affordable Care Act (ACA) required individuals to have healthcare coverage. The ACA's focus is on improving access and quality of healthcare by expanding insurance coverage, using payment reform strategies, and increasing quality reporting (Patient Protection and Affordable Care Act, 2010). Although the goal is to have patients contact their physicians for guidance prior to presenting to the ED so that they can be directed to other, more cost-effective locations, early reports are that 82% were instructed to continue on to the ED.

A recent poll conducted by the American College of Emergency Physicians queried members about ED volumes since January 2014. Seventy-five percent of the respondents indicated that patient volumes have increased (some significantly) since January 2014, and that they are spending a significant amount of time coordinating care for follow-up (American College of Emergency Physicians, 2015). The increase in patient visits, coupled with the increased amount of time ED physicians are spending in an attempt to coordinate the patient's ongoing care, create more challenges to ED throughput and patient satisfaction.

Telemedicine

Telemedicine shows great promise for multiple uses in the ED. For years, many hospitals have taken advantage of tele-radiology services as an after-hours resource to obtain digital X-ray readings for patients. Hospitals lacking specialty consultants in areas such as neurology and psychiatry have found the use of telemedicine to be an excellent option to obtain consultation. Current studies are examining the feasibility and value of using a remote emergency physician to help expedite patients through the ED during times when the department gets busy and patients are backing up. By utilizing this approach, the remote back-up physician is immediately available and may provide assistance to multiple hospital EDs at once.

When telemedicine is used in the ED, you must first verify the patient's consent to be treated by a remote physician. You also need to stay with the patient throughout the course of the examination to facilitate the call and serve as the physician's hands when conducting the patient's assessment. The remote physician is responsible to guide you with specific instructions during the exam. Although it's still in its infancy stages, telemedicine promises to provide an enhancement to the quality and timeliness of care provided in the ED. What remains unknown at this time is the degree of liability risk you're exposed to while assisting a remote physician.

Use of Scribes

A *scribe* is an unlicensed physician extender used in many EDs to assist with clerical activities required of ED physicians. They are generally employed by the emergency medical group through a direct hiring process and vary in their backgrounds, training, and experience. Direct oversight of the scribes and review of all documentation entered into the EMR is the responsibility of the emergency physician. As a general rule, scribes record the information elicited by the physician during the initial assessment of the history of present illness, past medical history, review of systems, medications, social and family history, and allergies. Some scribes are also tasked with gathering data such as lab and radiology reports so that everything is ready for the ED physician's review and disposition.

Although there are many ways for scribes to help with patient flow through the ED, there are definite limitations to their involvement with patients and documentation. Scribes may *not* do the following:

- Independently interview patients to obtain a review of systems, past medical or family history.

- Relay a verbal order given by an MD to another licensed person.

- Document lab or radiology results called in to the department.

- Relay medical information or give medical advice to patients or families.

- Engage in direct patient care (assist with removal of patient from backboard, position patient for procedure, set up suture tray, etc.).

- Provide discharge instructions to patients.

Electronic Communications

Electronic communication (e-communication) is rapidly becoming a part of standard business operations in healthcare. Texting, email, and electronic medical records are the types of e-communications most frequently seen at hospitals. Devices such as smartphones and tablets are commonplace in the ED setting. Although these tools have much to offer healthcare providers who are constantly on the move, they come with inherent risks (see Figure 12.4).

Unintended consequences may occur when using electronic devices in the healthcare setting. One example is that the electronic devices add another layer of distraction to those already present on the unit. The ECRI Institute identified distraction as one of the top ten health technology hazards in 2013. Patient injuries occur when distractions interfere with the performance of complex tasks, especially when first starting or finishing the task. A heightened awareness of the hazards inherent with the use of e-communication in the ED allows providers to implement measures to reduce those risks.

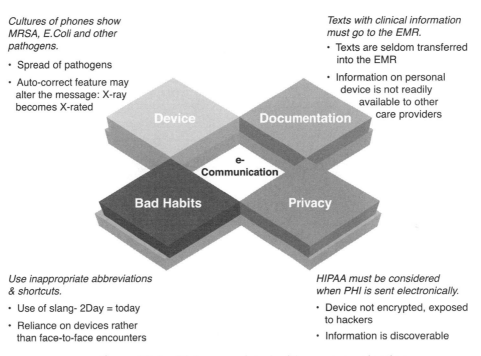

Cultures of phones show MRSA, E.Coli and other pathogens.

- Spread of pathogens
- Auto-correct feature may alter the message: X-ray becomes X-rated

Texts with clinical information must go to the EMR.

- Texts are seldom transferred into the EMR
- Information on personal device is not readily available to other care providers

Device

Documentation

e-Communication

Bad Habits

Privacy

Use inappropriate abbreviations & shortcuts.

- Use of slang- 2Day = today
- Reliance on devices rather than face-to-face encounters

HIPAA must be considered when PHI is sent electronically.

- Device not encrypted, exposed to hackers
- Information is discoverable

Figure 12.4 Risks associated with e-communication.

Summary

Many of the forces at work in the ED create unavoidable hazards to patient safety. Staff has no direct control over the numbers of patients arriving, timing, and acuity. As a result, you must take advantage of regulations, research, and guidelines designed to minimize the hazards of the work environment and improve the quality and safety of patient care. Armed with an understanding of liability exposures and available resources to combat them, you can deliver competent, safe, and compassionate care that can lead to greater personal job satisfaction and enhance the patient's experience.

References

45 CFR §164.506. (n.d.). Federal Register. Retrieved from http://www.ecfr.gov/cgi-bin/text-idx?SID=fba47e77f90ace599e46ee1451201529&mc=true&node=se45.1.164_1506&rgn=div8

American College of Emergency Physicians. (2015). 2015 ACEP poll affordable care act research results. Alexandria, VA: Marketing General Incorporated.

American College of Emergency Physicians; American Geriatrics Society; Emergency Nurses Association; Society for Academic Emergency Medicine; Geriatric Emergency Department Guidelines Task Force. (2014). Geriatric emergency department guidelines. *Annals of Emergency Medicine, 63*(5), e7–25. doi: 10.1016/j.annemergmed.2014.02.008. Retrieved from http://www.ncbi.nlm.nih.gov/pubmed/24746437

American College of Emergency Physicians (2013). The Uninsured: Access to Medical Care Fact Sheet. Retrieved from http://newsroom.acep.org/index.php?s=20301&item=30032

American Hospital Association (AHA). (2015). *Always there, ready to care: The 24/7 role of America's hospitals.* Chicago, IL: American Hospital Association.

American Nurses Association (ANA). (2014). *Nurse staffing plans & ratios.* Retrieved from http://www.nursingworld.org/MainMenuCategories/Policy-Advocacy/State/Legislative-Agenda-Reports/State-StaffingPlansRatios

Bagley, S. C. (2013). Identifying patients at risk for suicide: Brief review (NEW). *Making health care safer II: An updated critical analysis of the evidence for patient safety practices.* Rockville, MD: Agency for Healthcare Research and Quality.

Brenner, I. R. (2010). *How to survive a medical malpractice lawsuit: The physician's roadmap for success.* San Francisco, CA: John Wiley & Sons.

Buckley, J. (2014). The real cost of caring or not caring. *Journal of Emergency Nursing, 40*(1), 68–70.

California Health and Safety Code 1799.102; 16 Del.C. §6801 (a); Ariz. Rev. Stat. §9-500.02; 210 ILCS 50/3.150; Minn. Stat; § 604A.01. (n.d.). Retrieved from http://www.leginfo.ca.gov/cgi-bin/displaycode?section=hsc&group=01001-02000&file=1799.100-1799.112

Campbell, S. G., Croskerry, P., & Bond, W. (2007). Profiles in patient safety: A "perfect storm" in the emergency department. *Academic Emergency Medicine, 14*(8), 743–749.

Carayon, P., & Wood, K. E. (2010). Patient safety: The role of human factors and systems engineering. *Studies in Health Technology and Informatics, 153,* 23–46.

Carroll, R., & Nakamura, P. B. (Eds.). (2011a). *Risk management handbook for healthcare organizations: The essentials* (6th ed., Vol. 1). (pp. 3–9, 27–32, 54–62). San Francisco, CA: John Wiley & Sons.

Carroll, R., & Nakamura, P. L. B. (Eds.). (2011b). *Risk management handbook for healthcare organizations: The essentials.* (6th ed., Vol. 2). (pp. 8, 17–18). San Francisco, CA: John Wiley & Sons.

Centers for Disease Control and Prevention. (2011). *National Hospital Ambulatory Medical Care Survey: 2011 Emergency Department Summary Tables.* Atlanta, GA: Centers for Disease Control and Prevention.

Centers for Medicare & Medicaid Services (CMS). (1986). Conditions of Participation §482.24(c). Retrieved from http://www.ecfr.gov/cgi-bin/text-idx?SID=fba47e77f90ace599e46ee1451201529&mc=true&node=se42.5.482_124&rgn=div8

Centers for Medicare & Medicaid Services (CMS). (2014). *HCAHPS: Patients' perspectives of care survey.* Retrieved from http://www.cms.gov/Medicare/Quality-Initiatives-Patient-Assessment-Instruments/HospitalQualityInits/HospitalHCAHPS.html

Chassin, M., Loeb, J., Schmaltz, S., & Wachter, R. (2010). Accountability measures—Using measurement to promote quality improvement. *New England Journal of Medicine, 363*(7), 683–688.

Cline v. William H. Friedman & Assoc., 882 S.W. 2d 754 (Mo. Ct. App. 1994).

CRICO Strategies. (2015, May 26). *Nursing*. Retrieved from http://www.rmfstrategies.com/Clinician-Resources/Specialty-Reference-Tag/Nursing

Department of Veterans Affairs. (2011). *VHA national patient safety improvement handbook* (VHA Handbook 1050.1). Washington, DC: U.S. Department of Veterans Affairs.

Emergency Nurses Association. (2011). *Staffing and productivity in the emergency department*. Des Plaines, IL: Emergency Nurses Association.

Figley, C. R. (1995). *Compassion fatigue: Coping with secondary traumatic stress disorder in those who treat the traumatized*. New York, NY: Brunner.

Flarity, K., Pate, T., & Finch, H. (2013). Development and implementation of the Memorial Emergency Department fall risk assessment tool. *Advanced Emergency Nursing Journal, 35*(1), 57–66.

Graber, M .L. (2014). Minimizing diagnostic error: 10 things you could do tomorrow. *Inside Medical Liability*. Rockville, MD: PIAA.

Henry J. Kaiser Family Foundation. (2015, May 26). *State health facts: Total number of professionally active nurses.*. Retrieved from http://kff.org/other/state-indicator/total-registered-nurses/

Hoffman, J. (2014). *Malpractice risks in the diagnostic process* [Annual benchmarking report]. Retrieved from https://www.rmf.harvard.edu/Clinician-Resources/Article/2014/SPS-Malpractice-Risks-in-the-Diagnostic-Process

Institute for Healthcare Improvement. (2009). The Triple Aim: Optimizing health, care and cost. *Healthcare Executive*, 64–66.

Institute of Medicine (IOM) Committee on Quality of Health Care in America. (2001). *Crossing the quality chasm: A new health system for the 21st century*. Washington, DC: National Academies Press.

The Joint Commission. (2010). *A comprehensive review of development and testing for national implementation of hospital core measures*. Retrieved from http://www.jointcommission.org/assets/1/18/A_Comprehensive_Review_of_Development_for_Core_Measures.pdf

The Joint Commission. (2014). *Sentinel event policy and procedure*. Retrieved from http://www.jointcommission.org/Sentinel_Event_Policy_and_Procedures/default.aspx

The Joint Commission. (2015, May 23). *History of The Joint Commission*. Retrieved from http://www.jointcommission.org/about_us/history.aspx

Kipnis, A., Rhodes, K.V., Burchill, C. N., & Datner, E. (2012). The relationship between patients' perceptions of team effectiveness and their care experience in the emergency department. *The Journal of Emergency Medicine, 45*(5), 733–738.

Kohn, L. T., Corrigan, J., & Donaldson, M. S. (Eds.). (2000). *To err is human: Building a safer health system*. Washington, DC: National Academies Press.

Lembitz, A., & Clarke, T. J. (2009). Clarifying "never events" and introducing "always events." *Patient Safety in Surgery, 3*(26). doi: 10.1186/1754-9493-3-26

Logan v. Greenwich Hosp. Assoc., 191 Conn. 282, 302, 465 A.2d 294, 305 (1993); Shilkret v. Annapolis Emergency Hosp. Association, 349 A.2d 245 (Md. 1975).

Lombardo, B., & Eyre, C. (2011). Compassion fatigue: A nurse's primer. *Online Journal of Issues in Nursing, 16*(1). Retrieved from http://www.nursingworld.org/MainMenuCategories/ANAMarketplace/ANAPeriodicals/OJIN/TableofContents/Vol-16-2011/No1-Jan-2011/Compassion-Fatigue-A-Nurses-Primer.html

Lubarsky, S., Dory, V., Duggan, P., Gagnon, R., & Charlin, B. (2013). Script concordance testing: From theory to practice: AMEE Guide No. 75. *Medical Teacher, 35*(3) 184–193.

Monte, A. A., Anderson, P., Hoppe, J. A., Weinshilboum, R. M., Vasilliou, V., & Heard, K. J. (2015). Accuracy of electronic medical record medication reconciliation in emergency department patients. *The Journal of Emergency Medicine*. Retrieved from http://dx.doi.org/10.1016/j.jemermed.2014.12.052

Najjar, N., Davis, L. W., Beck-Coon, K., & Doebbeling, C. C. (2009). Compassion fatigue: A review of the research to date and relevance to cancer-care providers. *Journal of Health Psychology, 14*(2), 267–277.

National Patient Safety Forum. (2011). *Serious reportable events in healthcare—2011 update: A consensus report.* Washington, DC. Retrieved from www.qualityforum.org/Publications/2008/10/Serious_Reportable_Events.aspx

National Practitioner Data Bank (NPDB). (2015). *Location by practitioner type.* Generated May 26, 2015using the Data Analysis Tool at http://www.npdb.hrsa.gov/analysistool

National Transportation Safety Board. (1994). *Safety study: A review of flight crew-involved, major accidents of U.S. air carriers, 1978 through 1990.* Springfield, VA: Department of Commerce National Technical Information Service.

The Patient Protection and Affordable Care Act, Pub L No. 111-148, 124 Stat. 855 (March 2010).

Peasah, S. K., McKay, N. L., Harman, J. S., Al-Amin, M., & Cook, R. L. (2013). Medicare non-payment of hospital-acquired infections: Infection rates three years post implementation. *Medicare & Medicaid Research Review, 3*(3). Washington, DC. Retrieved from https://www.cms.gov/mmrr/Downloads/MMRR2013_003_03_a08.pdf

Pennsylvania Patient Safety Authority (PPSA). (2011a). *Risk management review: Emergency medicine January 1, 1985—December 21, 2010.* Rockville, MD: Physician Insurers Association of America.

Pennsylvania Patient Safety Authority (PPSA). (2011b). Medication errors in the emergency department: Need for pharmacy involvement? *Pennsylvania Patient Safety Authority, 8*(1), 1–7.

Physician Insurers Association of America (PIAA). (2011). Risk management review: Emergency medicine January 1, 1985–December 21, 2010. Rockville, MD: Author.

PricewaterhouseCoopers. (2006). Patients or paperwork? The regulatory burden facing America's hospitals. *American Hospital Association.* Retrieved from http://www.aha.org/content/00-10/FinalPaperworkReport.pdf

Rasmussen J. (1990). The role of error in organizing behaviour. *Ergonomics, 33*(10/11), 1185–1199.

Reason, J. (2000). Human error: Models and management. *BMJ: British Medical Journal, 320*(7237), 768–770.

Sanchez, C., Valdez, A., & Johnson, L. (2014). Hoop dancing to prevent and decrease burnout and compassion fatigue. *Journal of Emergency Nursing, 40*(4), 394–395.

Schloendorff vs. Society of NY Hospital; 211 N.Y. 215 (1914).

Sentinel Event Statistics Data—Root Causes by Event Type (2004 - 2nd Quarter 2015) Retrieved October 15, 2015 from http://www.jointcommission.org/sentinel_event.aspx

Sheeley v. Memorial Hosp., 710 A.2d 161, 167 (Rhode Island, 1998); Vergara v. Doan, 593 N.E.2d 185 (Ind. 1992).

Shilkret v. Annapolis Emergency Hosp. Association, 276 Md. 187, 349 A.2d 245 (1975); Pederson v. Dumouchel, 72 Wash. 2d 73, 431 P.2d 973 (1967).

Tarasoff v. Regents of the University of California, 529 P2d 553 (Cal Supreme Ct 1974/1976). https://scholar.google.com/scholar_case?case=2632319346734705 61&q=Tarasoff+v.+regents+of+the+university+of+california&hl=en&as_sdt=2006 Accessed October 15, 2015. Accessed May 26, 2015.

Thompson v. County of Alameda, 27 Cal. 3d 741, 614 P.2d 738, 167 Cal. Rptr. 70 (1980).

United States Code, Title 42, Section 1395dd (a). Retrieved from http://www.ssa.gov/OP_Home/ssact/title18/1867.htm

U.S. Commission on Civil Rights. (2014). *2014 statutory report: Patient dumping.* U.S. Commission on Civil Rights Publication. Washington, DC: U.S. Government Printing Office.

Watkins v. U.S., 589 F.2d 214, 219 (5th Cir. 1979); Zavalas v. State Department of Corrections, 861 P.21 1026, 1027 (Or. Ct. App. 1993); Kaiser v. Suburban Transportation System Corp., 398 P. 2d 14,16 (Wash 1965); Schuster v. Altenberg, 424 N.W. 2d 159, 161 (Wis. 1988).

Weichenthal, L., & Hendey, G. (2011). The effect of mandatory nurse ratios on patient care in an emergency department. *The Journal of Emergency Medicine, 40*(1), 76–81.

Widgery, A. (2014, April). Overdose deaths trigger state action. *State Legislatures, 40*(4). Retrieved from http://www.ncsl.org/Portals/1/Documents/magazine/articles/2014/SL_0414-Fin.pdf

Wilson, C. C. (2013). Patient safety and healthcare quality: The case for language access. *International Journal of Health Policy and Management, 1*(4), 251–253. doi:10.15171/ijhpm.2013.53

Young v. Cerniak, 467 N.E.2d 1045 (Ill. App. Ct. 1984).

EMERGENCY NURSING THROUGHOUT THE LIFESPAN

–Gayle Walker-Cillo, MSN/Ed, RN, CEN, CPEN, FAEN; Renee Semonin Holleran, PhD, FNP-BC, CEN, CCRN (emeritus), CFRN, CTRN (retired), FAEN; and Jeff Solheim, MSN, RN-BC, CEN, CFRN, FAEN

One of several things that differentiate emergency nursing from other fields of nursing is that emergency nurses must be prepared to care for nearly any type of patient. An emergency nurse could potentially care for a traumatically injured pregnant woman, a critically ill infant, a dying elderly patient, and a middle-aged man with a simple fracture, all in the same hour. This variety draws many people to the field of emergency nursing, but this variation and the knowledge base it requires also make this field of nursing so challenging.

As patients pass through the lifespan, nearly everything about their care changes. They're physiologically different, developmentally different, and socially different. The way that you assess and treat patients must be adapted to these differences. This chapter looks at three stages in the lifespan—pregnancy, childhood, and old age—and briefly discusses some of the modifications that you must consider when caring for each age group.

The Pregnant Patient

The interaction between the emergency department (ED) and the obstetrical department can be complex. During pregnancy, a woman's body changes, and what is normal outside of pregnancy may not be normal during pregnancy. The staff of the obstetrics department may be more familiar with these changes, and you might think that the obstetrical department is therefore better qualified to care for the pregnant patient and her unborn child. Yet pregnant women experience illnesses and traumatic injuries exactly as they would if they were not pregnant; the ED may be better prepared to care for these illnesses and injuries. Many emergency nurses dread caring for pregnant patients because of their unique physiological needs, but as an emergency nurse, you must recognize that the pregnant patient and her unborn child rely on your knowledge and expertise, in conjunction with the knowledge and expertise of the obstetrical department, to provide collaborative and holistic care.

In Pennsylvania alone, there were 20 reports of ineffective interactions between the ED and obstetrics that potentially had negative consequences on the pregnant patient and her unborn child in a single year. Thirty percent of these cases involved delays in instituting fetal monitoring for OB patients in the ED, while 45% of the cases involved pregnant patients being cared for in the obstetrical department for complaints that clearly needed the expertise of the ED. A review of these cases indicated that 50% of the negative outcomes arose from ineffective communication between the staff of the ED and the obstetrics department (Patient Safety Authority, 2008). Although you're not expected to be an expert in care of the obstetrical patient, you need to recognize that pregnant patients have illnesses and injuries that require your expertise. You must also lean heavily on the knowledge base of the obstetrics department and work collaboratively with them to meet the unique challenges of the pregnant patient and her unborn child.

EDs and their staff need to be prepared to care for obstetrical emergencies throughout the continuum of pregnancy. The ED must also care for pregnant women who have life-threatening conditions or injuries while trying to prevent adverse outcomes for both mother and baby. Sometimes the physiological changes of pregnancy itself are what cause such complications—changes that include alterations in cardiac output, blood volume, oxygen consumption, fluid shifts, glomerular filtration rate, anemia, smooth muscle relaxation, hypercoagulability, and displacement of organs.

The first question most women of childbearing age should be asked in the ED is the date of their last menstrual period (LMP). Although the answer to this question is not definitive to rule a pregnancy in or out, it can be very helpful. Even if a patient can recall her LMP, a bedside urine pregnancy test may be done to confirm or rule out pregnancy because of the differences in approach to diseases, radiology exams, and medications in the pregnant patient.

Complications of Pregnancy

The potential for pregnancy-related emergencies increases with the number of pregnancies a patient has had (parity), the age of the pregnant patient, high blood pressure, and smoking or alcohol or drug use. These factors should be part of the assessment of all pregnant patients. The goal of treatment throughout pregnancy is for both the mother and the fetus/newborn to remain healthy and viable. In the emergency environment, you may be called on to care for patients who have medical conditions while pregnant or who experience complications due to pregnancy. Each trimester of pregnancy comes with its own complications and symptoms (Benzoni, 2014; Gaufberg, 2014):

- **First trimester:** *Complications include:*

    - Ectopic pregnancy

    - Spontaneous abortion (miscarriage)

    - Molar pregnancy

    Symptoms include: Vaginal bleeding with abdominal pain or presence of tissue from the vaginal canal

- **Second trimester:** *Complications include:* Threatened abortion (miscarriage)

    Symptoms include: Vaginal bleeding

- **Third trimester:** *Complications include:*

    - Placental abruption (placenta pulls away from uterine wall)

    - Placenta previa (placenta implanted low in the uterus)

    - Uterine rupture

    Symptoms include:

    - Abdominal pain with dark red vaginal bleeding

    - Painless, bright red vaginal bleeding, specific to placenta previa

- Significant vaginal bleeding

- Fetal distress (abnormal fetal heart tones or changes in fetal movement)

- Expulsion of fetus, specific to a uterine rupture

- **All trimesters:** *Complications include:*

  - Hypertension

  - Gestational diabetes

  - Pre-eclampsia (>20 weeks)

  - Eclampsia (pre-eclampsia with seizures or coma)

  - Blunt and penetrating trauma

Symptoms include:

- Blood pressure greater than 140/90 mm Hg

- Proteinuria (protein in the urine)

- Edema

- Oliguria (reduced urinary output)

- Headache

- Vision changes

Trauma During Pregnancy

The leading cause of maternal death is trauma caused by either accidental injuries or violence. Between 5% and 20% of pregnant woman incur a traumatic injury while pregnant (Schwaitzberg, 2013). Sadly, much of this trauma is intentional in the form of intimate partner violence. The rate of intimate partner violence is grossly increased, with injury to the abdominal area especially high (battering, kicking, stabbing, inflicting gunshot or stab wounds, and other forms of assault directly to the gravid abdomen). Murphy and Quinlan (2014) report that 1 in 12 pregnancies is complicated by trauma, which they categorize as unintentional or intentional (see Table 13.1). For more information on intimate partner violence, see Chapter 15, "The Emergency Nurse and the Abused Patient."

Table 13.1 Traumatic Injuries to Pregnant Women

Mechanism of Injury	Percentage of Pregnant Traumatic Injuries	Type of Trauma
Motor vehicle crash	48	Unintentional
Falls	25	Unintentional
Intimate partner violence	17	Intentional
Suicide	3.3	Intentional
Homicide and gunshot wounds	4	Intentional

Source: Murphy & Quinlan, 2014.

Emergency nurses are called to care for pregnant trauma patients with both minor and major traumatic injuries. Many do not report pain, vaginal bleeding, fluid loss, or a loss or decrease of changes in fetal movement. It's important to note that pregnant women also have a 30% to 50% increase in fluid volume, so they are very late to show signs of shock. Ruffolo (2009) reports that more than 2 liters of volume loss can occur before any appreciable changes in cardiovascular status may be noted in the pregnant patient. Ruffolo goes on to note the importance of ensuring that all pregnant trauma patients should go to a tertiary trauma center. Trauma care of pregnant patients follows the same algorithms as others who experience similar trauma, with evidence-based recommendations. These clinical recommendations for pregnant trauma patients are (Ruffolo, 2009; Schwaitzberg, 2013):

- Assess fetal heart tones as soon as possible during the secondary survey.

- Monitor patients whose pregnancy is greater than 20 weeks gestation with minor trauma for a minimum of 4 to 6 hours by tocodynamometry.

- Draw a Kleihauer-Betke test for all women who sustain major trauma (detects fetomaternal blood transfusion to determine hemorrhage). The Rh- negative patient should receive Rh-immune globulin.

- Perform a perimortem Cesarean section delivery after maternal cardiac arrest if gestational age is more than 20 weeks or the fundus is 3 to 4 centimeters above the umbilicus (may improve maternal or fetal outcomes).

- Utilize preventive care, such as encouraging pregnant women to wear seat belts correctly and leave air bags on, and screening for intimate partner violence.

Other Considerations for the Pregnant Patient

It's important in the ED to realize that there are times when the patient or family is not aware of the patient being pregnant when an emergency occurs. Consider the following examples:

> A 15-year-old girl complains of severe abdominal pain in her right lower quadrant and is unable to stand up straight in triage. She thinks her last period was 7 weeks ago. Her parents are worried she may have appendicitis, but the emergency nurse is worried about an ectopic pregnancy.

> A young woman comes in with new onset status epilepticus that cannot be controlled by normal avenues. She is found to be pregnant and suffering from eclampsia.

> A peri-menopausal woman comes in complaining of "squeezing abdominal pain" that has been on and off all night. She is surprised to find out she is in labor.

Patients may be in denial, abused, victims of incest, having affairs, or just not knowledge-able about their own bodies and the changes associated with pregnancy. It's essential to frame discussions with these patients in a way that creates a certain level of trust. It's also imperative that you know both federal and state laws and statutes that govern the care of pregnancy, especially as it relates to pregnancy in the minor patient. In certain situations, teenagers can be registered anonymously and treated for pregnancy and other sexually related complaints without their parents' consent or knowledge. For additional information on consent, see Chapter 11, "Common Challenges Faced by Emergency Nurses."

The Pediatric Patient

In 2012, 12% of children living in the United States had at least one visit to the ED (Bloom, Jones, & Freeman, 2012). The management of children who are ill or injured can present a unique challenge because few EDs specifically care for pediatric patients. The majority of pediatric patients are seen in an ED that cares for all ages.

Why Pediatric Patients Are Seen in the Emergency Department

The most common diagnoses for pediatric patients in the ED include acute respiratory infections, otitis media and Eustachian tube disorders, fractures, and asthma. Even though two of the most difficult scenarios related to pediatric emergency are cardiopulmonary arrest or sudden death, it's not a common event in the ED. Approximately 16,000 children suffer a cardiopulmonary arrest in the United States annually (Hsieh et al., 2015).

The most common diagnoses for pediatric patients in an ED are (Centers for Disease Control and Prevention [CDC], 2015):

- Acute upper airway respiratory infections

- Otitis media and Eustachian tube disorders

- Contusion with intact skin surface

- Open wound of the head

- Asthma

- Fractures, excluding the lower limb

- Fractures of the lower limb

- Superficial injuries

- Pneumonia

- Cellulitis

- Conjunctivitis

- Poisonings

Injury continues to be the leading cause of mortality and morbidity in children in the United States (Albert & McCaig, 2014). In 2009 and 2010, there was an annual average of 11.9 million injury-related visits made by children and adolescents aged 18 years and under to the ED in the United States. Injuries occurred more often in male children. The leading causes of injuries included falls and striking against or being struck unintentionally by objects or another person (Albert & McCaig, 2014).

What's important is to understand the differences between a pediatric and adult patient and be familiar with warning signs of a serious illness or injury (Lancaster, 2005).

Preparing the Emergency Department for the Pediatric Patient

Pediatric patients comprise about 20% of the patients who are seen in EDs. However, 92% of these patients' visits are to community EDs, which may not be adequately prepared to care for ill or injured pediatric patients (Barata, Brown, Fitzmaurice, Griffin, & Snow, 2015).

In 2009, a joint policy statement, *Guidelines for Care of Children in the Emergency Department,* outlined recommendations for the preparation of EDs to care for ill or injured pediatric patients and their caregivers (American Academy of Pediatrics, Committee on Pediatric Emergency Medicine, American College of Emergency Physicians, Pediatric Committee, and Emergency Nurses Association Pediatric Committee, 2009). This document contains essential elements for the care of the ill or injured pediatric patient in the ED. It includes recommendations for staffing, staff education, and training and the equipment, supplies, and medications needed for pediatric care. A free copy of these guidelines is available at https://www.aap.org/en-us/advocacy-and-policy/aap-health-initiatives/Children-and-Disasters/Documents/Checklist_ED_Prep.pdf.

There are multiple courses available to help deal with pediatric emergencies. These include Pediatric Advanced Life Support (PALS) offered by the American Heart Association; Advanced Pediatric Life Support (APLS) presented by the American Academy of Pediatrics (AAP) with the American College of Emergency Physicians (ACEP); and Neonatal Resuscitation Program (NRP) and Pediatric Education for Prehospital Professionals (PEPP), both courses offered by AAP. One course developed for emergency nurses is the Emergency Nursing Pediatric Course (ENPC), which is coordinated by the Emergency Nurses Association (ENA).

Pediatric Emergency Assessment

Pediatric emergency assessment requires a specific set of knowledge and skills. You should be familiar with pediatric growth and development, which includes the anatomical and physiological differences seen in children, and the role of the family. Equipment and resources need to be available to manage the care of the ill or injured pediatric patient, including recognizing when the child should be transferred to a higher level of care, along with where and how to accomplish transfer.

A basic understanding of growth, anatomical and physiological differences, and developmental changes that occur in children is important when assessing, planning, and providing care for pediatric patients in the ED. Generally, children should be gaining weight and height as they age, but race, sex, and ethnicity influence differences in growth.

Development is gradual and continuous and may be influenced by the culture and environment in which the child is raised (ENA, 2013; Visser, Montejano, & Grossman, 2015). Table 13.2 contains a summary of some of the anatomical and physiological changes, and Table 13.3 contains a summary of some of the developmental changes to expect in the pediatric patient.

Table 13.2 Anatomical and Physiological Changes in the Pediatric Patient

Assessment Parameter	Unique Anatomical Findings	Clinical Significance
Airway	Large tongue	More likely to cause airway obstruction
	Obligate nose breathers	Nasal secretions and nasal trauma can cause respiratory distress
	Airway smaller in diameter	Small amounts of vomitus, blood, secretions, edema, or other foreign objects may cause obstruction
	Larynx more anterior	May be more difficult to intubate
	Short neck	Makes assessments of the neck for jugular venous distension or tracheal placement more challenging
Breathing	Chest wall more cartilaginous	Underlying structures are less protected and more vulnerable to injury
	Chest wall thinner	Breath sounds are transmitted differently
	Children rely on the diaphragm for breathing	Diaphragmatic breathing is normal and gastric distension may lead to respiratory distress
Circulation	Larger circulating blood volume than the adult	Hypovolemia will manifest differently in children
	Rapid heart rate is how children maintain their cardiac output	Tachycardia is an early indicator of cardiovascular compromise in children
	Hypotension is a late sign of failed compensatory mechanisms for a child in shock	Indications such as tachycardia should be noted and treated before hypotension develops
	Infants have immature renal function	Urinary output is not always an accurate reflection of cardiovascular status
Disability	Babinski reflex normal until the child starts to walk	Alters the neurological assessment
	Depending on the child's development, may be hard to determine the level of consciousness	Utilize pediatric-specific neurological assessments
Exposure	Because of body size and skin thinness, heat can easily be lost	Hypothermia more common in children

Source: ENA, 2013.

Table 13.3 Developmental Changes in the Pediatric Patient

Age	Developmental Changes
Neonate and Infant	Crying is primary form of communication Should be gaining weight and height Around 6 to 8 months, infant is afraid of strangers
Toddlers 1 to 3 years	Explorers Concrete thinkers Fear of separation and loss of control
Preschool 3 to 5 years	Magical thinkers Asks questions May see illness or injury as a punishment Fear of the dark, mutilation, and being left alone
School-aged 5 to 11 years	Developing logical thought processes Understand consequences of illness and injury May hide their thoughts or feelings Honesty is important
Adolescents 11 to 18 years	Experimentation and risk-taking Peers and body experience important Seeking independence

Source: ENA, 2013.

Family-Centered Care

When a child presents to the ED, he or she will more than likely be with a family member or caregiver. An important concept in pediatric nursing is family-centered care, which may include allowing family presence for invasive procedures or resuscitation. The process of family presence begins with an assessment of the family to determine whether they want to be present for the procedure or resuscitation and whether their presence is appropriate. Once this step is done, assess for potential barriers to family presence, and then provide clear explanations of what will happen at the bedside during the procedure or resuscitation. A dedicated member of the staff should support the family throughout the procedure or resuscitation (ENA, 2013).

 Family presence—The process of allowing significant others to remain at the bedside during invasive procedures or resuscitative efforts. Ideally, institutional policies and procedures are in place before family presence is undertaken.

Initial Assessment of the Pediatric Patient

The initial assessment of the ill or injured child is based upon the performance of a primary and secondary assessment, keeping in mind the anatomical and developmental differences in the pediatric patient. The primary assessment includes evaluating the child's airway, breathing, circulation, disability (neurological), exposure, and environmental control.

A useful tool to perform a quick primary assessment is the *Pediatric Assessment Triangle (PAT)*; see Figure 13.1 (Dieckmann, Browstein, & Gausche-Hill, 2010; ENA, 2013). The PAT focuses on the child's general appearance, his or her work to breath, and the circulation to the skin. The more components of the Pediatric Assessment Triangle that are altered or abnormal, the more likely the child is to be experiencing a significant illness or injury. For example, an ambulatory child who must be carried by the caregiver, who is rapidly breathing with sternal retractions, and whose skin is pale are signs that the child is very ill and requires rapid assessment and interventions.

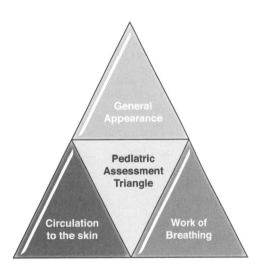

Figure 13.1   Pediatric Assessment Triangle.

The secondary assessment includes obtaining a full set of vital signs, facilitating family presence, considering the need for focused adjuncts such as advanced monitoring or urinary catheters, giving comfort measures such as pain management or emotional support, history (discussed in the next section), head-to-toe assessment, and inspection of the posterior surfaces.

A critical part of both the primary and secondary assessments is the initiation of interventions needed to manage any problem that has been identified. Tables 13.4 and 13.5 contain a summary of some of the red flags that you may identify in the primary and secondary assessments that could require rapid assessment and priority interventions.

Table 13.4 Red Flags in the Primary Assessment

Primary Assessment	Red Flag
Airway	Totally obstructed airway
	Inability to speak or cry
	Partially obstructed airway
	Stridor
	Child with a special healthcare need that affects the airway
Breathing	Lack of respiratory effort
	Nasal flaring
	Retractions
	Expiratory grunting
	Head bobbing
	Accessory muscle use
	Position of the child to breathe
	Child with special need who has a disorder of breathing
Circulation	Pulseless
	Lack of palpable peripheral pulses
	Cyanosis
	Pale or mottled skin color
	Hypotension
	Hypertension
	Tachycardia
	Irregular heart rate
	Capillary refill > 2 seconds
	Uncontrolled bleeding
	Lack of adequate urinary output
Disability (Neurological Assessment)	Altered level of consciousness
	Responsive to only verbal or painful stimuli
	Unresponsive
	Abnormal muscle tone for age
	Exposure
	Open wounds
	Bone deformities
	Signs of abuse

Source: ENA, 2013.

Table 13.5 Red Flags in the Secondary Assessment

Secondary Assessment	Red Flag
Full set of vital signs	Abnormal vital signs for age
Family considerations	Evidence of maltreatment
Give comfort measures	Inability to console the child Intractable pain

Source: ENA, 2013.

The need to consider transfer of the ill or injured pediatric patient is a significant part of the patient assessment. Not all EDs have the expertise or equipment to care for critically ill or injured pediatric patients. The sooner that you recognize that a child needs a higher level of care, the earlier the child can be transferred to the level of care needed to provide the most effective management for the injury or illness.

Obtaining a Pediatric History

In the ED, obtaining a history requires a rapid, focused method. Depending on the age of the child and stage of development, the child's ability may be limited to answer questions or understand what is being asked of him. The person bringing the child to the ED may not be the primary caregiver. The CIAMPEDS mnemonic provides a focused framework to gather important components of a child's history. Table 13.6 contains CIAMPEDS definitions.

Table 13.6 CIAMPEDS Mnemonic

Acronym	What It Stands For	What It Means
C	Chief Complaint	Reason why the child was brought to the ED
I	Immunizations and Immunocompromise	Has the child received recommended immunizations for that age? Does the child have a history of being immunocompromised?
I	Isolation	Exposure to a communicable disease that they have not been vaccinated for? Does the child have an active disease that requires isolation?
A	Allergies	Medications or foods Environmental
M	Medications	Prescribed Over-the-counter Alternative or integrative treatments Potential poisoning

continues

Table 13.6	CIAMPEDS Mnemonic	(continued)
Acronym	What It Stands For	What It Means
P	Past medical history	General medical history
		Medical history related to the chief complaint
		Focused history of the neonate should include birth history
P	Parent or caregiver's impression of the child	What does the parent/caregiver feel about the child's condition?
		Consider cultural differences related to illness or injury
		Consider children with special healthcare needs
E	Events surrounding the illness or injury	Time and date of onset of symptoms
		Use of mnemonics such as MIVT (M: mechanism of injury; I: injuries; V: vital signs before coming to the ED; T; treatment before arrival in the ED)
		Is this a revisit for the same problem?
D	Diet	Has the child been eating and drinking?
		When was the last intake of food or fluids?
		Is the infant breast-fed?
		Special diet required?
		Cultural influence related to diet, e.g., vegetarian
D	Diapers	Intake and output before arrival to the ED
		How many wet diapers?
		Bowel movements—color, amount, consistency
S	Symptoms associated with the illness or injury	Specific symptoms such as fever or chills, nausea or vomiting
		Pain

Source: ENA, 2013.

Care of the Ill or Injured Pediatric Patient

The ill or injured pediatric patient may require diagnostic procedures such as laboratory or radiology testing. It's important to plan and implement these procedures recognizing the influence of growth and development on the child. Fear of pain is common, especially if the child has been through the procedure before. Allowing the child some amount of control, explaining what is going to happen in simple terms, and providing an opportunity for the caregiver to be involved may help to decrease fear and pain and elicit cooperation from the pediatric patient.

The appropriate-sized equipment and protocols should be available for pediatric resuscitation. Endotracheal tube size for children 1 to 10 years of age may be calculated using a formula or a length-based tape. Intraosseous needles should be used when an intravenous access cannot be rapidly obtained. Fluid and pharmacological resuscitation are based on weight in kilograms. Because of children's larger body surface area to body weight, they are at risk of becoming hypothermic. Warm blankets and overhead warming lights need to be available.

Determine the appropriate-sized endotracheal tube by taking the child's age in years and dividing by 4. Add 4 to the result. The resulting number is the recommended diameter of an uncuffed endotracheal tube. (For example, the correct size for an uncuffed endotracheal tube for a 4-year old patient is 5.0. Divide the child's age [4 years] by 4 and add 4, which results in a size of 5.0.) If a cuffed endotracheal tube is to be used, the child's age is divided by 4, and the resulting number is added to 3.5 (American Heart Association, 2010).

The Older Adult

The number of people over the age of 65 years is predicted to increase by 20% in the United States by the year 2030. Between 2009 and 2010, over 19 million people 65 years and older were seen in the ED (Albert, McCaig, & Ashman, 2013). Patients over the age of 75 were found to have the highest rate of ED usage (Latham & Ackroyd-Stolarz, 2014). Based on the current statistics collected by the CDC and the aging of the population, the elderly are forecasted to make up an increasing share of the patients who come to the ED.

Many terms are used in the literature to describe adults over the age of 65. These include *older adult, elderly,* and *geriatric.* In this section, the term "elderly" has been chosen. Because the population is globally aging, one definition that has been proposed to describe the elderly is 65–75 years of age *young old;* 76–85 years of age *middle old;* and 86 years and above *old old.*

The focus of this section is to identify some of the reasons why older patients present to the ED, discuss the physiological changes related to aging, and explain the impact of these changes on the management of the ill and injured elderly patient. Transition of care, end-of-life care, and palliative care as they relate to the care of the elderly will also be described.

The Elderly Patient Who Presents to the Emergency Department

There are many reasons why elderly patients turn up in the ED for care. The most frequent complaints are (ACEP, AGS, ENA, SAEM, 2013; ENA, 2014; Gallagher et al., 2015; Latham & Ackroyd-Stolarz, 2014):

- Pain: chest, abdominal, generalized

- Urinary tract infections

- Gastrointestinal issues: nausea, vomiting, and diarrhea

- Altered mental status including dementia and delirium

- Respiratory infections

- Trauma: ground-level falls, motor vehicle collisions, and maltreatment

- Dizziness

- Medication problems: interactions, reactions, adverse effects

- Failure to thrive

- Social issues

- End-of-life care

The older adults that come to the ED are more likely to arrive by an ambulance, need care for emergent conditions, and have a higher risk for admission to the hospital, particularly the intensive care unit (Birnbaumer, 2014). Many of these are also at great risk of returning to the hospital for readmission. The patients who are at greater risk for readmission include those suffering from heart failure, acute myocardial infarction, and pneumonia. Additionally, patients discharged from the ED without appropriate follow-up or social resources are also likely to come back.

Elderly patients have unique needs that can be challenging to emergency nurses. Many of these patients have multiple comorbidities, cognitive and functional impairments, and complex social needs (Gallagher et al., 2015). The highest demand for care was found in patients who presented to the ED multiple times in a short time frame, suffered from multiple chronic illnesses, and had comorbid conditions such as limited mobility and dementia (Gallagher et al., 2015). Many times, these patients were transferred to the ED from care facilities with little or no information about these issues.

Physiological Changes of Aging and Their Effect on the Elderly Patient

Growth and development is a linear process. Just as in the young, there are physiological changes that occur with aging that will affect the management of an ill or injured older patient in the ED. As an emergency nurse, it's important to focus your primary and secondary assessment with these differences in mind and understand how the care of the elderly patient may vary because of these changes. Table 13.7 summarizes the physiological changes of aging and their effect.

Table 13.7 Physiological Changes of Aging and Their Impact

System	Physiological Change	Effect
Respiratory	Decreased vital capacity Decreased airway and lung compliance Decreased ventilatory drive Reduced ability to cough	Increased airway resistance Increased risk of hypoxia Presence of chronic obstructive pulmonary disease Increased risk of respiratory failure requiring intubation, barotrauma, and ventilator-associated pneumonia Obstructive sleep apnea
Cardiovascular	Increase in heart size and thickening Increase in arterial stiffening Decreased sensitivity to catecholamines Poor peripheral circulation Increased peripheral vascular resistance Increased difficulty in excreting fluid overload, which can lead to dilutional hyponatremia	Normal blood pressures are not normal in the elderly In those over 60 years of age, a systolic blood pressure of 150/90 may be acceptable Insufficient cardiac output can cause a state of hypoperfusion and shock not easily recognized, and patient may be under-resuscitated Underlying heart failure Hypertension Anemia
Nervous	Decreased number of neurons Slower nerve transmission Decrease in neurotransmissions Impaired control of body temperature	Baseline defects such as dementia Slower reactions Pain response is different Vision changes Pupillary changes Peripheral neuropathy Increased risk of developing hypothermia and hyperthermia Greater fall risk Arrhythmia development: atrial fibrillation, complete heart block

continues

Table 13.7 Physiological Changes of Aging and Their Impact   (continued)

System	Physiological Change	Effect
Integumentary	Thinning of the skin Decreased collagen content	Prone to wounds from low impact energy Slow healing Development of decubitus: importance of good skin care, frequent change in position
Hepatic Function	Decrease in hepatic cell mass Decrease in hepatic blood flow Alterations in microsomal enzyme activity	Alteration in pharmacokinetics and how medications may or may not affect the patient Increased risk of adverse medication effects
Renal Function	Decreased thirst response Decreased cell mass	Dehydration Decreased drug elimination Alteration in pharmacokinetics and how medications may or may not affect the patient Increased risk of adverse medication effects
Gastrointestinal (GI)	Decrease in blood flow to the GI tract Decrease in epithelial cell regeneration	Increase bleeding tendencies Longer healing times

Source: Birnbaumer, 2014; Flaherty & Resnick, 2014; Shea & Hoyt, 2015.

The resuscitation of an ill or injured elderly patient must be conducted with attention to the physiological changes that occur with aging and the effects those physiological changes can have. For example, fluid resuscitation, medication administration, and immobility can have serious consequences if not closely calculated and monitored.

Comorbidities

Many elderly patients have significant comorbidities that need to be considered when providing emergency nursing care in the ED. These comorbidities may have a direct influence on the patient's illness or injury, and you need to be sure that these are included in the initial assessment and history of the elderly patient. These are summarized in Table 13.8.

 Comorbidity—The simultaneous presence of two or more diseases or conditions.

Table 13.8 Medications and Comorbidities That May Affect the Care of the Elderly Patient in the ED

Medications	Diseases
Analgesics	Dementia
Anticoagulants	COPD
Anticonvulsants	Hypertension
Antipsychotic medications	Tinnitus
Benzodiazepines	CVA
Beta-blockers	Arthritis
Calcium channel blockers	Cataracts
Calcium containing antacids	Autoimmune diseases
Chemotherapy	Substance abuse
Cholinesterase inhibitors	Urinary incontinence
Diuretics	Vertigo
Insulin	Grave's disease
NSAIDs (e.g., ibuprofen)	Fecal incontinence
Opioid medications	Heart failure
Oral hypoglycemic	Renal failure
Polypharmacy	Diabetes
Sedative/hypnotics	Cancer
SSRIs	Dizziness

Source: Semonin Holleran, 2015.

Dementia and delirium can be particularly challenging when the patient and the family present in crisis. The management of delirium is discussed in Chapter 14, "Challenging Patient Populations Encountered by the Emergency Nurse."

Adverse reactions to medications may lead to ED visits more frequently than expected. Physiological changes that occur with aging, such as altered renal and hepatic function, affect the efficacy of many medications. The American Geriatric Society maintains the *AGS Beers Criteria for Potentially Inappropriate Medication Use in Older Adults,* which can assist in deciding which medications are useful or may have harmful side effects. This list is available at http://www.americangeriatrics.org/files/documents/beers/BeersCriteriaPublicTranslation.pdf.

Anticoagulants and Antiplatelet Medications

Anticoagulants and antiplatelet medications are prescribed to many elderly patients. Indications for the use of these drugs include atrial fibrillation, post-myocardial infarction, deep vein thrombosis, pulmonary embolus, and post–joint replacement surgeries. A list of some of these medications are:

- **Anticoagulants:** warfarin, enoxaparin, rivaroxaban, apixaban

- **Antiplatelets:** aspirin, clopidogrel, prasugrel

Patients who are on these medications are at a greater risk of suffering a gastrointestinal or intracerebral hemorrhage. A history of dark black stool or a fall should be a red flag for patients who are on these medications. Management of these patients is directed by the type of medication the patient is on and the risk/benefit of reversing or decreasing the effectiveness of the anticoagulation or antiplatelet medication.

Transition of Care

Transition of care is always an important component in the ED, but it can be critical in the care of the elderly. Whether the patient is admitted, sent back to a care center, or discharged home, certain elements should always be in place. These should include a summary of what happened in the ED, updated problem list, updated medication list, and a summary of the current medical and functional assessments of the patient. Ideally, this should be communicated both verbally and in written form. The *Geriatric Emergency Department Guidelines* contain recommendations and examples of ways to provide safe and competent transition of care (ACEP, AGS, ENA, SAEM, 2013).

To access the *Geriatric Emergency Department Guidelines,* visit http://www.acep.org/geriEDguidelines/.

End-of-Life Care

In 2012, Smith et al. published a study that found that half of patients age 65 and older enrolled in a longitudinal study between 1992 and 2006 visited the ED in the last month of life. Repeat visits to the ED before death were also quite common. The reasons given by patients and families for these visits included pain and worsening symptoms. The study pointed out end-of-life care in the ED is very expensive and generally not where patients and family wanted to be as death neared.

End-of-life care involves care that is provided to an imminently dying patient, for example, extubation and terminal sedation (Lamba & Mosenthal, 2010). However, many patients are brought to the ED for symptom management. One of the primary purposes of palliative care is symptom management.

Palliative care has become a familiar type of care provided in the ED. Palliative care has been described as care to prevent and relieve suffering and support the best quality of life for the patient and family (Lamba & Mosenthal, 2010). Palliative emergencies may include acute medical issues that could potentially be reversed, such as a bowel obstruction, and symptom management for symptoms such as pain, anxiety, constipation, nausea and vomiting, and terminal oral secretions (Rosenberg, Lamba, & Misra, 2013).

Emergency nurses need to be familiar with documents such as Physician Orders for Life Sustaining Treatment (POLST) that reflect patient and family wishes at the end of life. This can be difficult to honor but is an ethical part of emergency nursing practice.

Many emergency nurses are also experts at managing end-of-life symptoms, helping patients and families to identify goals of care and coordinate hospice care transition when indicated (Rosenberg, Lamba, & Misra, 2013). End-of-life and palliative care will continue to be a part of the care of the elderly in the ED.

Summary

Emergency nurses must be prepared to care for nearly any type of patient. As patients pass through the lifespan, nearly everything about their care changes. This chapter addressed three groups you can encounter in the ED that require specialized treatment: pregnant women, children, and the elderly. You should also know when to access additional resources and seek additional help to ensure that patients of any age group receive quality care.

References

Albert, M., & McCaig, L. (2014). Injury-related emergency department visits by children and adolescents: United States, 2009-2010. *NCHS Data Brief, 150,* 1–7. Hyattsville, MD: National Center for Health Statistics.

Albert, M., McCaig, L., & Ashman, J. (2013). Emergency department visits by persons aged 65 and over: United States, 2009–2010. Retrieved from http://www.cdc.gov/nchs/data/databriefs/db130.htm

American Academy of Pediatrics, Committee on Pediatric Emergency Medicine, American College of Emergency Physicians, Pediatric Committee, and Emergency Nurses Association Pediatric Committee. (2009). *Pediatrics, 124,* pp. 1233–1243.

American College of Emergency Physicians (ACEP), American Geriatric Society (AGS), Emergency Nurses Association (ENA), and Society of Academic Emergency Medicine (SAEM). (2013). *Geriatric emergency department guidelines*. Dallas, TX: American College of Emergency Physicians.

American Heart Association. (2010). Pediatric basic and advanced life support: 2010 international consensus on cardiopulmonary resuscitation and emergency cardiovascular care science with treatment recommendations. *Circulation, 122*, S466–S515.

Barata, I., Brown, K., Fitzmaurice, L., Griffin, E., & Snow, S. (2015). Best practices for improving flow and care of the pediatric patient in the emergency department. *Pediatrics, 135*(1), pp. e273–e283. doi: 10.1542/peds.2014-3425

Benzoni, T. E. (2014). *Labor and delivery in the emergency department*. Retrieved from http://emedicine.medscape.com/article/796379-overview

Birnbaumer, D. (2014). The elder patient. In J. A. Marx, R. S. Hockberger, & R. M. Walls (Eds.), *Rosen's emergency medicine concepts and clinical practice* (pp. 2351–2355). Philadelphia, PA: Elsevier Saunders.

Bloom, B., Jones, L. I., & Freeman, G. (2012). Summary health statistics for U.S. children: National Health Interview Survey. *Vital Health Statistics, 10*(250), 1–80.

Centers for Disease Control and Prevention (CDC). (2015). *National Hospital Ambulatory Medical Care Survey: 2010 emergency department summary tables*. Retrieved from http://www.cdc.gov/nchs/data/ahcd/nhamcs_emergency/2010_ed_web_tables.pdf

Dieckmann, R., Browstein, D., & Gausche-Hill, M. (2010). The pediatric assessment triangle: A novel approach for the rapid evaluation of children. *Pediatric Emergency Care, 26*(4), 312–315.

Emergency Nurses Association (ENA). (2013). *Emergency nurse pediatric course*. Des Plaines, IL: Author.

Emergency Nurses Association (ENA). (2014). *Collaborative care for the older adult*. Retrieved from https://www.ena.org/practice-research/Practice/Documents/OlderAdultTopicBrief.pdf

Flaherty, E., & Resnik, B. (Eds.). (2014). *Geriatric nursing review syllabus*, 4th ed. New York, NY: American Geriatric Society.

Gallagher, R., Gallagher, P., Roche, M., Fry, M., Chenoweth, L., & Stein-Parbury, J. (2015, March 28). Nurses perspectives of the impact of older persons on nursing resources in the emergency department and their profile: A mixed methods study. International Emergency Nursing. doi: 10.1016/j.ienj.2015.03.006

Gaufberg, S. V. (2014). *Early pregnancy loss in emergency medicine*. Retrieved from http://emedicine.medscape.com/article/795085-overview

Hsieh, T-C., Wolfe, H., Sutton, R., Myers, S., Nadkarni, V., & Donoghue, A. (2015). A comparison of video review and feedback device measurement of chest compressions quality during pediatric cardiopulmonary resuscitation. *Resuscitation, 93*, 35–39. doi: 10.1016/j.resuscitation.2015.05.022

Lamba, S., & Mosenthal, A. (2010). Hospice and palliative medicine: A novel subspecialty of emergency medicine. *Journal of Emergency Medicine, 43*(5), 849–853.

Lancaster, L. (2005). Mission impossible: Minimising the terror of pediatric resuscitation for staff in the ED. *Aci Emerg Nurs, 13*, 24–28.

Latham, L., & Ackroyd-Stolarz, S. (2014). Emergency department utilization by older adults: A descriptive study. *Canadian Geriatrics Journal, 17*(4), 118–125.

Murphy, N. J., & Quinlan J. D. (2014). Trauma in pregnancy: Assessment, management, and prevention. *American Family Physician, 90*(10), 717–721.

Patient Safety Authority. (2008, September 5). Triage of the obstetrics patient in the emergency department: Is there only one patient? *Pennsylvania Patient Safety Advisory, 5*(3), 96–99.

Rosenberg, M., Lamba, S., & Misra, S. (2013). Palliative medicine and geriatric emergency care: Challenges, opportunities, and basic principles. *Clinics in Geriatric Medicine, 29*, 1–29.

Ruffolo, D. (2009). Trauma care and managing the injured pregnant patient. *Journal of Obstetric, Gynecologic, and Neonatal Nursing, 38,* 704–714.

Schwaitzberg, S. (2013). *Trauma and pregnancy.* Retrieved from http://emedicine.medscape.com/article/435224-overview#a7

Semonin Holleran, R. (2015). Elderly trauma. *Critical Care Nursing Quarterly, 38*(3), 298–311.

Shea, S., & Hoyt, S. (2015). *Pocket reference guide for emergent/urgent ambulatory care.* New York, NY: Springer Publishing.

Smith, A., McCarthy, E., Weber, E., Cenzer, I., Boscardin, J., Fisher, J., & Covinsky, K. (2012). *Health Affairs, 31*(6), 1277–1285.

Visser, L. S., Montejano, A. S., & Grossman, V. A. (2015). *Fast facts for the triage nurse.* New York, NY: Springer Publishing Co.

14

CHALLENGING PATIENT POPULATIONS ENCOUNTERED BY THE EMERGENCY NURSE

–Gayle Walker-Cillo, MSN/Ed, RN, CEN, CPEN, FAEN; Renee Semonin Holleran, PhD, FNP-BC, CEN, CCRN (emeritus), CFRN, CTRN (retired), FAEN; and Jeff Solheim, MSN, RN-BC, CEN, CFRN, FAEN

The emergency department (ED) is truly a cross-section of society. Every person ultimately becomes ill or is injured, and, especially after regular business hours, there is only one place for individuals to meet their acute healthcare needs—the emergency department. At any given time, an ED may have patients from every end of the social spectrum—from a very influential person such as a politician or sports figure to a homeless, impoverished individual that is virtually alone in this world. In the ED, the very rich sit next to the very poor, the acutely ill may arrive simultaneously with the minimally ill, and people who would never interact with one another outside of the ED may find themselves side by side.

It's against this backdrop that the emergency nurse works every shift. One of the challenges that you face is providing equal care to a diverse patient population. It would easily be possible to write an entire book or even multiple books on the various patients that frequent the ED and the special needs that each one brings. This chapter provides a broad overview on some of the most challenging of these patient types and approaches to consider for each population.

Recidivism

EDs are the safety net for our communities and our medical systems. Several pieces of federal legislation affect the role the ED plays within this system. The Emergency Medical Treatment and Active Labor Act (EMTALA) legally compels the ED to see all patients who wish to be seen regardless of their ability to pay, provide them a medical screening exam to rule in or out an emergency medical condition, and, if one exists, to provide stabilizing care.

The Balanced Budget Act of 1997 further clarified that "...an emergency medical condition is one with recent onset and severity, including but not limited to severe pain that would lead a prudent layperson, possessing an average knowledge of medicine and health, to believe that his or her condition, sickness, or injury is of such a nature that failure to obtain immediate medical care could result in placing the patient's health in serious jeopardy, cause serious impairment to bodily functions, serious dysfunction of any bodily organ or part, or in the case of a behavioral condition placing the health of such person or others in serious jeopardy" (Veteran's Health Administration, n.d., p. 1).

In 2012, the Affordable Care Act created further legislation mandating insurance coverage (Centers for Disease Control and Prevention [CDC], 2012). For more information on legislation affecting emergency care, see Chapter 11, "Common Challenges Faced by Emergency Nurses," and Chapter 12, "Risk Management and Quality Issues Affecting the Emergency Nurse."

The CDC (2012) reported that the number of ED visits in the United States increased 34% between 1995 (97 million visits) and 2010 (130 million visits). Furthermore, because of the difficulties, conditions, and financing in healthcare, the supply of EDs has dropped 11% during the same time frame (CDC, 2012). As the baby boomers' age and life expectancy increases, the number of people with chronic illnesses such as cancer, stroke, and heart disease will continue to climb.

Recidivism—The utilization of the ED for four or more visits per year. Sometimes patients who practice recidivism are referred to as *frequent flyers* in the ED. It's a derogatory term that may bias emergency nurses negatively toward this population and should not be used by the professional emergency nurse.

As the number of EDs dwindles, the number of ED visits climbs, and more legislation is passed making the ED the safety net for everyone seeking medical care, the demand for emergency services continues to grow. Putting further pressure on an already overloaded system is a practice known as *recidivism*.

Common misperceptions of recidivism are that these patients are uninsured, not really sick, complex psychiatric patients, drug seekers looking for a "high," or the homeless wanting free food and shelter. Sadly, stereotyping this population may result in inadequate care with dismal outcomes. In fact, LaCalle and Rabin (2010), as well as Weiss, Wier, Stocks, and Blanchard (2014), found frequent users of the ED tended to be sicker, have national insurance, were more likely to be transported via ambulance, and have symptomology based on chronic illnesses such as cardiac disease, renal disease, sickle cell disease, and legitimate pain. These authors also found that patients who are frequent users of the ED often use other parts of the healthcare system such as outpatient clinics, homecare, and primary care physicians. In fact, 93% of patients identified as recidivists have primary care physicians, and many have had inpatient admissions in the past 3 months.

Patients who frequent the ED constitute a high risk for numerous reasons. They frequently have legitimate healthcare problems, which they feel (either subjectively or objectively) that they cannot meet within the constraints of the traditional healthcare system and need to utilize the ED to meet those needs. If the ED does not assist in meeting those needs, the patient's underlying medical condition may exacerbate. Attitudes of healthcare workers toward the well-known patient may harden over time, and this lack of compassion may breed carelessness and a callous attitude. This may not only leave the patient's condition undertreated but can also cause the patient to feel vulnerable with few options to seek relief from his or her underlying problem.

Patients Experiencing Psychiatric Illnesses

Patients who are suffering from psychiatric, behavioral, or substance use disorders are commonly seen in the ED. In the United States, approximately 8.4 million people suffer from mental health or substance use disorders including alcohol or illicit drugs (Heslin, Elixhauser, & Steiner, 2015). Approximately 4 million children and adolescents suffer from a serious mental disorder that affects their daily lives (National Alliance on Mental Illness [NAMI], 2015). Half of all lifetime mental disorders occur before the age of 14 (NAMI, 2015).

The ED has increasingly become the safety net for patients with mental and substance use disorders. Patients with mental health and substance use disorders frequently require more staff time and resources and experience an increased length of stay in the ED that can affect patient flow and lead to ED overcrowding (Stephens, White, Cudnik, & Patterson, 2014). Many EDs do not have dedicated places for these patients, whose propensity to violence is often greater than other patient populations. The patient's safety, as well as the safety of the staff, other patients, and visitors, may be at risk. In some parts of the United States, it may take days to find an appropriate place to transfer these patients.

Patients with a psychiatric emergency are very taxing to emergency nurses. In 2015, Wolf, Perhats, and Delao published a mixed-methods study that looked at perceptions of the challenges related to the care of a patient with behavioral health problems. The emergency nurses who participated in the study noted that a lack of education, resources, and treatment options affect providing safe patient care for these patients in the ED (Wolf et al., 2015). Utilizing staff specially trained to manage behavioral health problems and specific protocols could improve the care and transition of these patients from the ED (Wolf et al., 2015).

This section addresses some of the common psychiatric emergencies that present to the ED. We include the assessment and interventions essential to provide safe care to these patients and facilitate a timely transition to the care that they need, whether it be hospital admission or follow-up in their community.

Psychiatric Emergencies

There are many types of mental and substance use disorders that may present to the ED. The top five mental and substance use disorders admitted through the ED in 2012 are summarized in Table 14.1.

Table 14.1 Top Five Mental and Substance Use Disorders Admitted Through the ED in 2012

Mental Disorders	*Substance Use Disorders*
Mood disorders	Alcohol-related disorders
Schizophrenia and other psychotic disorders	Drug-induced mental disorders
Anxiety disorders	Opioid-related disorders
Adjustment disorders	Cocaine-related disorders
Impulse disorders	Hallucinogen disorders

Drug overdoses, as well as suicidal behaviors, are also common causes of crises that may present to the ED. In 2013, prescription drug overdoses were the leading cause of injury death in the United States, overtaking motor vehicle collisions. Seventy-one percent involved opioid painkillers, and about 30% involved benzodiazepines (CDC, 2015).

Illicit drug use has been increasing. In 2013, 24.6 million Americans aged 12 and older had used some sort of illicit drug, the most common being marijuana (Drug Facts, 2011). Illicit drug use can increase the symptoms of mental disorders as well as trigger a psychotic episode (Drug Facts, 2011).

In 2013, 41,149 people committed suicide. Firearms, hanging, and poisoning were the top three causes of death. Suicide was noted as the tenth leading cause of death overall (American Association of Suicidality, 2015). The majority of the time when an adverse event occurs related to substance use, or the patient attempts suicide, the patient will be brought to the ED for treatment.

Initial Assessment

When the patient presents to the ED for treatment of a mental or substance use disorder, begin assessing the patient by determining the risk for violence and ensuring the safety of the patient and the ED staff. Risk factors for the possibility of violence include male gender, police custody, prior history of violence, and drug or alcohol use (Heiner & Moore, 2014).

If the patient is combative or uncooperative, measures need to be taken to provide a safe environment. All patients should be screened for weapons and all belongings removed/ secured if patients are determined to be a danger to themselves or others. The patient should be undressed and quickly assessed for the presence of an injury or illness that may explain the precipitating factor for the aggression and anxiety. For example, is the patient hypotensive or febrile, has the patient been shot or stabbed and lost blood, or has the patient taken an overdose of medication?

You can employ several methods to manage the combative patient so that you can safely assess him or her and offer needed interventions. When possible, try verbal management first. Many times, directly addressing the patient's reasons for seeking care can decrease his or her anxiety and aggression. Other methods to use are:

- Be honest

- Offer patient some comfort such as a chair, food, and drink (as appropriate)

- Be non-confrontational

- Speak softly

- Be attentive and listen

- Keep calm

- Ask the patient why he or she has come to the ED

- Screen for suicidal ideation

For the combative patient, physical restraints may be indicated to prevent harm to staff, the patient, or others. Damage by the patient to the immediate environment is another indication for physical restraint. Specific ED protocols must be in place to initiate and continue the use of physical restraints. It must be determined that the patient does not have a medical condition that may contradict the use of physical restraints; for example, the patient isn't at risk for vomiting and aspirating. When you use physical restraints, you should:

- Determine that it is safe to restrain the patient.

- Not use restraints for convenience or punishment.

- Use physical restraints on an approved ED protocol.

- Explain the purpose of the restraints to the patient.

- If the patient is female, have a female care provider in attendance during the application of the restraints.

- Monitor the patient closely and change his or her position frequently.

- Completely document the reason for restraints and patient assessment while in the restraints; there's usually a standard form.

All staff members must be trained in the indications and use of physical restraints. The Joint Commission offers information about the use of restraints at http://www.jcrinc.com/. For more information on the use of restraints in the ED, see Chapter 11.

Chemical restraints are indicated for patients who may harm themselves or others. Chemical restraints can help facilitate a medical evaluation, especially if a medical condition that requires rapid intervention is suspected as the cause of the patient's combativeness. Remember, these medications are not without side effects, including altered mental status, respiratory depression and hypotension, prolonged QT intervals on the electrocardiogram, extrapyramidal side effects, and neuroleptic malignant syndrome. Some medications used for chemical restraint are (Heiner and Moore, 2014):

- **Benzodiazepines:** Lorazepam and midazolam

- **Antipsychotic medications:** Haloperidol, droperidol, olanzapine, ziprasidone

History

The evaluation of the patient with a psychiatric emergency should include a history and focused physical assessment for any organic causes of the patient's behaviors. When obtaining a history of mental and substance use disorders, begin with what caused the patient to seek care in the ED. Is there a history of mental illness or substance use? Is the patient currently being treated for either of these problems? Has there been a suicide attempt in the past? What has the patient done before presenting to the ED? Has the patient started any new medications? Has the patient suffered any recent traumatic events? The history is also used to identify pertinent risk factors. Specific questions that may help with collecting information related to psychiatric emergencies are (Montejano, 2015):

- Suicide:

    - Are you thinking of killing yourself?

    - Do you have a plan?

    - What are you going to do to harm yourself?

    - Have you attempted suicide before?

    - Do you feel down or hopeless?

    - What medications are you taking?

    - Do you have a family history of suicide or mental illness?

    - Have you lost someone close to you?

    - Do you have any chronic illness?

    - Have you been diagnosed with a new illness?

    - Have you been abused or mistreated?

    - Are you depressed?

- Psychosis:

    - Do you hear voices?

    - Are you seeing things?

    - What medications are you taking?

    - When did you last take your medications?

- Do you feel that someone is going to harm you?

- Do you feel someone or something is watching you?

- **Manic Behavior:**

  - Have you been able to sleep?

  - When was the last time that you slept?

  - What are you currently experiencing?

- **Overdose:**

  - What did you take before you came to the ED?

  - When did you take it?

  - How much did you take?

  - Why did you take it?

  - What did you do before you came to the ED?

  - Were you trying to hurt yourself?

Physical Assessment

The physical assessment of the patient with a psychiatric emergency is based on the same priorities as other patients (maintenance of airway, breathing, circulation, and neurological status). The safety of the patient, staff, and visitors is a priority, including ensuring that the patient does not have a weapon and has no intention of harming himself or others. If the patient has taken an overdose or caused physical harm, then initiate appropriate interventions to stabilize the patient.

Diagnostic Testing

Laboratory and radiographic studies should be ordered based upon the history of what brought the patient to the ED. In general, vital signs should be measured on a patient with an altered mental status. Organic causes of behavioral symptoms such as hypoxia, hypotension, and hypoglycemia should be quickly ruled out. A toxicology screen may be ordered if you suspect a substance disorder. Other studies to consider include serum electrolytes and thyroid function. A lumbar puncture may be performed in the febrile patient if infection is suspected.

Radiological studies such as a computerized tomography of the brain may be indicated if the patient has a history of recent trauma. The elderly patient, especially one on anticoagulants with a recent fall and an abrupt change in behavior, may benefit from this evaluation.

Management of Psychiatric Emergencies

Mental and substance use disorders continue to increase in all populations across the United States and even the world. EDs can generally manage the combative patient safely, intervene and treat overdose patients, and manage injuries from suicide attempts, but the aftercare of patients with psychiatric emergencies continues to challenge EDs daily. Interventions that have been used by some EDs include (Boudreaux et al., 2011; Stephens et al., 2014; Wolf et al., 2015):

- Developing specific areas for the treatment of these patients

- Using psychiatric-educated emergency nurses

- Making appointments for patients with mental health professionals

- Using case managers to assist the patient with a plan of care

- Setting up networks for community referrals

- Following up with phone calls to patients and families

The Homeless Patient

When the word "homeless" is used, many people conjure up a vision of an unkempt man sitting on the street in the shadows holding a bottle of alcohol disguised in a paper bag. Although this may capture some homeless people, it's essential not to stereotype this population. On a single night in January 2014, 578,424 people slept in some place other than a home (National Alliance to End Homelessness, 2015a). This may have been in a car, a shelter, somewhere outside, or any other place imaginable (or perhaps unimaginable). Many of these people come from lives that at one time or another may not have been much different from yours. A loss of job or other catastrophic life event forced them into temporary poverty, and they are left without the means to support themselves. Many of them are embarrassed by their situation and feel hopeless to find a way to escape. Some basic demographics for the homeless are (Karaca, Wong, & Mutter, 2013; National Health Care for the Homeless Council, 2013):

- 73.7% of homeless people admitted to the hospital are admitted through the ED.

- 16.1% of homeless individuals admitted to the hospital are under the age of 15.

- Homeless patients seen in the ED are 60.2% White, 22.5% Black, 10.6% Hispanic.

- Homeless patients admitted to hospital are 19.5% White, 33.2% Black, 15.1% Hispanic.

The majority of homeless people lack insurance and the means to pay for healthcare, so the ED is their link to the healthcare system. The only encounter they may have with healthcare comes with illness or injury. They are usually unable to adequately deal with chronic healthcare problems, and preventative medicine is almost certainly beyond their means. They are more likely to visit the ED, have a higher rate of admissions, and have longer hospital stays than other patients. Without insurance, they are unlikely to receive healthcare from most other sources. Karaca et al. (2013) noted that a variety of factors affected the rate of ED use among the homeless, including the amount of homelessness (stable versus unstable shelter), being victims of crime, arrests, mental illness, substance abuse, medical illness, or injury. Some facts regarding insurance and the homeless patient (Karaca et al., 2013; National Health Care for the Homeless Council, 2013):

- 28.1% of homeless patients admitted as an inpatient are uninsured.

- 42.8% of homeless patients in the ED are uninsured.

- 48.2% of homeless patients admitted to the hospital are covered by Medicaid.

- 34.7% of homeless patients treated and released from the ED are covered by Medicaid.

A review of homeless patients with mental disorders treated in the ED revealed that (Karaca et al., 2013; National Health Care for the Homeless Council, 2013):

- 49.0% were treated and released from the ED.

- 22.4% were admitted to inpatient units.

- 33.8% of inpatients with schizophrenia and other psychotic disorders were homeless.

- 52.8% of homeless people treated and released had alcohol-related disorders.

 Not all homeless people have a mental illness, yet many do. According to the National Alliance to End Homelessness (2015b), 40% of homeless people have a serious mental illness or conditions related to chronic substance abuse. Over the years, funding for the institutionalization of the mentally ill has declined dramatically, leaving this vulnerable population with nowhere to go.

With inadequate resources and lack of access to healthcare, health conditions in the homeless population tend to worsen and compound. Foster, LeFauve, Kresky-Wolff, & Richards (2010) noted that 52% of homeless people have a minimum of two chronic-health-related diagnoses. Common illnesses include mental illness, substance abuse, cardiovascular disease, arthritis, hypertension, diabetes, respiratory diseases, HIV/AIDs, hepatitis C, sexually transmitted infections, and dental problems.

The ED and only the ED is bound by federal law to see all patients and treat them until they are completely stable. Stability includes not only stabilization of physical ailments but also mental stability and sobriety.

EMTALA (Emergency Medical Treatment and Active Labor Act)—A law requiring hospitals with EDs to provide a medical screening examination to any individual who comes to the ED and requests such an examination, and prohibits hospitals with EDs from refusing to examine or treat individuals with an emergency medical condition (EMC) to ensure public access to emergency services regardless of ability to pay (Centers for Medicare and Medicaid Services [CMS], 2010).

Providing appropriate care for the homeless patient can be complex. It usually requires more than the standard treat and release that may be appropriate for patients with adequate resources. If, for example, a dressing is applied to the wound of a homeless patient, who will provide dressing changes after discharge from the ED? If the patient does not have a place to keep her belongings, any dressing supplies given to her may not be kept clean. If the patient is homeless, how will she cleanse the wound at the time of the dressing change? Where will any soiled dressings that she removes be discarded safely? Something as simple as a dressing can become a complex issue for these patients at the time of discharge.

If the patient requires admission or follow-up care, the situation can become increasingly complicated. What if the patient has a pet or a storage container for belongings, neither of which would be appropriate to bring to the inpatient unit on admission? These may be that individual's only worldly possessions and may have the same meaning to her as a home or car has for patients who are not homeless. You may have to implement creative strategies to gain the trust of the homeless individual and to solve her unique needs. This often requires the assistance of social work and outside agencies that provide relief to this population.

The other challenge you must deal with when caring for the homeless population is your personal attitude. Over time, it's easy to look at this population as utilizing the ED for free food ("They are only here for a sandwich"), shelter ("Why is it that their illness only flares up when it is cold or rainy outside?"), and free services ("I'll bet she will want a taxi cab voucher when we discharge her"). Sometimes, ED staff may actually resist providing this population with food, shelter, and services to discourage them from utilizing the ED. These attitudes may cross ethical lines, and you must constantly reassess your attitude and maintain the compassion that likely drew you to the profession of nursing in the first place. The homeless individual endures hardships that likely dwarf those of most individuals in society and deserves the same care and compassion as all patients.

Finally, you must understand the resources available to the homeless population in each community. What time does the shelter close? What time do they have to be out of the shelter each morning? Some transitional housing requires patients provide a urine sample before they can come back in the door; if the patient receives narcotics in the ED, the patient must have a note of explanation on discharge. Is there a shower for them to use somewhere? Is there any family that can provide temporary shelter?

For additional information on the homeless population, visit the following online resources:

- National Clearinghouse for Alcohol and Drug Information: http://www.samhsa.gov/nctic

- Homelessness Resource Center: http://www.nrchmi.samhsa.gov/

- U.S. Department of Health & Human Services page for the homeless: http://www.hhs.gov/homeless/

- Health Care for the Homeless Information Resource Center: http://bphc.hrsa.gov/

- Affordable Care Act: https://www.hudexchange.info/aca/

- Veterans Administration page for homeless veterans: http://www.va.gov/homeless/

Patients With Altered Mental Status

Although altered mental status or altered level of consciousness is not categorized as a specific disease, it's not uncommon among ED patients. Mental status changes can occur in relation to something as basic as hypoglycemia to something as complex as a stroke.

An alteration in mental status creates numerous challenges for the entire emergency team. Legal issues surrounding consent and the ability to determine a patient's wishes become problematic. Ascertaining a patient's identity and obtaining an accurate medical history is sometimes impossible. Determining the cause for the altered level of consciousness and developing an appropriate treatment plan can be challenging when the patient's history is not known.

Normal mental status consists of both a wakeful state *(arousal)* and cognition. Arousal is controlled by the reticular activating system (RAS) housed in the brainstem. For example, if you suspect a patient is having a hemorrhagic stroke and the patient is unarousable to painful stimuli, the hemorrhage is most likely located in the brainstem, in both hemispheres, or the bleed is so large it is causing systemic effects related to increased intracranial pressure. Cognition, on the other hand, is controlled by the cortical hemispheres and is more likely to be caused by head injuries, seizures, tumors, amnesia, hallucinations, delirium, and dementia.

Care of the Patient With an Altered Level of Consciousness

Initially, care of the patient with an altered level of consciousness is identical to any patient, with focus on maintaining the airway, supporting breathing and circulation, assessing neurological status (disability), and looking for clues regarding the cause of the condition. Table 14.2 presents a brief overview of the initial care of the patient with an altered level of consciousness.

Table 14.2 Initial Care of the Patient With an Altered Mental Status

Parameter	Assessment	Intervention
Airway	Loss of ability to independently protect the airway Loss of gag reflex Airway obstruction Uncontrollable vomiting/aspiration risks	Open airway (spinal mobility restriction stabilization if trauma suspected) Suction Nasopharyngeal airway Oropharyngeal airway (only with absent gag reflex) Endotracheal intubation
Breathing	Respiratory distress Retractions Abnormal respiratory/chest wall movements or sounds Hypoventilation Hypoxia Cyanosis Air hunger Abnormal breath sounds	High flow oxygen, or assist ventilation with bag-mask device if needed If breath sounds absent, decompress the chest or place chest tube Endotracheal intubation and mechanical ventilation as needed Pulse oximetry Capnography

continues

Table 14.2 Initial Care of the Patient With an Altered Mental Status   (continued)

Parameter	Assessment	Intervention
Circulation	Alteration in pulse rate or quality Abnormal blood pressure Prolonged capillary refill Abnormal skin color and temperature Altered electrocardiogram; obvious sources of hemorrhage Abnormal heart sounds	Intravenous access with initiation of fluid resuscitation as needed Cardiac monitoring Treat dysrhythmias appropriately Cardiopulmonary resuscitation as needed Defibrillation as needed Control of bleeding sources Bedside ultrasound
Disability	Pupil size and reaction Presence of papilledema, retinal hemorrhage, nystagmus, or extraocular movements Assess level of consciousness Assess for hypoglycemia Focal or lateralizing neurological deficits (lack of movement to one side points to stroke, lack of movement below a certain level points to spinal cord injury, repetitive movement points to seizure) Movement normal or abnormal Assess for potential toxicological emergencies Look for signs of trauma Measure Glasgow Coma Score	Administer dextrose In overdoses, administer reversal agents (slowly!): Opioids – naloxone; benzodiazepine – flumazenil Consider benzodiazepines for seizure activity Consider computerized tomography and fibrinolytics for stroke Consider interventions to reduce intracranial pressure for head injuries
Exposure	Remove clothing and view the entire patient (look for transdermal patches which may explain changes in level of consciousness) Look for indications of trauma, infections, rashes, liver failure, intravenous "track marks"	Remove drug patches Minimize heat loss Control bleeding

Source: Han & Wilber, 2013; Morrissey, 2013.

When utilizing the Glasgow Coma Score, patients are assigned a number that corresponds to a response in each area (eyes, verbal response, and motor response). The numbers from the three areas are totaled. A score of 13–15 is considered a normal or mild brain injury, a score of 9–12 is considered a moderate brain injury, and a score of less than 9 is considered a severe brain injury. Table 14.3 is an overview of the Glasgow Coma Score.

Table 14.3 Glasgow Coma Score

Parameter	Scoring
Eye opening	4 – Opens eyes spontaneously
	3 – Opens eyes in response to voice
	2 – Opens eyes in response to painful stimuli
	1 – Does not open eyes
Verbal response	5 – Oriented, converses normally
	4 – Confused and disoriented
	3 – Inappropriate words
	2 – Incomprehensible sounds
	1 – Makes no sounds
Motor response	6 – Obeys commands
	5 – Localizes painful stimuli
	4 – Flexion/withdrawal to painful stimuli
	3 – Abnormal flexion to painful stimuli (decorticate posture)
	2 – Extension to painful stimuli (decerebrate response)
	1 – Makes no movement

Source: Christensen, 2014.

Emergency Differential Diagnosis Approach

When treating the ED patient who presents with an alteration in consciousness, you must recognize that many times the level of consciousness will not improve until the true cause is revealed and treated. That is why it's important, with such a vast number of potential causes, to have a systematic approach to not only your assessments but also the categories you can rule in or out. See Table 14.4.

Table 14.4 Differential Diagnosis for Patients With Altered Level of Consciousness

Factor	Cause	Diagnostics
Systemic	Infection/sepsis	Laboratory blood work
	Inadequate pain control	Blood, urine, and other cultures as appropriate
	Trauma	Blood glucose
	Dehydration	Computerized tomography (CT) scan
	Hypo/hyperthermia	Rectal temperature
	Hypertension	Blood pressure
		Radiologic exams of traumatic injuries

continues

Table 14.4 Differential Diagnosis for Patients With Altered Level of Consciousness   (continued)

Factor	Cause	Diagnostics
Metabolic	Wernicke's encephalopathy	Administration of thiamine
	Hepatic failure	Laboratory blood work
	Renal failure	Serum osmolality
	Hypo/hypernatremia	Serum electrolytes, BUN/creatinine
	Hypo/hypercalcemia	Thyroid function tests
	Hypo/hyperglycemia	Serum cortisol levels
	Thyroid dysfunction	Arterial blood gases
Central Nervous System	Meningitis/encephalitis	Lumbar puncture (after computerized tomography)
	Cerebrovascular accident	Laboratory blood work
	Diffuse axonal injury	Blood glucose level
	Intracerebral hemorrhage	Computerized tomography (CT) scan
	Subarachnoid hemorrhage	Neurological consultants
	Subdural/epidural hemorrhage	Neurosurgical consultants
		Cranial nerve exam
	Tumors	Electroencephalogram (EEG)
	Status epilepticus	Magnetic resonance imaging (MRI)
	Neurological infections (focal abscess/toxoplasmosis)	Carotid/vertebral ultrasound
		Descent from altitude
	Acute mountain (altitude) sickness (cerebral edema)	Oxygen/hyperbaric/dexamethasone
	Dementia	
Cardiopulmonary	Acute myocardial infarction	Laboratory studies
	Heart failure	Blood glucose level
	Outflow obstructions	Computerized tomography (CT) scan
	Hypoxemia	Arterial blood gases
	Hypercarbia	Pulse oximetry
	Hypertensive encephalopathy	Indwelling catheter for output measurement
	Shock	Radiologic exams
	Urine output	Echocardiogram
Toxicology	Medications (sedatives, analgesics, anticonvulsants, narcotics, hypoglycemics)	Laboratory blood work
		Blood glucose
		Computerized tomography (CT) scan
	Recreational drug use	Urine drug screen
	Withdrawal	Blood alcohol level
	Steroids	Medication levels
	Alcohols	Arterial blood gases
	Household poisons	
	Polypharmacy	

Iatrogenic	Surgeries or procedures	Laboratory blood work
	Indwelling catheters/lines	Blood glucose levels
	Retained products or equipment	Computerized tomography (CT) scan
		Radiologic exams

Source: Han & Wilber, 2013; Morrissey, 2013; Harris & Pittman, 2014.

Older Patients With Altered Mental Status

The ED is commonly the point of entry and safety net for the older population. In the United States, 18 million patients who are 65 years and older are seen in the ED yearly. Delirium, dementia, stupor, and coma are alterations in levels of consciousness that occur in all ages but are particularly common in this age group. The most severe alterations in level of consciousness are considered to be stupor and coma, which occur in 5% to 9% of older patients. These medical emergencies require rapid evaluation because of the possibility for rapid decompensation as well as concerns for staff and patient safety. Like other alterations in level of consciousness, it is essential to determine the cause for stupor and coma and treat the cause rather than the symptom. Is the patient's condition the result of a urinary tract infection or the effect of a new drug the patient is taking?

One of the most difficult issues to tease out during an emergency visit is whether the change in mental status is new or part of an ongoing process. Delirium is an alteration in mental status related to a physiological imbalance and frequently has a rapid onset. Dementia is a chronic, non-reversible alteration in cerebral functioning that has a slower onset. But if the patient presents with an alteration in mental status, it is challenging to gather a history and differentiate these two conditions. Further complicating the issue is the patient with dementia who becomes delirious. The dementia may mask the delirium, and serious treatable medical issues may be missed.

Delirium is divided into two stages (Han & Wilber, 2013; World Health Organization [WHO], 2015). The first stage is the *hyperactive state* marked by symptoms such as:

■ Restlessness

■ Agitation

■ Anxiety

■ Combativeness

The second stage of delirium is also known as the *hypoactive state* with symptoms such as:

- Drowsiness

- Somnolence

- Lethargy

- Depression

- Fatigue

Sometimes patients with dementia may present with both hyperactive and hypoactive symptoms, referred to as *mixed dementia*.

Similarly, dementia is divided into three stages (Han & Wilber, 2013; WHO, 2015). The first stage, the *early stage*, includes symptoms such as:

- Forgetfulness

- Losing track of the time

- Becoming lost in familiar places

The second stage, the *middle stage*, is marked by symptoms such as:

- Forgetting recent events

- Forgetting people's names

- Becoming lost at home

- Increased difficulty with communication

- Needing help with personal care

- Behavior changes, including wandering and repeated questioning

The last stage of dementia, the *late phase*, is marked by symptoms such as:

- Becoming unaware of the time and place

- Difficulty recognizing relatives and friends

- An increasing need for assisted self-care

▣ Difficulty walking

▣ Behavior changes that may escalate and include aggression

Table 14.5 discusses additional methods to distinguish between the two.

Stupor—"Condition of deep sleep or unresponsiveness in which the patient can be aroused only with vigorous and continuous stimulation" (Han & Wilber, 2013, p. 2).

Coma—"A state of unresponsiveness in which the patient cannot be aroused with any stimuli" (Han & Wilber, 2013, p. 2).

Table 14.5 Separating Delirium and Dementia

Stage/Symptom	Delirium	Dementia
Onset	Rapid (hours or days)	Slow (months and years)
Course	Waxing and waning	Progressive
Vital signs/physical exam	Often abnormal	Usually normal
Focus	Inattention	Normal (except in severe dementia)
Level of consciousness	Altered	Normal (except in severe dementia)
Loss of cognition	Disorganized thought	Perceptual disturbances Disorientation Abnormal as disease progresses
Reversible cognitive decline	Usually reversible	Rarely reversible
Sleep-wake cycle	Disturbance	Normal (except in severe dementia)
Hallucinations or perceptual disturbances	May be present	Absent (except in severe dementia)
Causes	Organic	Organic (degenerative)
Safety risk	Yes, immediate	Yes
Prognosis	Positive if treated rapidly	Poor

Source: Han & Wilber, 2013; WHO, 2015.

For more information on delirium, visit www.americandeliriumsociety.org.

Summary

Emergency nurses truly see a cross-section of society, from repeat patients to patients suffering from psychiatric, behavioral, or substance use disorders; patients with altered mental states; and the homeless. Helping these patients requires extra care. This chapter offered an overview for these most challenging patient types and the approaches you should consider for each.

Remember that recidivist patients who frequent the ED often feel helpless to navigate the complex world of healthcare and usually have legitimate healthcare concerns that must be addressed. Take the time to discuss alternate avenues for obtaining healthcare, ensure that healthcare needs are met during the ED visit when possible, and enlist the assistance of other disciplines such as social services.

Psychiatric emergencies continue to increase in the United States, but the resources needed to manage them have not. Emergency nurses and EDs currently are one of the primary safety nets for these patients. However, long-term interventions are mandatory so that these patients can heal and live healthy lives.

Alterations in mental status complaints are both common and complex in the environment of the ED. Mental status changes may be affected from conditions as varied as abscesses to zygomatic fractures. The knowledge of prognostic assessment findings and their indications as clues to the cause or causes of the changes in mental status can be like a mystery novel. It's important to use a systematic approach to assessment, interventions, diagnostics, and treatment.

In the United States, 4.8 million people live in poverty; 6.4 million people pay more than 50% of their income to sustain a home (National Alliance to End Homelessness, 2015a). Sadly, some people end up homeless, helpless, and dependent on the ED to meet their healthcare needs and, to a certain extent, their emotional and even survival needs. You must remember the final line of the Florence Nightingale pledge, "…and devote myself to the welfare of those committed to my care."

References

American Association of Suicidality. (2015). *U.S.A. suicide: 2013 official final data*. Retrieved from http://www.suicidology.org/Portals/14/docs/Resources/FactSheets/2013datapgsv3.pdf

Boudreaux, E., Niro, K., Sullivan, A., Rosenbaum, C., Allen, M., & Camargo, C. (2011). Current practices for mental health follow-up after psychiatric emergency department/psychiatric emergency service visits: A national survey of academic emergency departments. *General Hospital Psychiatry*, 31, 631–633.

Centers for Disease Control and Prevention (CDC). (2012). *Chartbook: Special feature on emergency care*. Retrieved from http://www.cdc.gov/nchs/data/hus/hus12.pdf

Centers for Disease Control and Prevention (CDC). (2015). *Prescription drug overdose.* Retrieved from http://www.cdc.gov/drugoverdose/data/overdose.html

Centers for Medicare and Medicaid Services (CMS). (2010). *State operations manual.* Retrieved from http://www.cms.gov/Regulations-and-Guidance/Guidance/Manuals/Downloads/som107ap_v_emerg.pdf

Christensen, B. (2014). *Glasgow Coma Scale – Adult.* Retrieved from http://emedicine.medscape.com/article/2172603-overview

Drug Facts. (2011). *Addiction and other mental disorders.* Retrieved from http://www.drugabuse.gov/publications/drugfacts/comorbidity-addiction-other-mental-disorders

Foster, S., LeFauve, C., Kresky-Wolff, M., & Richards, L. D. (2010). Services and supports for individuals with co-occurring disorders and long-term homelessness. *Journal of Behavioral Health Services and Research, 37*(7), 239–251.

Han, J. H., & Wilber, S. T. (2013). Altered mental status in older emergency department patients. *Clinical Geriatric Medicine, 29*(1), 101–136.

Harris, S. N., & Pitman, J. (2014, June 10). Altitude illness: cerebral syndromes. *MedScape.* Retrieved from http://emedicine.medscape.com/article/768478-overview

Heiner, J., & Moore, J. (2014). The combative patient. In J. Marx, R. Hockberger, & R. Walls (Eds.), *Rosen's emergency medicine* (8th ed., pp. 2414–2421). Philadelphia, PA: Elsevier Saunders.

Heslin, K., Elixhauser, A., & Steiner, S. (2015). *Hospitalizations involving mental and substance use disorders among adults.* Rockville, MD: Agency for Healthcare Research and Quality. Retrieved from https://www.hcup-us.ahrq.gov/reports/statbriefs/sb191-Hospitalization-Mental-Substance-Use-Disorders-2012.jsp

Karaca, Z., Wong, H., & Mutter, R. (2013, March). *Statistical brief #152: Characteristics of homeless individuals using inpatient and emergency department services, 2008.* Retrieved from https://www.hcup-us.ahrq.gov/reports/statbriefs/sb152.pdf

LaCalle, E., & Rabin, E. (2010). Frequent users of emergency departments: The myths, the data and the policy implications. *Annals of Emergency Medicine, 56*(1), 42–47.

Montejano, A. (2015). Psychiatric emergencies. In L. Visser, A. Montejano, & V. Grossman (Eds.), *Fast facts for the triage nurse* (pp. 155–159). New York, NY: Springer.

Morrissey, T. (2013). *CDEM self-study modules: The approach to altered mental status.* Retrieved from http://www.cdemcurriculum.org/index.php/ssm/show_ssm/approach_to/ams

National Alliance on Mental Illness (NAMI). (2015). *Facts on children's mental health in America.* Retrieved from http://www.nami.org/Template.cfm?Section=Federal_and_State_Policy_Legislation&template=/ContentManagement/ContentDisplay.cfm&ContentID=43804

National Alliance to End Homelessness. (2015a, April 1). *Executive summary.* Retrieved from http://endhomelessness.org/library/entry/the-state-of-homelessness-in-america-2015

National Alliance to End Homelessness. (2015b, April 1). *Health care.* Retrieved from http://www.endhomelessness.org/pages/mental_physical_health

National Health Care for the Homeless Council. (2013, September). *Integrated care quick guide: Integrating behavioral health & primary care in the HCH setting.* Retrieved from http://www.nhchc.org/wp-content/uploads/2013/10/integrated-care-quick-guide-sept-2013.pdf

Stephens, R., White, S., Cudnik, M., & Patterson, E. (2014). Factors associated with longer length of stay for mental health emergency department patients. *The Journal of Emergency Medicine, 47*(4), 412–419.

Veteran's Health Administration. (n.d.). *Prudent layperson fact sheet.* Retrieved from http://www.pugetsound.va.gov/docs/prudentlaypersonfactsheet.pdf

Weiss, A. J., Wier, L. M., Stocks, C., & Blanchard, J. (2014, June). *Statistical brief #174: Overview of emergency department visits in the United States, 2011.* Retrieved from https://www.hcup-us.ahrq.gov/reports/statbriefs/sb174-Emergency-Department-Visits-Overview.pdf

Wolf, L., Perhats, C., & Delao, A. (2015). U.S. emergency nurses' perceptions of challenges in the management of behavioral health patients in the emergency department: A mixed methods study. *Australasian Emergency Nursing Journal, 18*(3), 138–148. Retrieved from http://dx.doi.org/10.1016/j.aenj.2015.03.004

World Health Organization (WHO). (2015). *Dementia.* Retrieved from http://www.who.int/mediacentre/factsheets/fs362/en/#

THE EMERGENCY NURSE AND THE ABUSED PATIENT

–Gayle Walker-Cillo, MSN/Ed, RN, CEN, CPEN, FAEN; Renee Semonin Holleran, PhD, FNP-BC, CEN, CCRN (emeritus), CFRN, CTRN (retired), FAEN; and Christi Thornhill, MSN, RN, ENP, ACNP-BC, CPNP-AC, CEN, CA-SANE, CP-SANE

You only have to switch on the news every day to realize that humans are frequently not kind to one another. This lack of kindness can be manifested in awful things people say to others; by showing disregard to someone else's feelings, belongings, or person; or by actually causing emotional and physical pain to another person, sometimes to the point of death.

Sadly, the emergency department (ED) is a frequent recipient of people affected by this lack of respect shown from one person to another. You'll feel some degree of pain and empathy for these cases, especially when it's a vulnerable member of our society, like a child or elderly person. Caring for victims of abuse is inherent to working in the ED.

But aside from caring for these individuals, you're also put in the unique role of being a guardian of the abused by recognizing it and offering the abused the assistance needed to escape the situation. This chapter looks at forms of abuse that may cause individuals to seek emergency treatment, symptoms of that abuse, and interventions that should be considered for these victims.

Child Abuse

Child abuse and neglect has always been a serious threat to children of all ages. It has only been in the last 60 years, however, that child abuse has been looked upon as both a social and medical issue that required legislation to protect children (Finn, 2011; Keenan & Leventhal, 2009). The Child Abuse Prevention and Treatment Act (CAPTA) is a key piece of legislation that originated on January 31, 1974, and provides guidance to protect children. It was most recently reauthorized on December 20, 2010 (Child Welfare Information Gateway, 2013).

All 50 states, the District of Columbia, and the U.S. territories have their own definitions of child abuse that are based on standards set forth by the CAPTA Reauthorization Act of 2010. The minimum definition of child abuse as set forth by the CAPTA Reauthorization Act of 2010 states that child abuse is (Child Welfare Information Gateway, 2013):

> "any recent act or failure to act on the part of a parent or caretaker which results in death, serious physical or emotional harm, sexual abuse or exploitation; or an act or failure to act which presents an imminent risk of serious harm"

Most states recognize four major types of child abuse (Black, 2012; Finn, 2011):

- **Neglect:** Failure to provide basic needs:

    - *Physical:* Includes failure to provide food, shelter, clothing, and adequate supervision.

    - *Emotional:* Includes neglecting mental health needs, making a child feel unsafe, belittling or humiliating a child in public, or exposing a child to domestic violence.

    - *Medical:* Includes refusal of healthcare or delay in seeking healthcare, including dental care.

    - *Educational:* Includes failure to enroll a school-age child in school, failure to ensure child attends school, and failure to address special educational needs.

- **Physical:** Infliction of physical injury including shaking, kicking, punching, biting, burning, hitting, beating, or any other mechanism that causes physical harm to a child.

- **Sexual:** Fondling a child's genitalia, penile-vaginal penetration, digital-vaginal penetration, digital-anal penetration, penile-anal penetration, oral copulation, exhibitionism, exploitation through sexual human trafficking or prostitution, exposure to pornographic materials, or the production of pornographic materials.

- **Psychological:** Acts or omissions that have or could cause serious behavioral problems, cognitive problems, emotional problems, or mental disorders.

 Nurses are mandated reporters for suspected child abuse and neglect.

Each state, the District of Columbia, and U.S. territories have laws that mandate certain professionals and institutions to report suspected child abuse to a child protective service (CPS) agency (Child Welfare Information Gateway, 2013).

Prevalence

The prevalence of child abuse is difficult to determine for many reasons, including lack of identification of abuse, lack of evaluation for abuse, and lack of reporting. A review of the literature reveals countless studies regarding risk factors, prevalence, and incidence of child abuse (Laskey, 2011).

According to Laskey (2011), the National Child Abuse and Neglect Data System (NCANDS) and National Incident Studies (NIS) are the two most commonly cited studies. NCANDS data is compiled by child protection agencies across the United States. Individual states construct a database with child-specific records for each report of alleged abuse and neglect that received a CPS response. This provides an enormous database with millions of data points. NCANDS, however, only gathers data on those children who come to the attention of CPS.

The NIS survey is a congressionally mandated research effort that occurs about every 10 years to assess the incidence of child abuse and neglect in the United States (Russell & Cooper, 2011). According to Laskey (2011), the goal of this study is to more accurately identify cases of child abuse and neglect in the community that do not come to the attention of CPS.

In 2013, according to the NCANDS annual report, 3.5 million referrals alleging abuse involving 6.4 million children were reported. Of these cases, 679,000 children were identified as having been abused. Of this 679,000, there were 1,520 fatalities. An estimated 70%

of the fatalities occurred in children under the age of 3 years old (Children's Bureau website, 2015). In 2014, a CDC (Centers for Disease Control and Prevention) study estimated the total lifetime costs associated with only 1 year of confirmed cases of child abuse is approximately $124 billion (CDC, 2014a).

More than 70% of the children who died as a result of child abuse or neglect were 2 years of age or younger (Child Help, n.d.).

It's believed that CPS reports of child abuse underestimate the true occurrence. A non-CPS study conducted in 2013 estimated that one in four children in the United States experience some form of child abuse in their lifetime (Finkelhor, Turner, Ormond, & Hamby, 2013).

"The United States has one of the worst records among industrialized nations—losing on average between four and seven children every day to child abuse and neglect." (Child Help, n.d.)

In 2012, 70% of the children who died from child abuse experienced neglect and 44% experienced physical abuse either exclusively or in combination with another form of abuse (CDC, 2014a). See Table 15.1 for the incidence of different types of child abuse.

Table 15.1 The Rate of Child Abuse by Type

Type of Abuse	Incidence
Neglect	78%
Physical Abuse	18%
Sexual Abuse	9%
Other*	11%

*Emotional, threatened abuse, parent's drug/alcohol abuse, or lack of supervision

Source: CDC, 2014a.

A child may suffer from only one form of abuse but frequently will suffer from more than one form.

Child abuse is not limited to specific socioeconomic classes, nor is it limited to specific religions, and it crosses ethnic lines. Table 15.2 provides an overview of the incidence of child abuse in various ethnic groups.

Table 15.2 Child Abuse Victims by Ethnic Group

Group	Percentage
African American	14.2%
American Indian/Alaska Native	12.4%
Multiracial	10.3%
Pacific Islander	8.7%
Hispanic	8.4%
Non-Hispanic White	8.0%
Asian	1.7%

Source: CDC, 2014b.

According to data obtained from the CDC, parents are the most frequent perpetrators of child abuse. (See Table 15.3.)

Table 15.3 Common Perpetrators of Child Abuse

Type of Perpetrator	Percentage
Parent	80.3%
Relative other than parent	6.1%
Unmarried partners of parent	4.2%

Source: CDC, 2014b.

Figure 15.1 lists common traits of perpetrators.

The Adverse Childhood Experiences (ACE) Study is a collaboration between the CDC and Kaiser Permanente's Health Appraisal Clinic in San Diego and is one of the largest investigations conducted to assess associations between child abuse and long-term health problems (CDC, 2014c). According to the ACE study, children who are abused are at long-term risk for ischemic heart disease, chronic obstructive pulmonary disease, liver disease, and other healthcare-related quality-of-life issues. These include risk for intimate partner violence, substance abuse at an early age, depression and suicide attempts, early initiation of sexual activity, multiple sexually transmitted infections, and unintended pregnancies. (See Figure 15.2.)

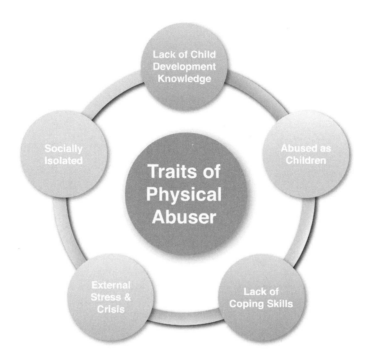

Figure 15.1   Characteristics of perpetrators of abuse.

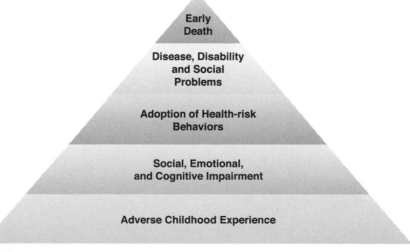

*Adapted from CDC, 2014c.

Figure 15.2   The ACE Pyramid conception.

Assessment

Rarely does a child present to the ED with a complaint of physical abuse or neglect. Caregivers of abused children frequently give false information regarding the child's medical history and mechanism of injury. A nonverbal child is unable to give a history as to what happened. A verbal child may have been threatened not to tell the truth about the circumstances related to the injury. All of these components add to the difficulty in identifying child abuse. For these reasons, it's imperative that you obtain a detailed history and perform a thorough head-to-toe assessment.

 It's essential that a child be completely undressed and gowned for the physical exam. Every aspect of the child's body must be assessed for signs of injury, including the genitalia.

It's imperative that a detailed medical history is obtained and documented. Ask a question, then more follow-up questions until enough details are known to be able to answer the questions: Who? What? When? Where? Why? How? The explanation given by the caregiver(s) should be consistent with the mechanism of injury. The explanation for the injury should remain consistent through repeated interviews and questioning. The child should be developmentally able to perform the action the caregiver attributes to the injury.

 The mechanism of injury must be consistent with the developmental ability of the child.

Conduct interviews in a private setting. Multiple healthcare workers may obtain information, including nurses, physicians, social workers, and pre-hospital care workers. Good communication among healthcare providers is essential to gather all aspects of the history. Also, interview caregivers separately. Verbal children should be interviewed alone when possible. Questions should be open-ended and non-leading. Document answers to questions in quotes when possible. If a language barrier is present, find a professional translator.

When performing an assessment for abuse, the following findings are concerning:

- No explanation or a vague explanation is provided for a significant injury

- An important detail of the explanation changes dramatically

- An explanation that is inconsistent with the pattern, age, or severity of injury/injuries

- An explanation that is inconsistent with the developmental capabilities of the child

- Different witnesses provide markedly different explanations for the injury/injuries

- Failure to disclose past injuries

- Delay in seeking medical care for injuries

 Child abuse is generally a crime of isolation. There usually will be one caregiver who knows what happened and another caregiver or family member who has been told what happened.

 Prior abuse is an indicator of future abuse.

In most incidences of child abuse with physical injuries, children exhibit symptoms as soon as the abuse occurs. It's important to obtain information in the history to develop a timeline to show when the child went from being "normal" to "not normal."

In addition to a detailed medical history, perform a thorough physical exam. The skin is the largest and most commonly injured body organ. Assess for abrasions, contusions, lacerations, cuts, burns, and bites. A study performed by Pierce, Kaczor, Aldridge, O'Flynn, and Lorenz in 2010 identified discriminating differences in abusive-type bruises versus accidental bruises. In this study, they stated that "bruising without clear confirmatory history for any infant who is not cruising and bruising to the torso, ear, or neck of a child 4 years or younger should be considered red flags and should serve as signs of possible physical child abuse" (Pierce et al., 2010, p. 73). *Cruising* is defined as a mobile infant that is crawling. Bruising and other soft tissue injuries are extremely uncommon in children younger than 6 months of age. Any bruising on an infant less than 6 months of age should be considered suspicious for abuse.

 If a child isn't mobile (at the least, crawling), he isn't old enough to bruise.

Bruising

All children get bruises. The age of the child and where the bruise occurs is key in determining if a bruise is accidental or abusive. Children move in a forward motion, so we expect to find bruises on the front plane of their bodies. Accidental bruises typically occur on the forehead and extremities, such as the elbows, knees, and shins. Abusive injuries are more likely if the bruises occur on different planes of the body, are in different stages of healing, have a central distribution, occur on the back, or are patterned-type injuries.

Contusions or bruises, especially to the face and neck, are the most common injury seen in abused children. Bruises to the face are an uncommon finding in non-abused children. Bruising from being slapped occurs in a linear fashion; the flesh between the fingers where tissue is squeezed or compressed bruises, but the area of the face impacted directly by the fingers is less likely to bruise.

Patterned bruises can include bruises inflicted from hand marks, switches or paddles, mini-blind rods, brooms, flyswatters, belts and belt buckles, ropes and cords, shoes, kitchen tools, as well as many other objects. Look for bruises that assume the pattern of a specific object. Pinch marks may appear as crescent-shaped bruises.

You must also be aware of medical and cultural causes of bruising. It's important that a medical condition, such as a clotting disorder, not be confused for physical abuse. The medical and cultural causes for bruising are:

- Idiopathic thrombocytopenia (a clotting disorder)
- Hemophilia
- Ehlers-Danlos syndrome (a genetic disorder)
- Mongolian spots
- Coining
- Cupping
- Leukemia

Bite Marks

Human bite marks may be an indicator of physical abuse and are often seen in sexual abuse but may easily be overlooked. Bite marks are ovoid in shape and may cause bruising, abrasions, or lacerations. According to Kellogg, the distance between human canine teeth is approximately 3 centimeters; therefore, an ovoid bruise that measures 3 centimeters in diameter should raise the index of suspicion for a possible bite wound (Kellogg & Committee on Child Abuse and Neglect, 2005). A bruise of smaller diameter, however, does not rule out a bite inflicted by an adult with a small mouth. If a bite mark is present, swab the area for saliva prior to cleansing to preserve possible genetic evidence.

Burns

According to Knox and Starling (2011), abusive burn injuries most often occur in children under the age of 6 years old, with most studies documenting a mean age between 2 and 4 years old. It's estimated that 20% of burns in children under the age of 3 years old are abusive. Table 15.4 compares characteristics of burns that are non-intentional with those that are intentional.

Table 15.4 Characteristics of Non-intentional Versus Intentional Burns

Non-intentional burns	Intentional burns
Splash or drip pattern	Distinct lines of demarcation
Non-patterned contact burn	Burns may assume the pattern of an object
Treatment is sought immediately	Delays in seeking treatment

Contact burns are caused when a hot object is placed upon the skin. These types of burns typically leave a distinct mark. These objects may include cigarettes, cigarette lighters, irons (household, curling irons, and flat irons), blow dryers, and heaters. Burns to the dorsum of the hand are indicative of abusive injury. Additionally, a child may sustain rope burns to the wrists, ankles, torso, or neck from being bound. With abusive burn injuries, there is frequently a delay in seeking care.

You need to be aware of medical and cultural causes of "burn" injuries as noted in Table 15.5. Education regarding cultural causes of burns and care of certain medical conditions such as diaper rash are an important aspect of care.

Stocking: Intentional burns of the feet and lower legs caused by dipping the child in a hot substance. There are clear lines of demarcation between the burned and unburned skin along the lower legs.

Glove: Intentional burns of the hands and lower arms caused by forcing a child's upper extremities into a hot substance. There are clear lines of demarcation between the burned and unburned skin along the lower arms.

Doughnut: Intentional burns to the buttocks caused by submerging a child into a hot tub of water. The area that is in contact with the tub may have less burning than the tissue around it, giving the appearance of doughnuts.

Table 15.5 Medical and Cultural Causes of "Burn" Injuries

Medical	Cultural
Cellulitis	Moxibustion
Contact dermatitis	Cao Gia (coin rubbing or coining)
Diaper rash	
Drug reaction	
Impetigo	
Staphylococcal scalded skin syndrome	
Phytophotodermatitis	
Psoriasis	

Abusive Head Trauma/Shaken Baby Syndrome

Abusive head trauma is a broad medical term that is inclusive of all mechanisms of injury, including shaking, that causes cerebral, spinal, and cranial injuries. The American Academy of Pediatrics (AAP) recommends using a less mechanistic term, such as *abusive head trauma* versus *shaken baby syndrome* (Christian, Block, & Committee on Child Abuse and Neglect, 2009). The CDC defines abusive head trauma as "an injury to the skull or intracranial contents of an infant or young child (< 5 years of age) due to inflicted blunt impact or violent shaking" (Parks, Annest, Hill, & Karch, 2012, p. 10). Excluded from that definition are unintentional injuries resulting from neglectful supervision and gunshot, stab wounds, and penetrating trauma.

Abusive head trauma occurs when a caregiver violently shakes a child or shakes and slams a child's head against an object, such as a bed, floor, sofa, or wall. There are often no external signs of injury, but there is injury to the brain and often to the eyes in the form of retinal hemorrhages. Abusive head trauma is the leading abusive cause of death in children under 2 years of age (Parks et al., 2012). Most head injuries in infants under 1 year of age are abusive in nature.

 Abusive head trauma, rather than *shaken baby syndrome,* is the medical terminology recommended by the American Academy of Pediatrics.

 Children rarely suffer fatal or life-threatening injuries from simple falls such as off couches, chairs, or even stairs (series of short falls).

Common findings for abusive head trauma are:

- History of minor trauma or perhaps a lack of traumatic history altogether

- History of a short fall (e.g., from a sofa or bed)

- Subarachnoid hemorrhages

- Axonal injuries

- Skull fractures

- Ligamentous injuries to the cervical spine

- Cerebral edema

- Subdural hematomas

- Retinal hemorrhages

- Rib fractures

- Metaphyseal lesions (fractures at the growth plate)

- May have no outward sign of injury

Crying is one of the most common "triggers" for shaking an infant. The Period of PURPLE Crying is a concept developed by Dr. Ronald Barr, MCDM, FRCPC, to explain to parents normal crying patterns that have in the past been called colic. According to Barr, a normal part of every infant's development begins at about 2 weeks of age and continues until about 3 to 4 months of age. During this time, an infant may cry more each week, with a peak at about 2 months of age, and then less by 3 to 5 months of age. Crying can come without reason. The infant may resist soothing. The infant may look like he is in pain when he is in fact not. The crying may last as long as 5 hours a day or more. The infant may cry more in the late afternoon and evening. This preventative program uses positive messages for parents and is based on almost 50 years of early infant development and crying research (Barr, n.d.). Figure 15.3 shows common triggers for abusive head trauma.

For more information on the Period of PURPLE Crying, visit www.purplecrying.info.

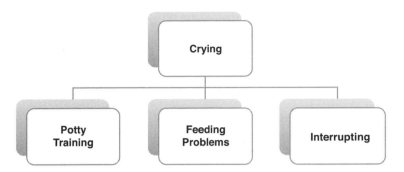

Figure 15.3   Common triggers for abusive head trauma.

Skeletal Injuries

Skeletal injuries are common in children. Because any fracture may be caused by abuse, it's essential that you obtain a thorough description of the mechanism of injury and determine if this is the likely cause of the fracture. Certain fractures have a higher specificity for inflicted injuries than others; see Table 15.6.

Table 15.6   Specificity of Radiologic Findings as Indicators of Abuse

Specifity	Signs of Abuse
High	Classic metaphyseal lesions or corner fractures
	Rib fractures, especially posterior
	Scapular fractures
	Sternal fractures
Moderate	Multiple fractures, especially bilateral
	Fractures in various stages of healing
	Epiphyseal separations
	Vertebral body fractures and subluxations
	Digital fractures
	Complex skull fractures
Low (most common)	Subperiosteal new bone formation
	Clavicle fractures
	Long bone fractures
	Linear skull fractures

Source: Kleinman, 1989, p. 9.

Abdominal Injuries

Abdominal injuries as a result of child abuse are often difficult to identify because they often have a delayed presentation and no outward signs of injury. Children with intentional abdominal injuries may have no history of trauma. Kicking, punching, or stomping can result in injuries to the solid or hollow organs. The lack of bruising is often due to the delay in presentation, as well as lack of bony prominences in the abdominal region. Children may present with subtle symptoms such as abdominal tenderness, rigidity, guarding, and fever as indicators of peritonitis. More severe signs include tachycardia, tachypnea, symptoms of hypovolemic shock, septic shock, and altered mental status.

Abusive abdominal trauma is rarely an isolated finding. Isolated abusive abdominal trauma is more common in older abusive victims.

Medical Child Abuse

The term *medical child abuse (MCA)* replaces what has been referred to as Munchausen syndrome by proxy (MSBP) (Roesler, 2011). Victims of MCA may present with symptoms that are only witnessed by the caregiver, such as excessive vomiting or apneic spells, or with symptoms that are inflicted, such as rashes, fevers, and bacteremia. Identification of MCA is often very difficult and requires the utilization of a multidisciplinary team and thorough review of medical records by a child abuse specialist. You can help identify victims of MCA by being aware of children who are frequently seen in the ED with vague symptoms, symptoms only witnessed by the caregiver, or frequent admissions. Table 15.7 outlines the clinical presentation for medical child abuse.

Medical child abuse—"A child receiving unnecessary and harmful or potentially harmful medical care at the instigation of a caretaker" (Roesler, 2011, p. 586).

Table 15.7 Some Clinical Presentations of Medical Child Abuse

Category	*Medical Findings*
Respiratory	Apnea, choking, cyanosis, sleep apnea, hemoptysis, asthma, respiratory infection, respiratory arrest
Cardiovascular	Bradycardia, cardiopulmonary arrest, hypertension, shock, cardiomyopathy
Gastrointestinal	Abdominal pain, anorexia, bleeding from nasogastric tube/ileostomy, celiac disease, Crohn's disease, diarrhea, feeding problems, vomiting, malabsorption syndromes

Genitourinary	Bacteriuria, hematuria, menorrhagia, nocturia, pyuria, renal failure, urine gravel
Neurologic/musculoskeletal development/psychiatric	Ataxia, cerebral palsy, developmental delay, headache, seizures, syncope, behavioral/personality disorders, hyperactivity, weakness
Skin	Abscesses, burns, eczema, excoriation, rashes
Infectious, immune, allergic	Fevers, immunodeficiency, osteomyelitis, septic arthritis, soft tissue infection, urinary tract infection
Abnormalities of growth, hematologic	Failure to gain weight, weight loss, anemia, bleeding from specific sites, easy bruising, leukopenia
Metabolic, endocrine, fluid and electrolyte	Acidosis, alkalosis, dehydration, diabetes, glycosuria, hyperglycemia, hypernatremia, hyperkalemia, hypoglycemia, hyponatremia, hypokalemia
Other	Abuse (physical, sexual, other), fatigue, foreign body ingestions, hypothermia, pain, poisonings

Source: Rosenberg, 2009.

Interventions

Children who have been abused require frequent assessments and re-assessments of the primary and secondary surveys. In addition to performing appropriate life-saving, medical, and psychosocial treatments, you must ensure the safety of the child, the caregivers, and the healthcare providers. Take these steps to provide care of a child you suspect or know to have experienced abuse:

1. **Conduct a primary assessment with life-saving interventions.**

    Check airway, breathing, circulation, and neurologic status.

2. **Perform a secondary assessment.**

    Conduct a full head-to-toe exam with child fully disrobed.

3. **Obtain a history.**

    This step includes a thorough medical and social history to include details regarding mechanism of injury.

4. **Conduct a skeletal survey.**

    This step is mandatory in cases where you suspect physical abuse in children under the age of 2 years old. There is limited value in children over 5 years old, but you can take it on a case-by-case basis with children 2 to 5 years old.

5. **Take further tests as needed:**

    ■ *Computerized tomography (CT) of the head:* Strongly consider in children less than 6 months old.

    ■ *Labs:* Complete blood count, clotting studies, liver function tests, amylase, lipase, and urinalysis

    ■ *Abdominal CT:* If liver enzymes, amylase, or lipase are elevated or there is a high index of suspicion by the provider for abdominal trauma, proceed with CT of the abdomen without lab.

    ■ *Chest CT:* If evidence of significant chest injury, consider chest CT.

    ■ *Ophthalmology consult:* If a closed head injury is present, consult ophthalmology as soon as possible to determine if retinal hemorrhages are present.

6. **Document all injuries.**

    Take photos at a distance, mid-range, and close up. Each photograph should contain an object to give size perspective and should be labeled with the patient's identifying information.

7. **Make appropriate reports to CPS and law enforcement.**

8. **Consult a child abuse specialist.**

    Talk to the child abuse team if available in your facility, or contact an outside child abuse specialist in your area (if available) for guidance.

9. **Document your findings.**

    Complete and thorough documentation of all findings and history is essential. Utilize direct quotes when documenting any history obtained.

A skeletal survey should be completed on children 2 years old and under if there are concerns of physical abuse. A systematic approach to obtaining a skeletal survey will ensure that all necessary views are obtained (see Table 15.8).

Table 15.8 Components of a Skeletal Survey

Appendicular Skeleton	*Axial Skeleton*
Humeri (anterior/posterior [AP] and lateral)	Thorax (AP and lateral)
Forearms (AP and lateral)	Oblique ribs
Hands (oblique PA)	Pelvis (AP with mid and lower lumbar spine)

Femurs (AP and lateral)	Lumber spine (lateral)
Lower legs (AP and lateral)	Cervical spine (lateral)
Feet (AP)	Skull (frontal and lateral)

Caregivers should be notified if you suspect child abuse that you're obligated by law to report the circumstances to both law enforcement and Child Protective Services. It's important that you maintain open communication with the caregivers. Children who are removed from caregivers will usually grieve and will require support to understand that they are not being punished and that it is not their fault that they cannot go home with their caregivers.

Children who present to the ED with fatal injuries secondary to abuse have usually suffered previous abuse that was not fatal. It's therefore incumbent on the emergency nurse to identify signs of abuse and initiate protection for the child to prevent continuing and escalating maltreatment.

Domestic Human Trafficking

Human trafficking is a global health problem that has been identified in more than 150 countries. Human trafficking includes sex trafficking as well as labor trafficking. Victims of sex trafficking may be found working in massage parlors, brothels, strip clubs, and escort services. Victims of labor trafficking may be found in domestic situations as nannies or maids, or in sweatshop factories, janitorial jobs, construction work sites, and restaurants. These are crimes that are difficult to detect; the idea that trafficking only occurs in the shady corners of city streets and dark motel rooms is a misconception. Human trafficking destroys a person's dignity and strips way an individual's humanity.

Prevalence

In 2009, Shared Hope International conducted undercover investigations utilizing a grant from the U.S. Justice Department and found that many children in America are being used in the commercial sex industry (Shared Hope International, 2012). Human trafficking is an approximately $150 billion per year business globally (International Labour Organization, n.d.). In the United States, human trafficking is an estimated $9.8 billion industry per year (Shared Hope International, 2012).

Sex trafficking—"The recruitment, harboring, transportation, provision, or obtaining of a person for the purpose of a commercial sex act, in which the commercial sex act is induced by force, fraud, or coercion, or in which the person induced to perform such act has not attained 18 years of age" (22, USC § 7102) (National Human Trafficking Resource Center [NHTRC], n.d.).

Labor trafficking—"The recruitment, harboring, transportation, provision, or obtaining of a person for labor or services, through the use of force, fraud, or coercion for the purpose of subjection to involuntary servitude, peonage, debt bondage, or slavery" (22 USC § 7102) (National Human Trafficking Resource Center [NHTRC], n.d.).

Domestic minor sex trafficking (DMST) is commercial sexual exploitation of children within the U.S. An estimated 1.68 million children run away each year. Of those 1.68 million, 100,000 are exploited and trafficked each year. The average age of the victim is 13 years old.

A commercial sex act is any sex act where anything of value is given or received by any person in exchange for the sex act. Things of value may include money, food, drugs, shelter, and car rides.

Trafficking victims tend to have parents who are single (85%) or incarcerated (56%). In addition, they have a history of sexual abuse, truancy, running away, drug abuse, poverty, and living in a foster family (Trafficking in Persons Report, 2012).

Most victims are teenage girls (98%) or come from the LGBTQ (lesbian, gay, bisexual, transgender, questioning) community. They might have tenuous family attachments and have had encounters with Child Protective Services (CPS) (Trafficking in Persons Report, 2012).

Children and teenagers are easily susceptible to the deception and manipulation of traffickers. Common places for traffickers to recruit are places that attract this age group, such as:

Schools	Group foster care homes
Youth sports events	Juvenile detention centers
Social network sites	Shelters
Shopping malls	Bus stops, train stations, or subway systems
Concerts	Courthouses
Gas stations/truck stops	Amusement parks
Tourist attractions	

Human trafficking and DMST is a form of child abuse and must be reported to Child Protective Services (CPS) and law enforcement. (See Figure 15.4.) Cases of abuse or neglect at the hands of a traditional caretaker are usually investigated by CPS. In some regions, these cases may be forwarded to a law enforcement team that specializes in human trafficking cases.

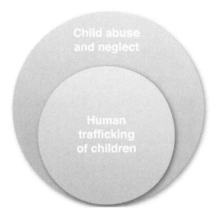

Figure 15.4   Human trafficking is a subset of child abuse and needs to be reported to Child Protective Services.

A *trafficker* is anyone who profits by receiving cash or other benefits in exchange for sex or labor. These criminals are sometimes referred to as *pimps*. Across the U.S., traffickers may be family members, friends, and "boyfriends." Up to 90% of victims are controlled by a trafficker (a pimp or handler). It's estimated that a trafficker may sell 20 to 800 individuals in his lifetime (Shared Hope International, 2012).

Some children are kidnapped and others are sold by their parents, but it's more common for children to be tricked by traffickers (De Chesnay, 2013). Traffickers are masters at manipulation. They will seduce children with the promise of a better life. They will shower them with compliments, gifts, attention, and "love." They will often entice children with offers of careers in things such as modeling, dancing, or music videos. After gaining the trust of the child, the trafficker will begin the process of inducting the child into the world of trafficking.

 The term "trafficking" implies that there is movement from one place to another, but 50% of traffickers operate at a local level (Shared Hope International, 2012).

After promising to care for the child, the trafficker will begin the process of dehumanizing and isolating the child. This often begins with sexual contact and sexual assaults to desensitize the child to commercial sex. The child may be transported to another town. The child may be left with other victims who will provide the child with instructions on how to behave, or the child may witness another child being violently beaten for intimidation. The child may be threatened that his or her family will be harmed. Children may be blackmailed with pornographic images of themselves taken by the trafficker. Often, the child will be branded or tattooed with the name or mark of the trafficker.

 Assess children for tattoos that may be indicators of trafficking. These tattoos are often the name of the trafficker, a diamond, a barcode, or a dollar sign. These tattoos show that the child is property of the trafficker.

Children who have been trafficked remain captive for many reasons. These children have been stripped of their identities, they are geographically isolated, they have been physically abused, and they are fearful or shameful. They may have no home to return to and are told by the trafficker how "bad it is out there." Often they are threatened that either their family members will be harmed or other children in the "stable" will be harmed.

According to De Chesnay (2013), a study of 1,142 female jail detainees found that running away had a dramatic effect on entry into prostitution as an adolescent but had little effect later in life. Being sexually abused as a child nearly doubled the odds of entry into prostitution not only as a child but also throughout their lives.

There are societal, community, relationship, and individual risk factors that increase the chance that a child will become the victim of DMST. Table 15.9 lists some of these risk factors.

Table 15.9 Social-Ecological Risk Factors for Being Trafficked

Societal	Community	Relationship	Individual
Lack of awareness	Social norms	Family conflict, disruption, or dysfunction	History of child abuse, sexual abuse, or neglect
Sexualization of children	Gang involvement	Peer pressure	Homeless, runaway, or "throw away"

Lack of resources	Under-resourced schools, neighborhoods, and communities	Unhealthy relationships	Stigma and discrimination
Glorification of pimp culture	Lack of willingness to address trafficking	Social isolation	History of being systems-involved (juvenile justice, criminal justice, foster care)
	Lives near transient male population		LGBTQ youth
	Adult prostitution		Truancy
	Criminalization of victim		Delinquency
	Tolerance of child-adult sexual relationships		Substance abuse
			Adolescent development
			Disability
			Poverty
			Mental health
			Low self-esteem

Assessment

Although human trafficking is one the fastest growing crimes globally, there is little research or evidence for the best practices for providing healthcare for the trafficking victim. The challenge for healthcare providers is being aware of what trafficking victims look like. Trafficking is a condition of life, not a clinical diagnosis (Crane, 2013).

Victims of trafficking will seek care in EDs, community health centers, primary care pediatrics, family practice clinics, mobile medical vans, public health clinics, school-based clinics, and urgent care centers. You'll see these victims in their interactions but will never know what they endure. You may be the only opportunity the victim has to speak to an outsider. Sadly, most healthcare providers have had no formal training in identification or treatment of a trafficking victim. The following table shows an overview of some of the warning signs and the traits of DMST that you should look for:

Significantly older boyfriend or girlfriend	Accompanying person dominates
Signs of trauma (physical or otherwise)	Patient defers or cowers before accompanying person
Travels with older male (not guardian)	Patient seems withdrawn, frightened, agitated, or anxious
Chronic runaway	Multiple delinquent charges
Homelessness	Special marked tattoo
Substance abuse	Companion attempts to control the interview
Vague or changing story of how injury occurred	Old injuries including bruises, poorly healed fractures, and abrasions
Evidence of self-mutilation, cutting	Poor dentition

Source: De Chesnay & Capponi, 2013 and Shared Hope International, 2012.

The safety of the staff and the patient are of utmost importance when a victim of trafficking is identified. Traffickers consider the victim a commodity to be bought and sold and will do what they feel necessary to protect their property. An underage girl will commonly sell for $400 per hour or more (Shared Hope International, 2012). It's unlikely a trafficker would harm the healthcare provider, but he may decline healthcare for his victim if pressed.

Attempt to interview and examine the patient alone. You might have to take the patient to another area for tests, such as radiographs or lab work. When interviewing the patient, establish a good rapport and speak to the patient respectfully and non-judgmentally. In a busy ED, there is likely little time for a lengthy interview. The following three questions can help you identify a victim of trafficking; only ask them out of the presence of the person accompanying the patient to the ED (De Chesnay & Capponi, 2013):

■ Can you come and go whenever you like?

■ Do you control your own money and ID?

■ Do you have to ask permission of anyone for how you spend your time?

If these questions raise flags about DMST, additional questions should include:

- How old are you?

- Who is the person accompanying you?

- Where do you live? Do you know what city you are in now?

- Are you in school?

- Have you been threatened?

- Have you ever been asked to have sex for money?

Victims of trafficking are at risk for many types of health problems, including physical complaints and psychological complaints. They may present with malnutrition, pregnancy-related issues, substance abuse issues, physical trauma, sexually transmitted infections, or other infectious diseases. These and other complaints common to trafficked victims are summarized in Table 15.10.

Table 15.10 Common Complaints, Signs, and Symptoms in Trafficked Victims*

Physical	Psychological
Sexually transmitted infections	Depression
Pregnancy	Anxiety
Vaginal or rectal trauma	Suicidal ideation
Urinary tract infection	Post-traumatic stress disorder
Soft tissue injuries (lacerations, bruises, bites, burns, strains, and sprains)	Addiction
Poorly healed fractures	Mood swings
Chronic back pain	Terror
Malnutrition, dehydration, exhaustion	Intense shame
Dental issues	Disorientation
Headaches, dizzy spells	Hostility
Abdominal pain	Panic attacks
Rashes, itching, skin sores	Impulse control disorder

*Not all-inclusive.

Source: De Chesnay & Capponi, 2013.

Interventions

Patients you identify as trafficking victims will require frequent assessments and re-assessments of the primary and secondary findings. In addition to performing appropriate life-saving, medical, and psychosocial treatments, you have to ensure the safety of the patient and the safety of other healthcare providers. The steps to treat a victim of trafficking are:

1. **Perform a primary assessment, including any life-saving interventions.**

    This includes airway, breathing, circulation, and neurovascular status.

2. **Perform a secondary assessment.**

    This should be a full head-to-toe exam with the patient fully disrobed, but respectful of privacy. Pay specific attention to weight, signs of injury, and signs of untreated illness.

3. **Obtain a medical history.**

    This includes treatment for any medical conditions or trauma, medications, surgeries, and allergies.

4. **Maintain the safety of the patient and staff by notifying security, law enforcement, and CPS as appropriate.**

5. **Perform an initial screening:**

    - *General testing:* CBC, complete metabolic panel, toxicology screen, pregnancy test

    - *Sexually transmitted infection testing:* Rapid plasma regain (RPR), human immunodeficiency virus (HIV), gonorrhea, chlamydia, hepatitis C

    - *Mental status exam:* Screen for acute psychosis, suicidal ideation, and post-traumatic stress disorder (PTSD)

6. **Consult with a forensic specialist/child abuse specialist.**

    After initial screening, a specialist should perform a forensic exam.

7. **Document all your findings.**

    Be sure the documentation is complete and thorough of all findings and history. Utilize quotes when documenting history.

You can intervene during the initial encounter with a suspected victim of trafficking. Prioritization and treatment of the patient's health problems are the most important part of the care given. It's not uncommon for victims of trafficking to decline help in the healthcare setting.

If the patient is an adult, offer to help, but be respectful of the patient's choice. Call the national trafficking hotline at 1-888-373-7888 for advice. This line is available 24 hours per day, 7 days per week, in more than 200 languages (Polaris, n.d.). The national hotline will often follow up with local authorities. If the patient is a minor, ensure that local law enforcement and CPS are notified and involved.

Find the National Human Trafficking Resource Center at http://traffickingresourcecenter.org/.

Intimate Partner Violence

Intimate partner violence (IPV) is a major public health problem throughout the world. The World Health Organization (WHO, 2013a, 2013b) reports that 35% of women worldwide have experienced physical or sexual intimate partner violence and 38% of women who are murdered are murdered by their intimate partners. Men are also victims of IPV. In fact, men who experience IPV are more likely to face significant threats of deadly violence, with 19% of male IPV involving a weapon (U.S. Department of Justice, 2013). Many times a victim of violence seeks healthcare in the ED rather than going through police. Emergency nurses need to be very adept at identifying at-risk injuries and behaviors, and then use screening tools to promote disclosure in a safe, non-confrontational way.

The U.S. Department of Justice (2013) found that male victims of IPV (39%) were more likely to suffer from serious violent crime from their intimate partner than female victims (34.6%). Women were more likely to be threatened prior to being injured and are more likely to seek medical treatment. Men (27%) were more likely than women (18%) to be attacked with a weapon (Breiding et al., 2014). When attacked with a weapon, men are more likely to be stabbed or shot, yet only 11% of male victims were medically treated for injuries sustained during IPV.

Conditions and Complaints

Many patients reporting to the emergency care environment with symptoms associated with IPV have complaints that are somatic, psychological, or difficult to discern in nature. The stories can have implausible explanations, repeated visits (recidivism) with no clear diagnosis, and obstructive partners present during examinations who further intimidate their victims. Chief complaints commonly associated with IPV are (WHO, 2013a, 2013b):

- Depression

- Anxiety

- Post-traumatic stress disorder

- Sleep disorders

- Suicidality

- Substance or alcohol abuse

- Unexplained chronic pain

- Unexplained chronic gastrointestinal symptoms

- Unexplained chronic genitourinary symptoms

- Chronic reproductive issues, including:

    - Multiple unintended pregnancies/terminations

    - Delay in care during pregnancy

    - Unexplained pelvic pain

    - Frequent vaginal bleeding

    - Frequent sexually transmitted infections (STIs)

- Traumatic injury—unexplained/vague/repeated/implausible

- Unexplained communication deficits, including:

    - Migraines/headaches

    - Cognitive problems

    - Stroke-like symptoms

    - Acute hearing or vision loss

The number and ways in which an IPV victim can present to the ED are plentiful. What is the best way to screen for IPV with so many at-risk complaints and patients passing through an ED daily? Many organizations utilize the "universal screening" of all patients at risk for IPV, while others use a more case-by-case basis. When screening at-risk patients, it's important to remember that not only women are at risk. Male and transgender patients can also be the victims of IPV, and as mentioned earlier, are more likely to experience IPV via weapons. Questions frequently used to screen for IPV include, "Does your partner ever hit, kick, hurt, or threaten you?" or, "Do you feel safe at home?"

Lesbian, Bisexual, Gay, Transgender, and Queer/Questioning Victims

IPV risk is increased with the intersections of class, transgender identity, race, and poverty (National Coalition of Anti-Violence Programs [NCAVP], 2013). The U.S. Department of Justice (2013) reported that 21.5% of men and 35.4% of women historically living with a same-sex partner had experienced physical abuse in their lifetimes, as compared to only opposite-sex cohabitation rates of 7.1% in men and 20.4% in women (Breiding et al., 2014; NCAVP, 2013).

First Line Support

Table 15.11 presents an excellent summary of things that can be done to support the potential or known victim of IPV in the ED.

Table 15.11 Chief Complaints Commonly Associated with Intimate Partner Violence

Women-Centered	LGBTQ
Consultation is done in private	Consultation is done in private
Ensure confidentiality (while informing of limits where mandatory reporting is required)	Ensure confidentiality (while informing of limits where mandatory reporting is required)
Non-judgmental, supportive, and validating approach	Non-judgmental, supportive, and validating approach
Practical care	Practical care
Don't pressure the individual to talk	Do not assume heterosexuality
Be careful with use of interpreters	Avoid labeling a patient as gay, lesbian, bisexual, or transgender unless prompted by the patient
Assist with access to resources	Make informed referrals to community services for LGBTQ patients experiencing IPV
Assist to safety	Verify with the patient the level of disclosure of sexual orientation or gender identity that is appropriate in any referrals to other professionals
Provide social support	
Refer to community-based services	
Immigrant women may feel at risk of being deported and may need additional support	

Source: Ard & Makadon, 2011; NCAVP, 2013; WHO, 2013a, 2013b.

Emerging Issues

Tweens and teens have more access to digital media, and the news has been riddled with stories of tween and teen IPV in the form of technology, sexting, stalking, rape, and sexual assault. These issues can happen after school hours when doctors' offices and therapy offices are closed. Bullied, distraught, and sometimes destroyed teens report to the ED as victims of IPV and partner bullying. These individuals can have all of the same subtle signs and symptoms of IPV as adult victims, including nondescript abdominal pain and headaches, but they can also be acutely suicidal, and each case must be assessed utilizing the nursing process. Remember that 12 to 19 year olds have the highest rates of rape and sexual assault and 18 to 19 year olds have the highest rates of stalking when compared with the population as a whole.

Tween—Generally defined as an individual between the ages of 9 and 13 who is not yet a teenager but is facing issues that may be associated with the teenage developmental stage.

With regard to sexting (Futures Without Violence, 2013):

- Half of those who sent nude photos felt pressured to do so

- 1 in 3 14–24 year olds have sexted

- 15% of 14–24 year olds sent naked videos or photos of themselves

- Teens who have sexted are 4 times more likely to consider suicide

- 15.9% of boys received nude/semi-nude pictures of someone from school

- 1 in 5 teen girls posted nude/semi-nude pictures of themselves

- 1 in 10 young teens (13–16) posted nude/semi-nude pictures of themselves

With regard to bullying/cyberbullying (Futures Without Violence, 2013):

- Bullying is a predictor of sexual harassment

- Men who were bullies when they were children are 3.82 times more likely to commit IPV

- Cyberbullied youth are 3.6 times more likely to experience electronic dating violence

- Cyberbullying youth are more likely to perpetrate dating violence

Sexual Assault

The Centers for Disease Control and Prevention (CDC) includes sexual assault within in its definition of sexual violence (2015). Sexual violence refers to sexual activity that has occurred without consent or when consent was not freely given (Black et al., 2011). Elements of sexual violence are (CDC, 2015):

■ Completed or attempted forced penetration of a victim

■ Completed or attempted alcohol/drug-facilitated penetration of a victim

■ Completed or attempted forced acts in which a victim is made to penetrate a perpetrator or someone else

■ Completed or attempted alcohol/drug-facilitated acts in which a victim is made to penetrate a perpetrator or someone else

■ Non-physically forced penetration that occurs after a person is pressured verbally or through intimidation or misuse of authority to consent or acquiesce

■ Unwanted sexual contact

■ Non-contact unwanted sexual experiences

The latest statistics collected from the CDC indicate that 1 in 5 women and 1 in 69 men have experienced an attempted or completed rape in their lifetime. Rape is defined as penetrating a victim by use of force or through the use of alcohol or drugs to facilitate the assault (Basilek, Smith, Breiding, Black, & Mahendra, 2014). Risk factors that contribute to sexual assault include:

■ Alcohol and drug use

■ Coercive sexual fantasies

■ Exposure to sexually explicit media

■ Hostility toward woman

■ Prior victimization or perpetration

■ Childhood history of physical, sexual, or emotional abuse

■ Poverty

■ General tolerance of sexual violence within a community and social norms that support sexual violence

Also, men who are gay, bisexual, in prison, and who have physical and mental illnesses are at greater risk to be assaulted.

Sexual violence continues to be underreported for numerous reasons, including fear that one may be attacked again, guilt, and shame. However, when the patient reports the incident to law enforcement, there is the presence of a life-threatening or serious injury, or the patient fears disease or possible pregnancy, the patient generally is transported to or voluntarily comes to the ED for care.

The Violence Against Women Act, which was passed in 1994 in the United States and renewed in 2013, helped set up federal funding for the care of sexual assault victims (SAV). Funding from this bill that became available in 2009 provides forensic guidelines for the management of SAV whether the incident was reported or not. This has posed problems for the storage and analysis of evidence because all SAV patients are guaranteed an exam even if they do not pursue legal action. As the news media and victims' advocates have noted, there is evidence that has never been analyzed. Currently, EDs and healthcare facilities do not have mandated regulations, accreditation, or quality management processes to handle evidence and for follow-up with SAV patients (Slaughter, 2014).

The ED has always been the place where most sexual assault patients present, and emergency nurses have always played a significant role in providing primary care, including identifying injuries, collecting or assisting in the collection of evidence, providing emotional support, and coordinating follow-up care. You play a pivotal role in the care of patients who have suffered physically and emotionally from sexual violence (Ledray, 2011).

Because patient advocacy is a major role of the emergency nurse, they have been pioneers in developing care for the victims of violence (Ledray, 2011). From this advocacy role came the sexual assault nurse examiner (SANE). Even though the SANE is a familiar role for many emergency nurses and departments, these resources are not available universally throughout the United States. You still need to be familiar with the triage assessment, forensic evidence collection, and post–emergency department treatment and resources to care for victims of sexual violence.

Assessment and Initial Management of the Victim of Sexual Violence

The initial presentation of the patient who has been sexually assaulted may range from a person who has suffered severe trauma to one who may quietly appear physically unharmed. The patient who has suffered significant trauma needs to be assessed and triaged to the appropriate area for stabilization, and the evaluation for sexual assault will have to be postponed until the patient is not in a life-threatening situation. However, just as with any other potential criminal act, when possible, collect and preserve all evidence.

Many EDs have elected to place patients with a reported assault to a higher triage category even if there is no acute evidence of life-threatening injury. This is done not only to protect patient privacy but also to ensure that the patient and at times even the staff are kept safe. It's important that you and other team members who work with the patient be comfortable and compassionate with victims of sexual violence.

Once the chief complaint of sexual assault has been established and the acuity of the patient has been addressed, an appropriate care provider such as a SANE may be contacted to provide care. Again, not all EDs have access to a SANE, and you may need to provide, or assist with, the exam.

If the patient was not brought in by law enforcement, the patient should be asked whether he or she would like to report the incident. Whether the patient chooses to report the incident should not influence how the patient is treated.

Consent for the exam should be obtained. Components of the consent form should include (Slaughter, 2014):

- A statement that hospitals and healthcare professionals are required to report the incident, but it can be reported without the patient's identification

- Information about victim compensation funds

- An explanation of what the physical exam and evidence-collection procedures entail

- The use of photography to document injury

- Where the information and evidence collected will be sent

- The fact that the patient can withdraw his or her consent at any time

- There should be no charge for the exam whether the incident is reported or not

- The patient should also receive information about what type of treatment may be recommended, such as medication for sexually transmitted diseases or pregnancy prevention

The history and physical exam of the SAV is focused not only on identifying and treating physical injuries but also collecting medicolegal information associated with a sexual assault. This must be done in a competent and compassionate way. Table 15.12 contains a description of medicolegal history that should be noted.

Table 15.12 Medicolegal History Taking

Category	Specifics to Ask
Past Medical History	Allergies
	Medications
	Medical/surgical history
	Vaccination status
Anogenital-urinary History	Last consensual intercourse
	Pregnancy history
	Contraception usage
	Last menstrual period
Event History	Actual/attempted acts
	Date and time of the event
	Location of the event
	Assailant information
	Use of weapons/restraints/threats
	Suspected drug-facilitated sexual assault
	Condom use
	Ejaculation
	Pain or bleeding associated with the acts
	Physical assault
	Potential destruction of evidence

Source: Poarch et al., 2013.

Some physical findings you might find related to sexual assault are (International Association of Forensic Nurses, 2013):

- Assessment of the patient's general appearance, demeanor, cognition, and mental status

- Assessment of clothing and other personal findings

- Assessment of body surface areas for injuries such as abrasions, lacerations, hematoma, gunshot wounds, petechiae

- Identification of normal anatomical variants

- Identification of patterns of injury potentially related to sexual assault

- Physical findings that can be misinterpreted as resulting from sexual assault

Some of the interventions that you can use to confirm physical findings that may indicate sexual assault include (International Association of Forensic Nurses, 2013):

- Positioning of the patient

- Labial separation/traction

- Speculum insertion

- Sterile water irrigation

- Colposcopic visualization

- Anoscopic visualization

- Toluidine blue dye application

- Foley catheter technique

- Wet to dry technique

- Peer review/expert consultation

Care of the Sexual Assault Victim

The care of the sexual assault victim in the ED is multifaceted. It begins with identifying the acuity of the patient and assigning him or her to the appropriate care area. A team approach is required that includes the collection of medicolegal data and providing the emotional support that is needed to get through a difficult and often invasive exam. Sometimes this support is provided by ED personnel or advocates that are specially trained to be a part of the responding team. A medicolegal evidence collection is then performed either by a SANE or a qualified emergency nurse.

Once the exam is completed and the evidence collected, the victim may need care of identified injuries as well as post-assault prophylaxis. Throughout the entire process, documentation must be completed and chain of custody must be maintained and the evidence appropriately stored or given to the correct law enforcement agency. Protocols should be in place in all EDs as to how to collect, document, store, and dispatch the evidence from a sexual assault exam.

Prophylaxis for sexually transmitted diseases as well as pregnancy prophylaxis should be offered and provided. The CDC provides guidelines as to what medications should be provided post sexual assault (CDC, 2010):

- Sexually transmitted diseases:

    - *Ceftriaxone:* 250 mg IM in a single dose or **Cefixime** 400 mg orally in a single dose. Plus **Metronidazole** 2 g orally in a single dose; **Azithromycin** 1 g orally in a single dose or Doxycycline 100 mg orally twice a day for 7 days

    - *Post exposure hepatitis B:* **Vaccination should be after at the time of the exam if the patient has never been vaccinated. Repeat vaccinations should be given 1–2 and 4–6 months after the first dose.**

- **Pregnancy prophylaxis:** Combined oral contraceptives, Progestin only, FDA-approved over-the-counter medications, Copper T IUD insertion

Encourage the patient to have repeated testing, especially if the patient refuses any prophylaxis treatment at the time of the exam. For example, repeated HIV testing is encouraged at 6 weeks, 3 months, and 6 months.

The care of a sexual assault victim requires a team approach. As part of the primary care team, you can provide information to the patient about resources for the long-term consequences of such a violent act. It was a nurse, Ann Burgess, and a social worker, Linda Holmstrom, who first described the impact of sexual assault as *rape trauma syndrome* (Ledray, 2011). The patient is at risk for developing anxiety, depression, fear, guilt, and shame. Suicidal ideation and long-term physical problems such as headaches, abdominal pain, and chronic nausea and vomiting may result and continue to manifest themselves throughout the patient's life. Each patient should be offered an advocate from a rape crisis center during the exam and provided information about assistance when the exam is over. As noted, this violence has both an immediate and long-term effect on the patient, and the emergency nurse and the ED play a key role in the recovery of these patients. Some resources you can provide a patient at discharge are:

- Information about the local rape crisis center, crisis center, social services, alcohol or drug counseling if indicated

- Information about national associations that can offer support such as the Rape Abuse and Incest National Network (www.rainn.org)

- Information about how lab results will be communicated to the patient and referrals for places to follow up such as Planned Parenthood or local health department

- A copy of all the medications that were administered or prescribed during the exam, including potential side effects

Elder Abuse

Elder abuse is the abuse of someone over the age of 60 by someone the victim trusts. This can be a family member, caregiver, or even someone who is responsible for the elder person's wellbeing in a care center. The CDC (2014b) has identified six types of elder abuse. Table 15.13 contains definitions and examples of each of these.

Table 15.13 Definitions of Elder Abuse

Type of Abuse	*Description*
Physical	Injury caused by physical violence such as being pushed, assaulted, or threatened with a weapon, or inappropriately restrained
Sexual abuse or abusive sexual contact	Any sexual contact without consent or understanding by the elder patient; intentional touching including through clothing of the genitals, groin, breasts, mouth, inner thigh, or buttocks
Psychological or emotional	Trauma after exposure to threatening or coercive acts; for example, humiliation, controlling behaviors, social isolation, or destruction of property
Neglect	Failure or refusal of the care provider to provide basic physical, emotional, or social needs of an elder person; for example, inadequate food, shelter, clothing, or healthcare
Abandonment	Willful desertion of an elderly person by the one responsible for his or her care
Financial abuse or exploitation	Unauthorized or improper use of an elder person's resources; examples include forgery, theft of money or possessions, and improper use of guardianship or power of attorney

Source: CDC, 2014b.

The population across the world is aging. It has been projected that by 2050, 20% of the people in the United States will be over 65 years of age. The fastest growing population is over the age of 85 (National Center on Elder Abuse Administration on Aging [NCEA], 2015). Even though the elder population continues to grow, it isn't clear how many people suffer elder abuse. The CDC (2014b) has estimated that about 500,000 elder people per year may suffer abuse. All 50 states in the United States have some sort of Adult Protective Services (APS) available, but not all require mandatory reporting of abuse. Unlike child abuse, there is not a federal law that requires mandatory reporting of elder abuse.

Risk Factors and History for Elder Abuse

Many patients who suffer elder abuse are treated in the ED. You should be aware of the risk factors and indications of potential elder abuse. Risk factors associated with elder abuse include cognitive impairment such as dementia or psychiatric illness, dependency, family conflicts, social isolation, financial distress or lack of understanding of available resources, physical impairments of the elder person (such as loss of vision, hearing, incontinence of bowel and bladder) and stressful family events (Powers, 2014; Tronetti, 2014; Young, 2014). It's important to interview the patient alone when possible and then the caregiver. Some questions to ask are (Anglin & Homeir, 2014; Flaherty & Resnick, 2014):

- Do you live alone?

- Do you feel safe where and with whom you live?

- Are you afraid of anyone?

- Who helps take care of you?

- Who makes your meals?

- Who helps you pay your bills?

- Have you ever fallen?

- Have you ever been slapped, kicked, or punched?

- Have you ever been locked in a room or the house?

- Has anyone ever touched you in a place on your body that made you feel uncomfortable?

- Has anyone ever threatened you?

- How often are you left alone or cannot find help when you need it?

- Has anyone ever taken any money from you without your permission?

- Where does your money come from?

- If someone lives with you, do you support them?

- Has anyone ever disagreed with your wishes for your healthcare?

Indications of Elder Abuse

To evaluate for the signs of abuse, perform a general and focused assessment. As with child abuse, patterns of behaviors and injury may indicate elder abuse. If the patient has suffered a life-threatening significant injury or medical emergency, the initial assessment is directed at identifying and intervening to support the patient's airway, breathing, and circulation. If the patient is agitated, uncooperative, or demonstrating unsafe behaviors, the initial assessment and care is directed at patient and staff safety. However, just as with the sexual assault victim, recognition and documentation of indications of abuse should not be ignored. Table 15.14 contains a summary of possible indicators of elder abuse that may help you screen for elder abuse.

Table 15.14 Questions to Collect Information About Elder Abuse

Category	Description
General Appearance	Clothing: inappropriate dress, dirty clothes, ill-fitting clothes Hygiene: dirty hair, fingernails, uncut nails—look at the patient's feet and toenails Altered nutritional status Skin integrity: open wounds, bruises
Indications of Abuse	Behaviors: fearful of or anxious around the care provider or family Bruises that may indicate abuse such as "grabbing patterns" on arms and legs Lacerations Fractures Frequent falls Frequent emergency department visits
Indications of Sexual Abuse	Sexually transmitted disease, vaginal discharge, bruising of the inner thighs, rectal and vaginal tears Statements from the patient indicating abuse
Neglect	Contractures Dehydration and malnutrition Depression Diarrhea and/or fecal impaction Failure to seek care for a life-threating injury or disease Inappropriate use of medication Poor hygiene, body odor Pressure ulcers Repeated hospital admissions Urine burns Statements from the patient about neglect

continues

Table 15.14 Questions to Collect Information About Elder Abuse (continued)	
Category	Description
Exploitation	Loss of money and property without explanation
	Reports of demand for money or other assets
Abandonment	Evidence that the patient is left alone unsafely
	Evidence that the patient is not being cared for

Care of the Victim of Elder Abuse in the Emergency Department

The care of the patient who is the victim of elder abuse begins with identifying the abuse. Again, if the patient has sustained a life-threating illness or injury, the primary focus is emergent management of these. Yet, you cannot overlook the context in which the event occurred. When possible, pictures and written documentation of indications of abuse or neglect should be a part of the written record of the care provided. Other interventions to consider when caring for the elderly patient who has been abused are summarized in Table 15.15.

Notify appropriate agencies, including law enforcement. All 50 states in the United States and many countries outside of the United States have resources for both immediate and long-term care of patients who have been abused. The National Center on Elder Abuse Administration on Aging (NCEA) has multiple resources to help healthcare providers care for the abused elder patient.

 This website has a map of the United States in which each state's elder-abuse resources are listed: http://ncea.aoa.gov/Stop_Abuse/Get_Help/State/index.aspx.

Table 15.15 Interventions for Victims of Elder Abuse	
Intervention	Description
Immediate Interventions	Assessment and treatment of life-threatening injury or illness
	If the environment is unsafe, get the patient to a safe place, which may require hospital admission or admission to another institution
	Report to appropriate law enforcement or Adult Protective Services directed by state regulations

Suspected Abuse	Development of a follow-up plan to include referral to home health if indicated
	Follow-up plan developed and documented which should include assessment of the patient's cognitive, functional, and medical status. This may also need to include the patient's caregiver if he or she is elderly, too
	Report to APS for further investigation
	Provide support for the caregiver
Resources for Caregivers	Information specific to the patient's illness or injury
	Community resources and eligibility for them
	Home health referral
	Group supports
	Senior centers
	Transportation
	Assistance with personal caregiver needs, medical and mental health

Summary

The emergency department is the place abuse victims come for refuge. With a focused, well-planned approach to treatment, you can positively affect their future and give them a good shot at recovery.

As an emergency nurse, you will encounter victims of abuse, sadly more than you will want to. Sometimes the abuse will be obvious; other times it may require keen assessment skills to detect. Unfortunately, there are many times when abused patients pass through the ED and are treated and released without the underlying abuse being detected.

It's essential that you're educated on signs of abuse and willing to ask potential victims the difficult questions needed to substantiate or rule out abuse. When abuse is detected, you're in a unique position to assist the abused individual to find an escape. Even if the individual chooses not to seek escape, you can provide temporary love and acceptance that the victim of abuse may not have outside the walls of the ED.

References

Anglin, D., & Homeir, D. (2014). Elder abuse and neglect. In J. Marx, R. Hockberger, & R. Walls (Eds.), *Rosen's emergency medicine* (8th ed., pp. 885–892). Philadelphia, PA: Saunders.

Ard, K. L., & Makadon, H. L. (2011). Addressing intimate partner violence in lesbian, gay, bisexual, and transgender patients. *Journal of General Internal Medicine, 26*(8), 930–933.

Barr, M. (n.d.). *What is the Period of PURPLE Crying?* Retrieved from http://www.purplecrying.info/what-is-the-period-of-purple-crying.php

Basilek, K., Smith, S., Breiding, M., Black, M., & Mahendra, R. (2014). *Sexual violence surveillance: Uniform definitions and recommended data elements.* Retrieved from http://www.cdc.gov/violenceprevention/pdf/sv_surveillance_definitionsl-2009-a.pdf

Black, A. (2012). Child maltreatment. In *Emergency nursing pediatric course: Provider manual* (4th ed., pp. 343–356). Des Plaines, IL: Emergency Nurses Association.

Black, M., Breiding, M., Smith, S., Walters, M., Merrick, M., Chen, J., & Stevens, M. (2011). *The national intimate partner and sexual violence survey: 2010 summary report.* Retrieved from http://www.cdc.gov/violenceprevention/pdf/nisvs_report2010-a.pdf

Breiding, M. J., Smith, S. G., Basile, K. C., Walters, M. I., Chen, J., & Merrick, M. (2014). Prevalence and characteristics of sexual violence, stalking, and intimate partner violence survey, United States, 2011. *Centers for Disease Control and Prevention: Morbidity and Mortality Weekly Report, 63*(8).

Centers for Disease Control and Prevention (CDC). (2010). *2010 STD treatment guidelines.* Retrieved from http://www.cdc.gov/std/treatment/2010/sexual-assault.htm

Centers for Disease Control and Prevention (CDC). (2014a). *Child maltreatment.* Retrieved from www.cdc.gov/violenceprevention/pdf/childmaltreatment-facts-at-a-glance.pdf

Centers for Disease Control and Prevention (CDC). (2014b). *Elder abuse.* Retrieved from http://www.cdc.gov/violenceprevention/elderabuse/index.html

Centers for Disease Control and Prevention (CDC). (2014c, May 13). *Injury prevention and control: Division of violence prevention.* Retrieved from http://www.cdc.gov/violenceprevention/acestudy/

Centers for Disease Control and Prevention (CDC). (2015, February 10). *Sexual violence: Definitions.* Retrieved from http://www.cdc.gov/violenceprevention/sexualviolence/definitions.html

Child Help. (n.d.). *Child abuse statistics and facts.* Retrieved from https://www.childhelp.org/child-abuse-statistics/

Child Welfare Information Gateway. (2013, November). *Mandatory reporters of child abuse and neglect.* Retrieved from https://childwelfare.gov/pubPDFs/manda.pdf#page=1&view=Professionals Required to Report

Child Welfare Information Gateway. (2013). *Definitions of Child Abuse and Neglect in Federal Law.* Retrieved from https://www.childwelfare.gov/topics/can/defining/federal/

Christian, C. W., Block, R., & Committee on Child Abuse and Neglect (2009). *Abusive head trauma in infants and children* [Policy statement]. Elk Grove, IL: American Academy of Pediatrics.

Crane, P. (2013). A human trafficking toolkit for nursing intervention. In M. De Chesnay (Ed.), *Sex trafficking: A clinical guide for nurses* (pp. 167–181). New York, NY: Springer.

De Chesnay, M. (2013). Sex trafficking as a new pandemic. In M. De Chesnay (Ed.), *Sex trafficking: A clinical guide for nurses* (pp. 3–21). New York, NY: Springer.

De Chesnay, M., & Capponi, N. (2013). Policy and procedures for emergency departments and community-based clinics. In M. De Chesnay (Ed.), *Sex trafficking: A clinical guide for nurses* (pp. 295–304). New York, NY: Springer.

Finkelhor, D., Turner, H. A., Ormond, R., & Hamby, S. L. (2013). Violence, crime, and abuse exposure in a national sample of children and youth: An update. *JAMA Pediatrics, 167,* 614–621.

Finn, C. (2011). Child maltreatment: Forensic biomarkers. In V. A. Lynch & J. B. Duval (Eds.), *Forensic nursing* (2nd ed., pp. 341–354). St. Louis, MO: Elsevier Mosby.

Flaherty, E., & Resnick, B. (Eds.). (2014). *Geriatric nursing review syllabus: A core curriculum for advanced practice geriatric nursing* (4th ed., pp. 97–101). New York, NY: American Geriatric Society.

Futures Without Violence. (2013a, February 26). *Emergency issues facing tweens and teens.* Retrieved from http://startstrong.futureswithoutviolence.org/wp-content/uploads/emerging-issues-facing-tweens-and-teens.pdf

International Association of Forensic Nurses (2013). *Sexual Assault Nurse Examiner (SANE) education guidelines.* Elkridge, MD: International Association of Forensic Nurses.

International Labour Organization. (n.d.). *Forced labour, human trafficking and slavery*. Retrieved from http://www.ilo.org/global/topics/forced-labour/lang--en/index.htm

Keenan, H. T., & Leventhal, J. M. (2009). The evolution of child abuse research. In R. M. Reece & C. W. Christian (Eds.), *Child abuse: Medical diagnosis and management* (3rd ed., pp. 1–18). Elk Grove, IL: American Academy of Pediatrics.

Kellogg, N., & Committee on Child Abuse and Neglect (2005). Oral and dental aspects of child abuse and neglect. *Pediatrics, 116*, 1565–1568.

Kleinman, P. K. (1989). *Diagnostic imaging of child abuse* (2nd ed.). Chicago, IL: Mosby.

Knox, B. P., & Starling, S. L. (2011). Abusive burns. In C. Jenny (Ed.), *Child abuse and neglect: Diagnosis, treatment, and evidence* (pp. 222–238). St. Louis, MO: Elsevier Saunders.

Laskey, A. L. (2011). Epidemiological issues in child maltreatment research, surveillance, and reporting. In C. Jenny (Ed.), *Child abuse and neglect: Diagnosis, treatment and evidence* (pp. 3–9). St. Louis, MO: Elsevier Saunders.

Ledray, L. (2011). Sexual violence: Victims and offenders. In V. Lynch & J. Barber Duval (Eds.) *Forensic nursing science* (2nd ed., pp. 380–396). St. Louis, MO: Elsevier Mosby.

National Center on Elder Abuse Administration on Aging (NCEA). (2015). *Elder abuse*. Retrieved from http://www.ncea.aoa.gov/Library/Data/index.aspx#problem

National Coalition of Anti-Violence Programs (NCAVP). (2013). *Lesbian, gay, bisexual, transgender, queer & HIV-affected intimate partner violence*. Retrieved from http://www.avp.org/storage/documents/ncavp_2012_ipvreport.final.pdf

National Human Trafficking Resource Center (NHTRC). (n.d.). *Human trafficking*. Retrieved from http://traffickingresourcecenter.org/type-trafficking/human-trafficking

Parks, S. E., Annest, J. L., Hill, H. A., & Karch, D. L. (2012). *Pediatric abusive head trauma: Recommendations for public health surveillance and research*. Retrieved from www.cdc.gov/ViolencePrevention/pdf/PedHeadTrauma-a.pdf

Pierce, M. C., Kaczor, K., Aldridge, S., O'Flynn, J., & Lorenz, D. J. (2010). Bruising characteristics discriminating physical child abuse from accidental trauma. *Pediatrics, 125*, 67–74.

Poarch, C. J., Wieczorek, K., Pierce-Weeks, J., Allen, E., Carson, J., Collette, R., ... Maguire, K. (2013). *Sexual assault nurse examiner education guidelines*. Elkridge, MD: International Association of Forensic Nurses.

Polaris. (n.d.). *NHTRC and BeFree hotlines*. Retrieved from http://www.polarisproject.org/what-we-do/national-human-trafficking-hotline/the-nhtrc/overview

Powers, J. (2014). Common presentations of elder abuse in health care settings. *Clinics of Geriatric Medicine, 30*, 729–741.

Roesler, T. A. (2011). Medical child abuse. In C. Jenny (Ed.), *Child abuse and neglect: Diagnosis, treatment, and evidence* (pp. 586–591). St. Louis, MO: Elsevier Saunders.

Rosenberg, D. A. (2009). Munchausen syndrome by proxy. In R. M. Reece & C. W. Christian (Eds.), *Child abuse: Medical diagnosis and management* (3rd ed., pp. 513–547). Elk Grove, IL: American Academy of Pediatrics.

Russell, J., & Cooper, T. (2011). *The NIS-4: What it all means (and doesn't mean)*. Reno, NV: National Council of Juvenile and Family Court Judges.

Shared Hope International. (2012). *Domestic Minor Sex Trafficking in the US*. Vancouver WA: Shared Hope International.

Slaughter, L. (2014). Sexual assault. In J. Marx, R. Hockberger, & R. Walls (Eds.), *Rosen's emergency medicine* (8th ed., pp. 855–871). Philadelphia, PA: Saunders.

Tronetti, P. (2014). Evaluating abuse in the patient with dementia. *Clinics of Geriatric Medicine, 30*, 825–838.

U.S. Department of Justice. (2013, November). *Intimate partner violence: Attributes of victimization, 1993–2011*. Washington, DC: Bureau of Justice Statistics.

World Health Organization (WHO). (2013a). *Global and regional estimates of violence against women: Prevalence of health effects of intimate partner violence and non-partner sexual violence*. Retrieved from http://www.who.int/reproductivehealth/publications/violence/9789241564625/en/

World Health Organization (WHO). (2013b). *Responding to intimate partner violence and sexual violence against women: WHO clinical and policy guidelines*. Retrieved from http://www.who.int/reproductivehealth/publications/violence/9789241548595/en/

Young, L. (2014). Elder physical abuse. *Clinics of Geriatric Medicine, 30*, 761–768.

THE EMERGENCY NURSE CARING FOR DIVERSE CULTURES AND ETHNICITIES

–Patricia L. Clutter, MEd, RN, CEN, FAEN

Emergency nurses have the potential to care for individuals from any culture or ethnic background. The world today has become so small, and multiple groups of people form many of the present-day communities. This chapter gives an overview of important cultural concepts that you may come across during your practice as an emergency nurse.

When patients from other backgrounds come to the emergency department (ED) for care, many concerns go through their minds. First, it's an emergency department! This is where people take your clothes off and stick you with sharp objects! Combine that with the fact that the person is from another culture and that the usual comfort zone of "home" is completely absent. Try to put yourself in the same position and imagine being in a foreign country, all alone and frightened when a crisis occurs. It may be a major trauma or it may be as minor as a splinter. Fear of the unknown and language barriers are constant reminders that this experience is far different from other medical issues they may have dealt with in comfortable settings at home or within their own countries.

Whose Viewpoint?

Everyone, including emergency nurses, have a certain way of viewing particular situations. Two transcultural linguistic terms can help you to understand this facet (Andrews & Boyle, 2011; Purnell, 2012):

- *Emic* is the viewpoint from the person experiencing the situation—the insider's view. It's your personal view and is a compilation of your knowledge gained from traditional, local knowledge that has been passed on to you, which is part of *enculturation*—how you were raised.

- *Etic* is the outsider's view. It encompasses knowledge that is gained through an educational process such as classes or reading. This is the healthcare professional's viewpoint.

These viewpoints can challenge each other or come under suspicion from the other's viewpoint. Consider a person who treats their child at home with *coining,* a common practice in Hispanic and Asian cultures that involves the use of a coin rubbed briskly over oiled bony prominences such as the anterior and posterior chest. This leaves ecchymotic areas that can mimic child abuse. The emic view is one of "caring for my child." The etic view is "You are hurting your child."

Major Points to Consider

You must always remember that there are often other ways to do things. These may be very different from what you're used to, and sometimes you may not fully agree with the process; however, it has validity to the individuals involved, and you must understand the behavior within its cultural context, a process known as *cultural relativism. Ethnocentrism* is the opposite and means that people believe their way is the only right way.

It's always in the best interests of your patients to attempt to understand the differences between these two concepts (Andrews & Boyle, 2011; Purnell, 2012). The following sections discuss a few viewpoints you need to consider while practicing.

Stereotypes

We've all been raised with old wives tales, folk remedies, and superstitions.

The first and foremost consideration must be given to the fact that as a healthcare professional, you must be careful not to stereotype individuals just because they belong to a particular ethnic group or come from a specific cultural base. When studying the phenomena of cultural differences, we look at folk rituals that people perform to treat illnesses; however, it's wrong to assume that all individuals from that population practice or believe in all of the studied traditions. You have to examine these commonly held beliefs but not fall into stereotyping. You can intellectually process generalizations about a culture, but labeling an individual and making assumptions is incorrect. You might think, "This person is from an Italian background. I wonder if they do indeed come from a large and all-inclusive family base." A stereotype would be the belief that all Italian families are large and extended (Galanti, 2008).

Always practice with the idea that it's to your advantage to understand long-held beliefs or to have an appreciation for their history and background in order to care for people, but always look at the person as a unique human being who is his own person. If you discuss and find out that the patient does practice certain cultural customs, then it's to your benefit to understand the cultural context under which these practices have occurred.

No matter what your cultural or ethnic foundation is based upon, you also have medically related idiosyncrasies within your personal norms. Whether an individual believes in the "evil eye" or that tying a white cotton sock infiltrated with aromatic rubs around the neck will help cure the common cold, everyone has culturally ingrained medical beliefs.

 Take a moment and consider what your own personal health idiosyncrasies might be. What did your parents or grandparents teach you?

In the United States, the number 13 is considered to be unlucky. Many EDs may actually skip room 13 and go from 12 to 14! In some Asian populations, the number 4 is associated with bad luck because it sounds very similar to the same word for death, while the number 8 is considered good fortune (Galanti, 2008).

When individuals have emigrated from their home country to the United States, the acculturation process is different for each of them. Many things affect how fast this process occurs. Some of these factors are (Andrews & Boyle, 2011; Galanti, 2008; Purnell, 2012):

- How long has the individual been in the U.S.?

- Does the individual have older individuals in the home who've immigrated with them? Or perhaps the older individuals came at a different time?

- How old was the individual when he or she entered the U.S.?

- What type of community did the individual come from?

- What type of community are they presently living in? (Is it an integrated or segregated community?)

- Is their original background urban or rural?

- What was their social or economic class in their home country? What is it now?

Each person is unique and processes information and languages in their own way and time. As the professional in the picture, you must help patients during their times of crisis and fear.

 Every person acculturates at his or her own speed!

Be especially careful with labeling. Not all Asian people are from one group; they can be from China, Japan, the Philippines, or Indonesia, for example. To assume that each of these groups of people has the same health practices, familial upbringing, or considerations is stereotypical. A person who comes from Singapore may be very distressed to be grouped together with those from China. These are distinct locales, and you can offend people by lumping them all together (Andrews & Boyle, 2011; Purnell 2012).

By the same token, not all people who speak Spanish are from a particular location. Some Spanish speakers are from Mexico, but others are from Spain or South America. Nor are all individuals who appear to be from the Middle East alike. There are multiple countries in the Middle East, and each has a well-defined cultural background. An individual from Jamaica came from a different world than an African American raised in the United States.

 For an interesting and thought-provoking look at cultural differences, consider reading the *Clan of the Cave Bear* novels by Jean Auel. In this series, two distinctive and well-defined tribes of people live physically close to each other, traversing the same terrain, but are very distinct in their beliefs of an omnipotent being, the manner in which they deal with the separate genders within the tribe, and their local medicinal rituals (Auel, 1983–1990).

Values

Just as people are dissimilar in their health beliefs, values can also be a point of dissension. For instance, in the United States, independence is highly valued. In some other cultures, independence is not highly valued, and the accepted norm is for children to remain in their parents' homes until they marry and begin their own families. These individuals then, after immigration to the United States, may find themselves at odds with their neighbors or when they are dealing with others in professional relationships. In a similar example, Americans value privacy, and many routines and policies are built around these Western-held beliefs. However, in some groups, privacy issues are not part of the family unit, and they may have large extended families that are important to them. They may have many visitors, and it is important to their recovery to have these people around them (Andrews & Boyle, 2011; Galanti, 2008; Purnell, 2012).

Another example involves generational differences; the mature population may prefer the use of the titles "Mr." and "Mrs." when being addressed. They may also have differing views of privacy than their younger counterparts. If appropriate titles are not used or privacy is not maintained, they may be left at odds with the younger generation.

Other distinct groups may not fit the traditional mold of ethnicities, such as the lesbian, gay, bisexual, transsexual, and queer/questioning community (LGBTQ). They often have differences in values and should be considered at high risk for prejudice and discrimination. Many organizations have still not addressed issues of consent, withdrawal of care, or visitation for the LGBTQ communities. Think of a place where you could be married but not visit your husband or wife in the critical care unit.

Prejudice and Discrimination

Prejudice and discrimination is another aspect that can play a role in how patients interact with emergency staff and in how you, as the healthcare professional, may deal with them. Even if you feel you have no bias or prejudice, you might actually harbor some aspect of this, however minor. The other side of this can play out in how patients may feel about the care they are about to receive based on long-held beliefs and stories that may have been passed down through the generations.

Consider an older African American who remembers when the federal government in Tuskegee, Alabama, told a group of Black men they were going to take care of those afflicted with syphilis. Researchers did not tell them that the pills they were receiving were placebos and that they were part of a research study (Galanti, 2008). This ethical debacle changed the way we do ethical research in the United States. Although more than 40 years have passed since this event, this injustice still resonates with some communities, adds to the distrust and antagonism toward medical providers, and provides insight into why some feel they are treated differently by the healthcare system.

 The movie *Miss Evers' Boys* depicts the story of those who lived through the syphilis studies in Tuskegee, Alabama, and can help you understand what happened.

 Be aware of prejudice and discrimination that may affect both you and the patient.

Alternative Treatments

Some groups need the satisfaction of having care provided by both a westernized healthcare team and their own healthcare practitioner. This can often enhance their recovery and should not be seen as a hindrance to care. In the country of Bolivia, it's not unheard of to have two offices in a medical clinic—one for the physician and one for the Kallawaya. These Kallawaya are the indigenous "medicine men" and are held in reverence. The sick individual may see either or both of these healthcare practitioners.

Native Americans also have their own shamans or medical providers and commonly utilize both. In some federally funded Native American hospitals, special rooms are available in which rituals can be carried out including the burning of sage, which is a purifying agent. The combination of using a preferred medical provider along with a westernized hospital can play a crucial role in the healing process (Andrews & Boyle, 2011; Purnell, 2012). But remember that these practices can sometimes come into conflict with one another, and you should always ask what things have been done to treat the illness prior to arrival in the ED.

Do not create bad feelings when people share with you that they have consulted their own "medicine man." Be confident in your own provision of care and understand that this is of very great value to them. As long as the rituals are not hurting or interfering with care the patient needs, allow them this level of control in their lives. Some other names that you might hear are curandero or yerbero for Hispanic populations, Braucher for the Amish, and Granny Woman in the mountains of Appalachia (Purnell, 2012).

 Allow your patients to appreciate care from medical people of their own culture and that of the westernized world!

Cultural Phenomena

You need to take into consideration these six cultural phenomena regarding cultural understandings. The following sections offer a brief explanation of each.

Communication

Communication is both verbal and nonverbal. When patients have language barriers, it's imperative to obtain some manner of communication with them. It's not acceptable for a child or other relative to translate for the patient. This can become problematic, and lawsuits have been filed and won by the patient when appropriate translators were not obtained or at least offered to them. Some relatives might feel uncomfortable talking about certain body parts or issues and the translation may be incorrect, which can lead to invalid assessments or treatment plans. Becoming comfortable with the mode of translators that your institution utilizes is imperative. If the patient refuses or declines to use a translation service, be sure to have the patient sign a consent form confirming the agreement.

When using a translator, be aware that some hints might make it easier for both parties. When you're not fluent but think you can understand the patient's or family member's language, problems can occur. In one case, an 18-year-old patient of Hispanic origin said the word *intoxicado* and was treated for a day and a half as a drug overdose until someone determined that this word can also mean "nauseated," and he was then correctly treated for a brain aneurysm (Weise, 2006). Here are a few tips on how to use a translator in the ED (Andrews & Boyle, 2011; Bridges, 2006; Galanti, 2008; Purnell, 2012):

- Determine which language is needed.

- Be aware of rivalries. Just because people speak the same language does not mean they are friendly toward each other in their home countries.

- It is usually good if the genders of the patient and the translator match.

- Ideally, the translator and the patient should be similar in age.

- Remember that you are not aware of what they are saying. Talk to the translator and ask the person to translate verbatim as much as possible.

- Be sure to utilize the correct level of translator. Sign language translators must have passed particular classes to be a medical translator. This is imperative with this group.

- The patient and translator may request some time alone.

- Social class disparities can make a difference. The translator may not translate everything if the translator thinks the patient is saying something "silly" or that the patient is being superstitious. The translator may be condescending, and often the patient or family members would rather attempt their own understanding of your language than deal with this type of embarrassment from someone who speaks their own language.

One trap people may fall into when speaking to someone with a language barrier is to speak louder. Speaking louder and slower does not fix the situation. The patient still doesn't understand you and now may think you are angry. Instead, use short sentences, forgo medical jargon, and keep thoughts and phrases simple. Watch for nonverbal interactions, and remember that small nuances in words can make a huge difference in the translated meanings, as well as the fact that some words in one language have a different meaning in another language.

Nonverbal communication is another significant issue. For some, such as Native Americans, the use of silence is embedded in their culture. Also eye contact, which for the average American is a key factor in psychological evaluations, may not be the norm for the patient for whom you are providing care. A Vietnamese individual might not maintain eye contact with a superior. Touching may also be a cultural consideration. An Orthodox Jewish or Muslim man may not touch a female healthcare provider, and even a simple handshake may be avoided. Gestures can also be problematic. The accepted circle created by touching the thumb and index finger together (often utilized to motion "OK" in the United States) may be considered rude and vulgar in some cultures. It would be inappropriate to signal to a member of the Vietnamese population with an upturned index finger moving back and forth as if to say "come here." And the long cherished "V" for victory sign sometimes used by Americans can be construed as vulgar in South Africa (Andrews & Boyle, 2011; Galanti, 2008; Purnell, 2012).

Also, sometimes in interpersonal interactions with patients, you might invade a patient's "intimate distance." Seek permission first before performing treatments or diagnostic tests that involve sensitive areas.

Social Organization

Social organization has to do with family structures. What is normal for one family unit may be different for another. This can become distressful for patients if you limit family members from rooms. Table 16.1 describes some common family units encountered in the ED.

Table 16.1 Types of Families

Family Unit	Description
Traditional Nuclear Family	Contains two distinct generations (can be biological or adopted children)
Nuclear Dyad Family	One generation is present (may occur after the death of an only child)
Extended Family	Includes many generations
Skip Generation Family	The middle generation is absent, such as when a grandparent is raising a grandchild or grandchildren
Alternative Family	Any family that does not fit the traditional definition of a family; examples include families with same-sex parents, or families with a single parent or unmarried parents
Single Parent Family	Includes two generations, but one parent is raising a child or children
Reconstituted/Blended Family	Two families have combined to become one

Source: Andrews & Boyle, 2011; Purnell, 2012.

Family structure also deals with whether a family is matriarchal or patriarchal. Often there are individuals who are very important decision-makers in the family. Be sure to ask to determine whether anyone else needs to be present to make decisions (Andrews & Boyle, 2011; Purnell, 2012).

Matriarchal—The woman plays the dominant role in the family.

Patriarchal—The male plays the dominant role in the family.

Religion

Obviously, religion plays a central role in many people's lives. There are multiple religions within the boundaries of the United States, and they run along a continuum from very liberal to very conservative. In the Jewish religion, the sect known as the Hasidic Jews are very strict in their beliefs, while other Jewish individuals may practice their religion in a less rigorous manner while still maintaining their Jewish identity. Every religion has different variations (from moderate to very strict) of beliefs, cultures, norms, roles, and behaviors (Galanti, 2008).

Time Orientation

Most people in the United States work from a *future time* orientation. This means that they consider future ramifications for activities that are presently being performed. They consider health and wellness activities to be essential and can see the importance of following up with appointments, having routine examinations (such as mammograms) and checkups. Those with *present time* orientation are concerned with what is going on now. Whatever is happening now is the most important thing. Therefore, wellness issues, such as caring for oneself now in order to avoid issues later, is not as important. They also may tend to be late for appointments because something else was occurring in their lives at the scheduled time.

Present-oriented patients may not seek preventative care or they may not even seek care for minor ailments because they do not see this as pertinent to their current situation. But when the condition becomes emergent, they seek care in the ED, and the condition may have deteriorated significantly by this time. Rigid hospital schedules do not fit well for these patients and family members. As a healthcare provider, you must be flexible and adaptable to meet the needs of your patients. It can be difficult when you're attempting to provide care or when you're working with another individual who is from a different time orientation than yourself. Past time orientation is also utilized by some cultures, while other groups may integrate the past, present, and future time orientation (Andrews & Boyle, 2011; Galanti, 2008; Purnell, 2012).

Environmental Control

Environmental control has to do with healthcare practices that are common for each person. These may deal with folk illnesses and remedies. One of the problems with folk illnesses is that when people diagnose members of their group with a folk illness and then treat it accordingly, they may not seek care from their physician or ED as early as they should. Another name for folk illnesses is *culture bound syndromes* or *cultural concepts of distress* (Correll, 2014).

Types of cultural practices that you may encounter in the ED are:

- **Efficacious:** Can be beneficial to the patient. An example is the hot/cold theory for someone who has gastroenteritis.

- **Neutral:** Has no effect, either beneficial or dysfunctional. An example is burying the placenta after birth.

- **Dysfunctional:** Harmful practices. An example is turning a baby upside down and shaking him or her to treat a "fallen fontanelle."

■ **Uncertain:** No determination has been made as to whether it is efficacious, neutral, or dysfunctional. An example is taping a quarter on the baby's umbilical area after the cord has fallen off.

 Folk illness—Health beliefs and practices shaped by the cultural conventions of a specific group of people.

Biological Variations

Many ethnicities have biological variations common to that ethnicity. It's important, though, to know that not everyone of that ethnicity is necessarily affected by the common biological variation. Examples of common biological variations include Inuit children being born with teeth, precordial T wave inversion for African-American males, Tay-Sachs disease in the Jewish population, increased risk of hypertension in the African-American population, and a predisposition for diabetes among Native Americans (Andrews & Boyle, 2011; Galanti, 2008; Purnell, 2012). It's essential to have an understanding of some of these variant changes that may be normal for populations that you see.

Summary

It would take a more lengthy discussion to truly delve into the fine points of cultural diversity. There are many books and classes available to help you understand how best to care for those who may be different from yourself. There are many mandates within society on how to understand each other, and while it is good that these directives exist, the most compelling reason to learn about others is because you want to care for patients with the utmost understanding. It is, after all, for them that you come to work each day.

The most important point in caring for individuals of different ethnic or religious backgrounds is respect. When patients are cared for with respect for their particular differences, both sides win. When confronted with someone who is different from you, ask questions. There is no way to remember every aspect of divergent practices among all peoples. It is great to learn and to continue to read and study the differences so that we can provide the best care possible, but simply show respect for those who were raised with beliefs and practices that are uncommon or dissimilar to your own.

References

Andrews, M., & Boyle, J. (2011). *Transcultural concepts in nursing care* (6th ed.). Philadelphia, PA: Lippincott, Williams and Wilkins.

Auel, J. (1983–1990). *The clan of the cave bear* [series]. New York, NY: Bantam Books.

Bridges, A. (2006, April 12). Health forum tackles race issues. *Springfield News-Leader,* p1B.

Correll, C. U., & Stetka, B. S. (2014, July). 20 more rare and unusual psychiatric syndromes. *Medscape Multispecialty.* Retrieved from http://www.medscape.com/features/slideshow/culture-synd

Galanti, G. (2008). *Caring for patients from different cultures* (4th ed.). Philadelphia, PA: University of Pennsylvania Press.

Purnell, L. D. (2012). *Transcultural health care: A culturally competent approach* (4th ed.). Philadelphia, PA: F. A. Davis Company.

Weise, E. (2006, July 20). Language barriers hinder hospitals. *USA Today, Springfield News-Leader*, p7A.

INDEX

M

Z

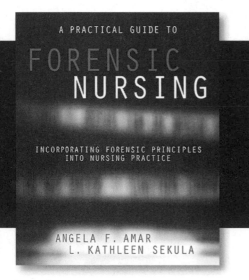
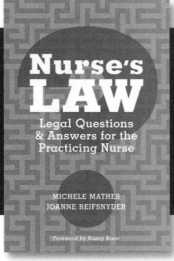
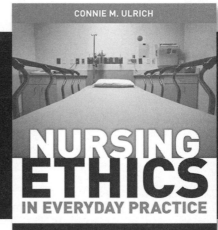

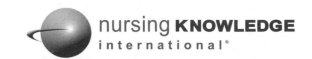

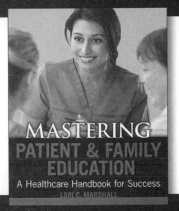
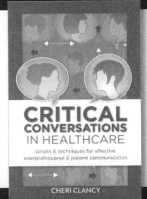
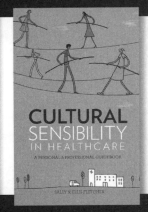
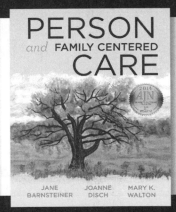

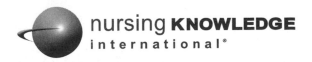

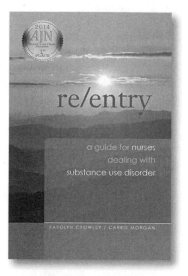
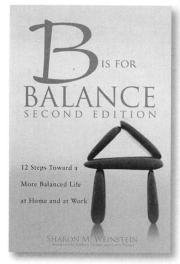
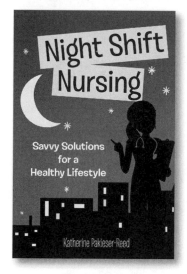
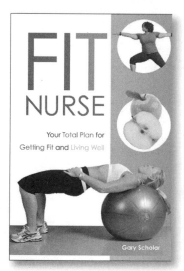

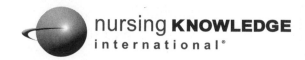